Toxic Chemicals, Health, and the Environment

THE JOHNS HOPKINS SERIES IN ENVIRONMENTAL TOXICOLOGY

Zoltan Annau, Series Editor

also in this series

Neurobehavioral Toxicology, edited by Zoltan Annau

The Toxicity of Methyl Mercury, edited by Christine U. Eccles and Zoltan Annau

Lead Toxicity, edited by Richard Lansdown and William Yule

Toxic Chemicals, Health, and the Environment

EDITED BY

Lester B. Lave, Ph.D.

James H. Higgins Professor of Economics
Graduate School of Industrial Administration
Carnegie-Mellon University

and Arthur C. Upton, M.D.

Professor and Director
Institute of Environmental Medicine
New York University Medical Center

THE JOHNS HOPKINS UNIVERSITY PRESS   BALTIMORE AND LONDON

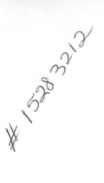

58879

RA
566
T69
1987

The Johns Hopkins University Press
701 West 40th Street
Baltimore, Maryland 21211
The Johns Hopkins Press Ltd., London

∞

The paper used in this publication meets the minimum requirements
of American National Standard for Information Sciences—
Permanence of Paper for Printed Library Materials, ANSI Z39.48-1984.

LIBRARY OF CONGRESS CATALOGING-IN-PUBLICATION DATA
Toxic chemicals, health, and the environment.

(The Johns Hopkins series in environmental toxicology)
Includes index.
1. Pollution—Toxicology. 2. Pollution—Environmental
aspects. 3. Environmental health. I. Lave, Lester B.
II. Upton, Arthur C., 1923- . III. Series.
[DNLM: 1. Environmental Health. 2. Environmental
Monitoring. 3. Environmental Pollution—prevention &
control—United States. 4. Toxicology. WA 670 T7562]
RA566.T69 1987 363.7′3 86-46276
ISBN 0-8018-3473-2 (alk. paper)
ISBN 0-8018-3474-0 (pbk. : alk. paper)

Contents

Contributors

Richard N. L. Andrews, Ph.D., Professor of Environmental Sciences and Engineering and Director, Institute for Environmental Studies, University of North Carolina at Chapel Hill

Angela D. Arms, Health and Safety Research Division, Oak Ridge National Laboratory

Robert U. Ayres, Ph.D., Professor, Department of Engineering and Public Policy, Carnegie-Mellon University

Scott Baker, Ph.D., Special Assistant to the Assistant Administrator, Office of Research and Development, U.S. Environmental Protection Agency

Michael Gallo, Ph.D., Associate Professor, Department of Environmental and Community Medicine, Rutgers Medical School, University of Medicine and Dentistry of New Jersey

Michael Gochfeld, M.D., Ph.D., Clinical Associate Professor, Department of Environmental and Community Medicine, Rutgers Medical School, University of Medicine and Dentistry of New Jersey

Bernard D. Goldstein, M.D., Professor and Chairman, Department of Environmental and Community Medicine, Rutgers Medical School, University of Medicine and Dentistry of New Jersey

Ronald D. Hill, Ph.D., Director, Hazardous Waste Engineering Research Laboratory, Land Pollution Control Division, U.S. Environmental Protection Agency

Lester B. Lave, Ph.D., James H. Higgins Professor of Economics, Graduate School of Industrial Administration, Carnegie-Mellon University

Steven P. Levine, Ph.D., Associate Professor, Occupational Medicine Program, University of Michigan School of Public Health

Morton Lippmann, Ph.D., Professor, Institute of Environmental Medicine, New York University Medical Center

Francis Clay McMichael, Ph.D., Walter J. Blenko, Sr., Professor of Environmental Engineering, Department of Engineering and Public Policy, Carnegie-Mellon University

Norton Nelson, Professor, Institute of Environmental Medicine, New York University Medical Center

Joseph O'Connor, Ph.D., Research Associate Professor, Institute of Environmental Medicine, New York University Medical Center

Samuel R. Rod, Department of Engineering and Public Policy, Carnegie-Mellon University

Bernard E. Saltzman, Ph.D., Professor, Department of Environmental Health, University of Cincinnati College of Medicine

Adel Sarofim, Ph.D., Professor, Department of Chemical Engineering, Massachusetts Institute of Technology

Steven R. Tannenbaum, Ph.D., Professor, Massachusetts Institute of Technology

Curtis C. Travis, Ph.D., Director, Office of Risk Analysis, Health and Safety Research Division, Oak Ridge National Laboratory

Alvis G. Turner, Ph.D., Professor, Department of Environmental Sciences and Engineering, University of North Carolina School of Public Health

Arthur C. Upton, M.D., Professor and Director, Institute of Environmental Medicine, New York University Medical Center

David Gordon Wilson, Ph.D., Professor, Department of Mechanical Engineering, Massachusetts Institute of Technology

Gerald N. Wogan, Ph.D., Head, Department of Nutrition and Food Science, Massachusetts Institute of Technology

Lily Young, Ph.D., Research Associate Professor, Institute of Environmental Medicine, New York University Medical Center

Foreword

Rene Dubos was a most remarkable man: a deep thinker and an inspiring speaker and writer. But above all, he was a lover of humanity and of this earth. He was one of the first environmentalists. What set him apart from many others claiming this title was his unshakable belief that we, humanity, can improve on nature and have the duty to do so. He was equally insistent that we should revere and love our earth, avoid misusing it if possible, and correct our mistakes when they occur. He conceived of the world as resilient and forgiving, a belief that I share.

This book springs from this most reasonable and benign philosophy of Dr. Dubos. Before his death, he established the Rene Dubos Center for Human Environments, in which I had the privilege to play a role for some time. In 1984, the center held a forum on toxic chemicals. People attended from all sectors of contemporary life—science, medicine, environmental groups, government, industry, labor, journalism, and, most important of all, the public. In workshops, the participants debated important issues relating to the toxicity of chemicals. These included the right of the public and of industry to have access to proprietary data; the role for risk assessment in risk management; the need for improved toxicological data and interpretive methods; the way decisions are made in the different sectors; and the communication of data and decisions to the various publics involved. One persistent theme emerging from the workshops was that better information must be developed and disseminated to our leaders and to the public. This volume addresses this need. State-of-the-art information is presented by a most distinguished group of authorities on the relationship of toxic chemicals to human health and to the environment. This book is written for those who have at least a minimum level of scientific training and a deep interest in these issues.

Chemicals, even those that are toxic, have been and will always be with us. The issue is not how to eliminate them, but rather how to control and use them effectively. How do we live with them with a reasonable degree of safety? Every material thing in our world, good or bad, is composed of chemicals; we cannot evade them. Moreover, all chemicals have the potential to harm us if taken into the body in sufficient quantity. We are increasingly discovering that, in addition to those acutely toxic natural substances that have always been regarded as poisons, many naturally occurring chemicals present hazards when low levels are encountered over time. Dr. Bruce Ames and others have pointed out forcefully, for example, that our daily diet is rife with potent natural carcinogens and mutagens. Fortunately, a lucky combination of our bodies' natural defenses and the healthful substances we ingest counteracts most of these dietary insults. But it is not possible or feasible for us to exist without daily taking in a substantial measure of naturally occurring toxic chemicals.

The same state of irreversible dependence applies to manmade chemicals. In street terms, we are hooked. Essentially all economic activity involves synthetically produced molecules. I'll wager it would be difficult to think of one thing useful in daily life that does not contain or was not grown with a substantial amount of synthetic chemicals. The secret of living with them successfully is simply to understand their effects and to prevent toxic exposures by limiting their access to our environment, just as our ancestors did when they discovered that certain animals or plants were dangerous and devised ways to avoid them or use them safely. And continuing to do so is also what this book on toxic chemicals is about.

I affirm Dr. Dubos's unbridled optimism about our ability to solve our problems. I marvel at the speed with which the field of toxic chemicals management changes as new scientific information and methods emerge. In fact, my ultimate hope is for the virtual disappearance of human concerns about toxic chemicals. I know this unabashedly optimistic outlook conflicts with that of many others who view our continued headlong pace toward worldwide industrialization as inevitably leading to our extinction by toxic chemicals. But I believe these analysts are selling short what science and humanity can do. Most certainly we will learn to minimize the production of toxic chemicals and to limit our exposure to those that remain. Beyond this, we may even develop an analog of antibiotics that would bolster our natural immunological defenses against toxic substances. After all, within my own lifetime infectious diseases were the major killers. Now, thanks to vaccination procedures and indeed to Rene Dubos himself, who in 1939 developed the first systematic method for the discovery of antibiotics resulting in their production commercially, infectious diseases are no longer the major causes of death in developed countries. The astounding rate of progress in the life sciences leads me to believe that medical defenses against toxic chemicals will one day be a part of our repertoire for managing them.

On this note of hope with which I'm sure Dr. Dubos would have concurred, I encourage you to read this excellent description of where we stand today.

JAMES F. MATHIS
Trustee, The Rene Dubos Center
Vice-President for Science & Technology, Exxon Corporation (retired)

Preface

Modern technology has clearly improved the quality of our lives in countless ways, but it has inevitably generated new risks fundamentally different in both character and magnitude from those encountered in the past.

Much effort has gone into calculations and estimates of various risks, but too little effort has been devoted to the question of acceptability of risk for the sake of socioeconomic values.
—Rene Dubos

In March 1984, some nine months before the Bhopal tragedy, the Rene Dubos Center for Human Environments sponsored a forum, "Environment and Human Health: Toxic Chemicals," to help policy makers and the lay public communicate on the subject of potential and real environmental health hazards. That prescient forum, hosted by Dr. Joshua Lederberg, President of the Rockefeller University, and the two subsequent Dubos forums, on "Managing Water Resources" and "Managing Land Use," were guided by a distinguished steering committee chaired by Dr. James F. Mathis, trustee of the center and the then vice-president for science and technology with Exxon. All contributed conceptually to *Toxic Chemicals, Health, and the Environment.*

For the past ten years, the Rene Dubos Center for Human Environments has provided facilities and opportunities for scientists, technologists, scholars, and decision makers with diverse, often conflicting interests to explore solutions to difficult environmental problems, based on the belief that the discussion of these problems is best carried out not in an adversary atmosphere but in a cooperative spirit. Whereas other organizations deal with the protection of the environment, the Dubos Center is primarily concerned with the impact of environmental problems on human health and the quality of life. The center complements the defensive policies of the environmental movement by emphasizing the creative aspects of human interventions into nature.

Founded by Rene Dubos, the eminent scientist/humanist and professor emeritus at the Rockefeller University, to focus on the humanistic and social aspects of environmental problems, the center's practical purpose is to help decision makers and the public-at-large formulate policies for the resolution of environmental conflicts and for the creation of new environmental values. To this end, the center, a nonprofit education and research organization based in New York City, maintains a library, including the archives of its founder; runs the Dubos Forum Program, which calls for national and international meetings involving policy makers; and mounts a range of activities that includes fellowships, college courses, and media, both electronic and print, to disseminate the information.

We wish to thank all of the members of the Dubos Forum Program steering committee, especially the following trustees: Dr. Paul F. Deisler, the then vice-president of health, safety, and environment of Shell Oil Company, for encouraging this work and suggesting that it be coedited by Dr. Lester Lave; Mrs. Rene Dubos, for her constant and untiring efforts devoted to evaluating the social and environmental philosophy of the program; Dr. Mathis, to whom the Dubos Center is indebted for his leadership, advice, and infinite patience in overseeing the diverse group of authorities involved in the Dubos Forum Program for over three years; Dr. Norton Nelson, Professor of Environmental Medicine at New York University Medical Center, often referred to as "the Dean of toxicology," for his wisdom and encouragement and comprehensive contribution to this book.

We are proud of this important work and grateful to Dr. Arthur Upton, coeditor, personal friend of Rene Dubos, and professor and Director of New York University's Institute of Environmental Medicine, for making it possible. We are equally grateful to Dr. Lester Lave, coeditor, James H. Higgins, Professor of Economics, Graduate School of Industrial Administration, Carnegie-Mellon University, for making it happen. And we thank each of the authors for the sum and substance of this book, which provides the best available information on this most critical and complex environmental issue.

RUTH A. EBLEN   WILLIAM R. EBLEN
Executive Director   President
The Rene Dubos Center for Human Environments, Inc.
New York, New York

Toxic Chemicals, Health, and the Environment

1. Introduction

LESTER B. LAVE AND ARTHUR C. UPTON

Toxic chemicals, both natural and manufactured, pervade the environment. Even before our industrial economies began turning out masses of chemicals, fuels, and products—indeed, before human activity—the environment contained radioactive substances such as uranium and radon gas, organic chemicals such as benzene and benzo(a)pyrene, and heavy metals such as lead and mercury. Human activities, particularly in industrial societies, introduced new toxic chemicals and vastly increased the possible exposure to such materials.

Many historical and current misfortunes indicate the danger of these substances. Thousands of people in Africa and Asia die from liver cancer each year as a result of ingesting aflatoxin; thousands of U.S. workers are killed by exposure to industrial chemicals; areas of Missouri have been rendered unsafe for human habitation because oil containing dioxin was spread on roads; all Americans have measurable levels of pesticides such as DDT (dichlorodiphenyltrichloroethane) in their bodies. In the 1960s, with the help of writers like Rachel Carson (1962), Americans awoke to the threats of harm from toxic chemicals that form the basis of our economy and way of life. Later, we learned about natural carcinogens in our food and environment.

Totally eliminating these toxic chemicals is not feasible. The naturally occurring toxins will persist to some degree despite our best efforts. Synthetic chemicals, because they form the basis of our economy, cannot be eliminated without destroying the foundation of our economic well being and even our medical care. According to Aaron Wildavsky (1979), such a cut in our standard of living would have grave health consequences, consequences much larger than those that might be averted by eliminating the toxic substances.

Thus this book rejects the simplistic notion that society can eliminate all toxic chemicals. A sufficiently small quantity of a toxic substance is assumed to be essentially harmless. Thus society's task is to protect humans and the environment against excessive exposures. Some chemicals are so toxic, and convey so little benefit in particular uses (e.g., carbon tetrachloride as a cleaning fluid), they should be banned for such uses. Other chemicals are highly toxic but highly valuable (e.g., vinyl chloride monomer); hence they must be used under strictly controlled conditions. Still other chemicals are relatively benign at the doses usually encountered but can be dangerous under particular circumstances (e.g., carbon monoxide).

This book is concerned with the management of these environmental toxic chemicals. The following chapters explore how they enter the environment; the control processes for their emission, their dispersion and biological reconcentration; the pathways by which people are exposed to them; the health effects of exposure, including recent techniques for measuring the effects of tiny levels of exposure; methods for monitoring these toxic chemicals in the environment and for cleaning up waste sites; and policy problems involved in managing toxic chemicals. The book seeks to help us understand the potential for human injury by toxic chemicals and how to prevent injury without sacrificing the benefits of our industrial economy.

Essentially, any chemical can cause death if taken into the body in sufficiently large amounts. But the chemicals of primary concern in environmental health are those which in small doses can cause an adverse health effect. For most adverse health effects, this dose is in excess of a certain threshold. For other effects, however (like cancer), there may be no threshold, i.e., there may be a slight risk of cancer even at miniscule doses (Office of Science and Technology Policy 1985).

Of the millions of chemicals known to scientists, and of the many thousands in commerce, relatively few have been characterized toxicologically. For the vast majority, too little information is available to allow assessment of toxicity (National Academy of Sciences 1984). Many substances not yet tested are likely to prove toxic. Identifying these toxic chemicals is urgent in order to quantify their risks and to take appropriate measures to protect against them.

In chapter 2, Andrews and Turner examine sources of toxic chemicals and methods of controlling their emission into the environment. They present basic data on the amounts of these substances released by production, transport, retail sales, consumer uses, and waste disposal, as well as the amounts of toxins originating from natural sources. The options for engineering control are presented, as well as options for safeguarding transport and for protecting people against local concentrations.

The generation of toxic chemicals is the subject of chapter 3. Ayres, McMichael, and Rod use the materials balance framework to show the potential release of substances into the environment and how to monitor control efforts. The method describes the magnitude of the potential problem and where control efforts need to be concentrated.

Saltzman describes the theory and practice of environmental monitoring in chapter 4. What types and levels of substances can be detected? What are the characteristics of a good environmental monitoring program?

A major source of human exposure is via food, as explained by Travis and Arms in chapter 5. What is particularly worrisome is the fact that some toxic chemicals are reconcentrated in the food chain, so that some people are exposed to increasing amounts of a chemical such as mercury, even though it is present in only minute quantities in the environment.

Other sources of human exposure are explored in chapter 6 by Lippmann. People come in contact with environmental chemicals in myriad ways, such as breathing them, touching them with their skin, and ingesting them via food and water. The potential for toxic chemicals to enter the human body through these various routes of exposure is described.

People exposed to toxic chemicals may react in measurable ways short of frank injury or disease, as explained by Wogan and Tannenbaum in chapter 7. Thus control programs should be designed to detect antecedent, short-term reactions so that corrective measures may be taken immediately. This rapidly evolving field seeks to characterize the level of exposure and to identify early warning signs of serious reactions, such as the beginning stages of disease.

Gallo, Gochfeld, and Goldstein characterize the biomedical aspects of environmental exposures in chapter 8. At a gross level, they describe the various ways in which different types of compounds are toxic. At a detailed level, they describe some of the mechanisms by which toxic chemicals perturb physiological processes to produce disease and death.

The dumping of wastes or simply the leaving of residuals in a factory or warehouse can create a contaminated site requiring cleanup. Nelson and his coauthors describe the process of cleanup in chapter 9, from appraising the need for cleanup to the methods available for rendering an area safe for human activities.

The focus of this book is on scientific aspects of the relationship between environmental chemicals and human health, but the objective of this book is to respond to concern for protecting people against toxic environmental chemicals. Chapter 10 sketches the associated policy issues, from the decision about which chemicals should be the target of concern to the role of science in public and private decision making. Each of the chapters presents the current state of knowledge, with the aim of influencing current approaches to controlling toxic chemicals in the environment. Some legislation of a decade ago is based on now outmoded scientific theories. Through an understanding of the latest theoretical and empirical work, policy makers can fashion better toxic substances policies.

References

Carson, R. 1962. *Silent Spring.* New York: Houghton Mifflin. National Academy of Sciences. 1984. *Toxicity Testing: Strategies to Determine Needs and Priorities.* Washington, D.C.: National Academy Press.
Office of Science and Technology Policy. 1985. Chemical carcinogenesis: A review of the science and its associated principles. *Federal Register* 50:10372–442.
Wildavsky, A. 1979. No risk is the highest risk of all. *American Scientist* 67:32–37.

2. Controlling Toxic Chemicals in the Environment

RICHARD N. L. ANDREWS AND ALVIS G. TURNER

Andrews and Turner introduce the many aspects of toxic chemicals in the environment: their release into the environment, their transport once in the environment, strategies for their control, and environmental decision making. In some cases, they report quantity of releases and discuss attempts to reduce their volume and toxicity. Decision making requires setting priorities and goals—prevention of chemical releases, particularly through designing the process so as to not produce toxic residuals, has obvious advantages over the complicated, expensive process of cleanup. Equity is also a paramount issue in making policy. The authors see the control of toxic chemicals as a complicated process, affected by increases in scientific knowledge and changes in public goals. They counsel focusing on reducing risks to people and the environment.

Toxic chemicals are substances that are harmful to living organisms. Some are harmful to other animals or plants but not to humans. The ideal pesticide, for instance, selectively kills only predator species, and such chemicals are used both by humans and by some plants and animals as defenses against predators. Others are poisonous to humans but not to some other species. A particular concern, for instance, is for substances that are toxic to humans but can be bioconcentrated in food chains, accumulating without lethal effects in species that are then used for human food. Of most concern are substances that are poisonous both to humans and to other species which maintain ecological conditions favorable for human habitation.

Actions to control toxic substances in the environment therefore have two basic purposes: (1) to protect human health; and (2) to protect the health of other animals and plants and the functioning of biological ecosystems.

This chapter begins with a framework for understanding the movements of toxic chemicals into and through the environment and for identifying the control options appropriate to each stage of this process. Later sections return to broader management issues, such as strategies for selecting and implementing control options, the role of government in encouraging implementation, and the problems of setting priorities and integrating control measures across multiple substances, processes, and objectives.

Points of Control

Figure 2.1 shows a simplified model of the flow of toxic chemicals. The substances originate in sources, which release them into the environment. These sources may be either manufactured or natural: radon gas, for instance, is an important hazard released primarily from natural sources. Many other toxic chemicals can be measured in the environment at background levels, which are assumed to be from natural sources and not harmful to human health or ecological stability.

Many toxic chemicals from manufactured sources are released into the environment deliberately as products. Pesticides are the most obvious example, but others include such products as tobacco, paints and solvents, and glues. Others enter the environment as residuals: materials emitted or thrown away as wastes, such as discharges of liquids and gases and solid wastes, or as a result of leaks or accidental spills.

Toxic chemicals may be released to any of three environmental media: air, water, or land. Once released, they may move and mix and react with those media in processes referred to as the *transport and fate* of pollutants in the environment. They may be transported to other locations, such as from land into groundwater, and they may move from one medium to another through deposition or volatilization. They may be diluted in the air

Figure 2.1. Sources, movements, and consequences of toxic chemicals in the environment.

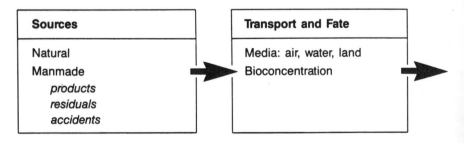

or water or transformed into other compounds that may be more or less toxic; and they may be absorbed and concentrated in living organisms through food chains. The magnitudes of these effects will vary with the characteristics of both the substance and the environment, but an understanding of how they move, and where and in what form they end up, is an essential step in designing controls.

As toxic chemicals move in the environment, they create risks of exposure, both for humans directly and for other species whose welfare concerns us. Exposure may occur as a single major dose of a single substance, as in the case of an accidental emission or chemical spill, but more typically it occurs as an individual's cumulative exposure to complex mixtures over longer periods of time. Recent studies, for instance, have shown higher exposures to toxic chemicals in indoor environments of "clean air" regions, such as North Carolina, than in outdoor environments even of "dirty air" regions such as the industrial complexes of New Jersey. Some people are exposed both at work and at home; some smoke; some use toxic consumer products. Exposure to toxic chemicals from any single source or in any particular environment must be assessed, therefore, in the context of the individual's total exposure, both to that substance and to other substances that may magnify its effects.

Finally, exposure to toxic substances may cause adverse health effects in the exposed individuals. These effects are the end points of our concern with toxic chemicals. Even here, however, there are important differences both in the degree and type of toxic effect and in the susceptibility of the individuals involved. Toxic chemicals vary widely in their potency. Some can cause cancer or genetic damage, but others are simply irritants whose effects will end when exposure ceases. Some cause acute poisoning; others cause damage only after prolonged exposure. The chosen controls must therefore be based on reasonable distinctions among types and degrees of toxicity.

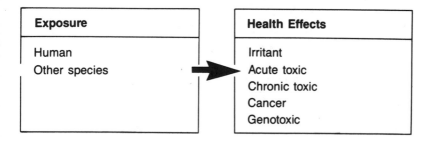

Individual people (and other organisms) also vary widely in their susceptibility to health damage as a consequence of exposure. Elderly people are more susceptible to lung infections than younger ones, while younger people are more susceptible to early-stage carcinogens than older people. Children, and especially fetuses, are more susceptible than adults to most toxic chemicals. Ecological toxicity also includes hazards to communities of organisms, such as proliferation of noxious species when an essential predator species is poisoned, and bioconcentration of sublethal toxic substances through food chains.

The chosen controls must therefore protect not only people of average health, at the threshold limit values used as occupational health guidelines, but also susceptible subgroups likely to be exposed. They must also take account of levels at which significant ecological damage may result, even though these levels may be below those at which any direct damage to human health might occur.

Sources of Environmental Toxic Chemicals

Toxic chemicals in the environment have their origins in society's activities and in naturally occurring sources. Naturally occurring toxins are usually from a single source. Anthropogenic toxicants, however, often have multiple origins.

▌ Natural Sources

Important natural sources of toxins include animals, plants, microorganisms, and minerals. Bruce Ames (1983) pointed out that "Nature is not benign. The human diet contains a great variety of natural mutagens and carcinogens."

Aflatoxin, for instance, a complex mixture of very toxic chemicals, has been found in corn, rice, sorghum, peanuts, and many other foods (Patten 1981). The source of this toxin is a fungus, *Aspergillus flavus. A. flavus* occurs worldwide, but it is especially common in warm countries, where crops such as peanuts and corn are allowed to become wet after harvest. Maximum production of the toxin occurs at 25°C on foodstuffs with a moisture content of 15–30 percent. Many naturally occurring plants are also sources of toxins. The toxicity of many species of mushrooms has been known for centuries. *Amanita phalloides* produces a general toxin and *A. muscaria,* a neurological toxin, which can be lethal if eaten in sufficient quantities (Bryan 1979). Plants such as jimson weed, hemlock, and oleander contain alkaloids that can cause acute illness if consumed.

Most of today's serious concerns about toxic chemicals, however, come from human activities that increase either the presence or the potency of such substances in places where living organisms may be exposed to them.

For instance, the association between skin cancer, the most common human cancer, and exposure to sunlight was recognized more than 100 years ago (Scott and Straf 1977). While this is a natural toxic exposure, its incidence has increased due to human behavior patterns such as sunbathing, and it is predicted to increase significantly in the future due to increasing human releases of chlorofluorocarbons (used in air conditioning, plastics production, aerosol sprays, and other compounds), which cause progressive and major destruction of the stratospheric ozone layer that shields people from these rays.

Environmental radon also has recently been recognized as a major source of public exposure to ionizing radiation. The occurrence of radon in water and air is associated with its parent nuclides, uranium and radium, in rock and soil. Uranium is widely distributed in the earth's crust, but uranium concentrations may vary considerably among rock bodies of the same type or even within a single formation. High radon concentrations have been measured in drinking water supplies (table 2.1). Human exposure has also been unwittingly increased by energy-saving measures that reduce ventilation in buildings where radon vapors are present from natural sources.

▌ Manufactured Sources

Most current concerns regarding toxic chemical contamination of the environment, however, arise from anthropogenic sources, either directly or indirectly related to human activity. As a nation we regularly use more than 62 thousand chemicals in industry, agriculture, and the home. Many of these chemicals are hazardous to human health. As knowledge about sources, fate, transport, and effects of environmental pollutants has increased, the need for valid data on exposures and doses has become more critical. It was not until the 1980s that we had much accurate field data on the actual exposures of populations to hazardous environmental residuals. Only recently have uniform methods been proposed for predicting future exposures of populations or for estimating how population exposures might change in response to different regulatory actions.

With few exceptions, anthropogenic sources of toxic chemicals in the environment can be generally classified under one or more of the following activities:

1. Mining or extraction of ores or biomass.
2. Production and manufacturing of goods, products, and energy.

Table 2.1. Radon in U.S. drinking water supplies, thirty-nine states

	Geometric Mean of Radon 222, Pico Curies per Liter of Water			
State	In Private Wells	Wells Sampled	In Public Groundwater	Groundwater Supplies Sampled
Alabama	120	22	70	132
Arizona		0	250	124
Arkansas	230	2	12	22
California	43	6	470	15
Colorado		0	230	76
Delaware		0	30	72
Florida	6,000	34	30	327
Georgia	2,100	2	67	225
Idaho		0	99	155
Illinois		0	95	314
Indiana		0	35	185
Iowa		0	220	85
Kansas		0	120	47
Kentucky	1,500	10	32	104
Maine	7,000	24		0
Massachusetts	1,000	8	500	212
Minnesota	1,400	1	130	233
Mississippi		0	23	104
Missouri	0	2	24	138
Montana	4,300	8	230	71
Nevada		0	190	57
New Hampshire	1,400	18	940	52
New Jersey		0	300	38
New Mexico	59	57	59	171
New York	1,500	4	52	292
North Dakota		0	35	133
Ohio		0	79	165
Oklahoma		0	93	33
Oregon	450	18	120	69
Pennsylvania	910	16	380	105
Rhode Island	6,500	69	2,400	575
South Carolina	1,100	23	130	384
South Dakota	4,300	2	210	155
Tennessee	0	2	12	98
Utah		0	150	195
Vermont	210	23	660	71
Virginia	560	42	350	284
Wisconsin	730	40	150	278
Wyoming		0	330	32

Source: Hess et al. 1985.

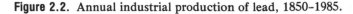

Figure 2.2. Annual industrial production of lead, 1850–1985.

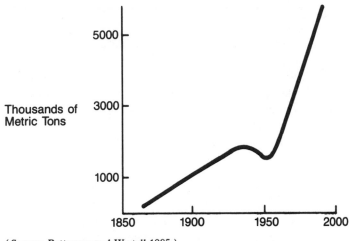

(*Source:* Patterson and Westell 1985.)

3. Transportation of raw materials, goods, products, and wastes.
4. Consumer uses of goods and products.
5. Disposal of wastes.

Mining

Concentrations of many toxic chemicals occur naturally only in ecological sinks—mineral deposits that are relatively isolated from living organisms. Examples include both toxic metals, such as lead, mercury, and cadmium, and substances whose combustion products are toxic, such as coal and oil. These substances exist naturally, but they do not become hazards until they are extracted for human use and thus reintroduced into the biologically active portion of the environment—air and water—where they may affect people, plants, and animals. Industrial production rates, therefore, provide important primary measures of anthropogenic toxic pollution.

Elevated levels of lead in air, drinking water, and foods provide a useful example of this source of toxic substances. American industry alone produces about 1.3 million tons of lead annually. Figure 2.2 shows industrial production of lead during the last 135 years. About 600 thousand tons of lead, which is toxic to humans, other animals, and plants, are released into the environment each year in the United States alone. While the combustion of coal adds small amounts of lead to the atmosphere and water, the most significant source is the burning of leaded gasoline in automobiles. The National Academy of Sciences (1980b) estimated that, in 1976, 217 thousand metric tons of lead were added to gasoline and 100 thousand metric tons were emitted into the environment from this source. As a result, the environment of the United States and of many other countries is contaminated with lead far above natural background levels.

Production and Manufacturing

Environmental releases of toxic chemicals may occur at numerous stages in production and manufacturing processes. They may be fugitive, such as emissions from compressor and pump seals, valves, spills, storage tanks, and pipelines, or they may be intentional releases into air and water of discharges and discarded solid wastes.

The industrial refining of crude oil into gasoline and fuel oils, and the conversion of this oil into petrochemical products, exemplify all these types of environmental releases. More than 90 percent of crude oil is refined into fuels. Most of it is then released into the air as combustion products, while the remainder is converted into petrochemical products. Elkin (1977) estimated that total hydrocarbon losses from petroleum refineries may range from 0.1 to 0.6 percent of crude throughput. The U.S. Environmental Protection Agency (1979) detected twenty-four toxic pollutants even in the treated effluents of petroleum refineries. These pollutants included one chemical (benzene) identified by the National Toxicology Program as a known carcinogen and four chemicals—1,2-dichloroethane, bis(2,3)ethylhexylphthalate, benzo(a)pyrene, and benzo(a)anthracene—identified as likely carcinogens. The major air pollutants from petroleum refineries include hydrogen sulfide, selenium, fluorides, and hydrocarbons. While the individual concentrations of these substances are often very small, together they add significant amounts to the pollutant load in the environment.

The leaking of petroleum products and other chemicals from underground storage tanks has contaminated groundwater. These releases were serious enough to result in a new program for regulating underground storage tanks. This program is spelled out in the Hazardous and Solid Waste Amendments of 1984 (Resource Conservation and Recovery Act).

Transportation

Spills and discharges involving the release of hazardous substances result from transportation accidents on land and in waterways, at industrial plants, and at hazardous waste disposal sites. The National Academy of Sciences (1983b) has estimated that 4 billion tons of hazardous materials are transported annually in the United States, one-half on highways. Very little information is available, however, about the amounts of hazardous materials lost in spills, the effectiveness of spill cleanup, the ultimate disposal of cleaned-up materials, or the amount of spilled material that threatens surface or groundwater.

Estimates of the number of spills vary. A contractor for the EPA estimated an average of 2,216 spills in excess of 100 gallons per year from 1978 through 1982 (Arthur D. Little, Inc., 1978). This projection included all hazardous chemicals except oil. The National Academy of Sciences (1983a) has estimated that approximately 16 thousand spills occur annually. EPA (1986) has also estimated that when hazardous materials are transported by truck, approximately 0.35 percent of them (slightly more than 38 gallons) are lost during each shipment of 200 fifty-five-gallon drums. North Carolina alone identified 709 spills reported to the state over a two-year period, 1982 to 1984; 56 percent of these spills occurred at industrial, commercial, or residential sites, while the remainder involved transport (Andrews et al. 1986). Fuel (diesel, gasoline, fuel oil) was the spilled material in 61 percent of the incidents, followed by alkalies (10 percent), acids (6 percent), and solvents (4 percent).

Consumer Uses

The use of hazardous substances by consumers, service businesses, and government agencies contributes significantly to the presence of these materials in the environment.

Approximately 1.43 billion pounds of pesticide end-use products, for instance, were manufactured in 1981 (Schaub 1983). Production of these chemicals has doubled since the mid-1960s. Aerial spraying accounted for 65 percent of all pesticide applications in 1978 (U.S. Department of Agriculture 1978).

Environmental contamination by pesticides can occur from common use, spills, accidents, disposal of excess materials, disposal of wastewater from equipment, and rinsing of empty containers. Movement of pesticides through soil and into groundwater depends on a number of factors, but groundwater contamination from the use of these substances in agricultural operations has been found in at least eighteen states (Cohen et al. 1984). Pesticide residues in food, drinking water, and the atmosphere are not uncommon.

It is paradoxical that one of our most widely used and beneficial chemicals can result in the formation of products that are carcinogenic for experimental animals. The chlorination of drinking water has been the most widely used method for disinfecting water supplies in the United States since 1908. However, it has now been shown that chlorine reacts with humic materials, which are ubiquitously present in natural waters, to produce trihalomethanes, which may be hazardous to human health (National Academy of Sciences 1980a).

Disposal of Wastes

Uncontrolled and careless disposal of wastes is a major source of toxic chemicals in the environment. The Council on Environmental Quality reported that 162 million metric tons of air pollutants (particulates, sulfur oxides, nitrogen oxides, volatile organic compounds, and carbon monoxide) from eighteen different mobile and stationary sources were emitted in the United States in 1981; 150 billion metric tons of solid waste were disposed of by manufacturing industries in 1980; 150 million metric tons of consumer solid waste were disposed of in 1978; 41 million wet metric tons of industrial hazardous waste was generated in 1980; and 2.5 million cubic meters of low-level radioactive wastes were buried in 1981 (Council on Environmental Quality 1982). These estimates do not include wastewater discharges, which in actual volume would far exceed the sum total of these wastes. It is very difficult to estimate the total volume, weight, or concentration of toxic chemicals discharged in waste streams.

Figure 2.3. Loci and categories of control options.

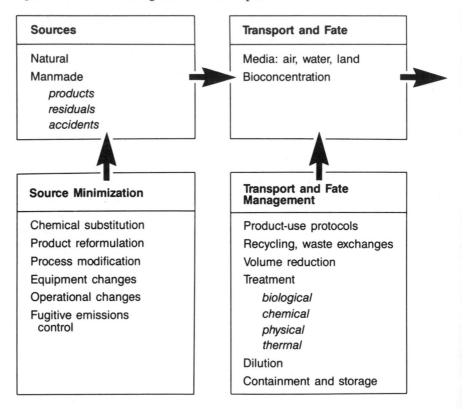

Control Strategies

At each point in the flows of materials, control strategies are available. Figure 2.3 shows the control options that can be applied at each of the stages shown in figure 2.1 (see also Kneese and Bower 1979; U.S. Congress, Office of Technology Assessment 1983; National Academy of Sciences 1985).

At the sources, the primary purpose of control is to minimize the production of toxic chemicals, both as products and especially as wastes (see especially Sarokin et al. 1986; Kohl et al. 1984; Kohl and Triplett 1984). *Chemical substitution* means changing the raw material inputs of the production process to less toxic materials (for instance, replacing a mercury that contains a biocide with one that does not). *Product reformulation* also offers many opportunities to reduce the spread of toxics in the environment, by making products less toxic in the first place. Current examples

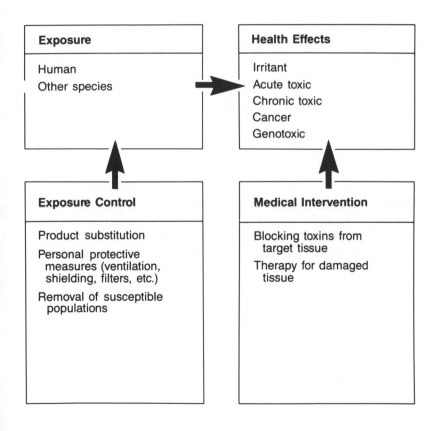

include phasing out solvent-based paints and substituting less toxic agents in wood preservatives. *Process modification* allows the manufacturer to make products in less hazardous ways. After the Bhopal disaster, for instance, several manufacturers noted that the same product can be produced by a process that synthesizes methyl isocyanate at the precise rate it is needed, thus eliminating the need to store or transport it.

Equipment and operational changes, such as changing from batch processing to continuous process and using separate piping for different chemicals, may substantially reduce toxic wastes. And *fugitive emissions control* can greatly reduce toxic pollution from dusts, vapors, spills, and storage tank leakage.

When toxic chemicals are not eliminated at the source, transport and fate management can reduce their potential harm in the environment. For products that are deliberately used because of their toxic effects, like pesticides, and where less toxic substitutes are not available, *product-use protocols* tell the user how to apply them so as to minimize excessive use or unintended side effects.

▌ Control Strategies for Source Minimization

A preventive program, including environmental monitoring, release detection systems, and contingency planning, can reduce the hazards and costs of toxic substance releases. Internal environmental audits of industrial and transportation operations can identify those areas that need attention and improved control management. Such approaches reflect not only sensible business planning but sound policies of corporate responsibility to the public.

Chemical Substitution

Solvent-borne inks are widely used in the printing industry. As these inks dry, large amounts of solvent vapor enter the air. Many of the solvents, which include toluene, methylethylketone, acetone, alcohol, and hexane, are toxic. Water-borne inks are not a perfect substitute, but their use greatly reduces solvent emissions, and waste solvents used in the cleanup of presses, rollers, and other equipment are eliminated.

Product Reformulation

Products themselves, of course, do not always require the toxic components that have been used in the past. High-octane gasoline, for instance, is now blended without lead additives. New blending components, such as tertiary butyl ether and ethyl alcohol, have replaced lead to meet octane requirements (Patterson and Westell 1985), and the EPA has projected a total ban on lead in gasoline in the 1990s. While these substances are themselves toxic, they are less so than lead and are more quickly broken down in the environment. The costs and benefits of lead reduction are shown in table 2.2. Similar changes have occurred in the removal of lead and solvents from many paints and in the substitution of less toxic components in wood preservatives.

Process Modification

Industries modify manufacturing processes to increase production efficiency, to improve products, and to reduce costs. Process modifications can also be used effectively to reduce toxic substances. As waste management costs increase, as regulations become more stringent, and as liability coverage grows more difficult to obtain, the minimization of both accidental and intentional releases of environmental residuals is becoming a primary purpose of process changes.

Generally, process modifications must be developed in the context of each specific plant or process, and they therefore require the active interest of engineers and managers at each facility.

A recent example of how process modification can reduce the generation of hazardous wastes in the chloralkali industry was reported by the U.S. Congress Office of Technology Assessment (1983). The chloralkali process is based on the electrolysis of brines to produce chlorine, hydrogen, and sodium hydroxide. One process uses a mercury cell, which results in a

Table 2.2. Costs and monetized benefits of alternative lead levels in 1986 (millions of 1983 dollars)

Effect	Lead Level (gplg)[a]				
	0.50	0.40	0.30	0.20	0.10
Monetized benefits	5,398	5,992	6,606	7,229	7,930
Children's health effects	466	504	539	571	602
Adult blood pressure	4,018	4,483	4,955	5,436	5,927
Conventional pollutants	278	278	278	278	278
Maintenance	517	608	706	808	933
Fuel economy	119	119	128	136	190
Refining costs	243	305	386	472	607
Net benefits	5,155	5,687	6,220	6,757	7,323
Net benefits excluding blood pressure	1,137	1,204	1,265	1,321	1,396

Source: Schwartz et al. 1985.
Note: Amounts are assuming that leaded gasoline is used in all vehicles designed to use it.
[a]Grams per leaded gallon of gasoline.

large concentration of mercury and a smaller concentration of chlorinated hydrocarbons discarded in process waste. A modification of this process uses a diaphragm cell instead of a mercury cell, which eliminates mercury contamination in process waste. Other modifications in the chloralkali process have also been made (table 2.3).

Equipment Changes

Reducing toxic emissions at the industrial source can often be achieved by redesigning or substituting equipment. The furniture industry provides an example.

Conventional airspray guns spray sealer and paint on furniture. This process emits toxic chemicals into both interior and exterior air and requires significant amounts of solvent to clean equipment and work surfaces. Substituting airless electrostatic spray units can reduce consumption of coating materials up to 20 percent and greatly reduces volatile organic solvent emissions, since there is less solvent lost to evaporation; solvent waste from cleaning the spray booth is also reduced (Kohl et al. 1984). Even though the electrostatic units are more expensive and require specially formulated coatings and sensitizers, these costs can often be recovered in as little as one year due to savings on coating material and solvent.

Operational Changes

Changing operational procedures can also reduce industrial waste streams and thus minimize the concentration of toxic substances released to the environment. A European organization of oil companies, CONCAWE, reported that replacing the once-through cooling cycle of older petroleum refineries by air or closed-circuit water cooling can reduce typical water use from 30 cubic meters per ton of crude oil processed to as low as 0.05 cubic meters (CONCAWE 1980). Since many toxic chemicals ap-

Table 2.3. Process modifications in chloralkali industry

Modification	Effect on Waste Stream	Reason for Modification
Diaphragm cell	Elimination of mercury-contamination	Preferred use of natural salt brines as raw material
Dimensionally stable anode	Elimination of chlorinated hydrocarbon waste	Increased efficiency
Membrane cell	Elimination of asbestos diaphragm waste	Reduced energy costs, higher quality product

Source: U.S. Congress, Office of Technology Assessment 1983.

pear in refinery wastewaters—heavy metals (lead, cadmium, chromium, iron, copper, manganese, nickel, mercury, and zinc), polynuclear aromatics, sulphides, and cyanides, for instance—reduction in the volumes of these wastewaters would significantly reduce environmental releases and allow more efficient treatment of the concentrated remainder.

Fugitive Emissions Control

Storage tanks, valves, flanges, and connectors are major sources of fugitive hydrocarbon emissions in the petroleum industry. Fritz and Hanzevack (1980) have estimated that hydrocarbon emissions from a typical refinery may range from 280 to 580 kilograms per thousand tons of crude oil processed (table 2.4). Using a floating roof on storage tanks can significantly reduce hydrocarbon emissions by restricting the amount of surface area exposed to the air (CONCAWE 1977). Other methods for controlling vapor losses from storage tanks include submerged filling or bottom loading, collection and recycling of emissions, cooling of the tank contents, and absorption of vapors into carbon beds.

Refineries must monitor atmospheric emissions if they expect to exert any control over these environmental pollutants. Once identified, abatement technologies, such as seal systems on running engines, valves and flanges, closed-process and surface water rundown systems, floating roofs, and vapor return lines, can be instituted.

▌ Control Strategies for Emissions and Wastes

For toxic substances generated as wastes rather than as useful products, several management measures are available. Recycling and waste exchanges, for instance, seek new markets for residuals (leftover material without obvious economic value) in economically useful processes. Volume

Table 2.4. Typical oil refinery hydrocarbon emissions

	Emissions	
Source	Kilograms per Metric Ton of Throughput	Percentage Loss
Fugitive leaks	70–200	0.007–0.020
Tanks	70–100	0.007–0.010
Truck loading	70–140	0.007–0.014
Effluent treatment, flares, and stacks	70–140	0.007–0.014
Total	280–580	

Source: Fritz and Hanzevack 1980.

reduction can be accomplished by separating toxic from nontoxic wastes, dewatering, compacting, or other means, thus concentrating waste. Physical, chemical, or biological treatments convert toxic materials into less toxic forms. Incineration and other thermal destruction processes use heat to achieve the same purpose. Careful attention must also be given to the residuals from the treatment processes themselves.

Recycling, Waste Exchange

The International Reclamation Bureau (BIR) defines recycling as "the whole system in which obsolete or redundant products and materials are reclaimed, refined or reprocessed, and converted into new, perhaps quite different, products once more" (Bureau International de la Recuperation 1980). BIR is a nonprofit organization founded in 1948, with a membership representing forty-four countries and 7,000 organizations, to promote international trade, exchange of information, recovery of secondary materials, and resource recovery.

Waste brokers buy or accept wastes, analyze their properties, identify potential uses, reprocess as needed, and sell them at a profit. Information brokers transfer information on available wastes or materials, usually through a regularly issued bulletin. Significant quantities of waste materials have been recycled, reused, and salvaged through these avenues over the past two decades (U.S. Environmental Protection Agency 1980).

Waste exchanges are often the least costly and most environmentally and socially sound options for managing waste materials once they have been removed from the generation source. However, these methods may also create or sustain a market for toxic substances, which discourages technological innovation that would reduce production of these substances in the first place (Caldart and Ryan 1985).

Volume Reduction and Treatment

Source segregation technologies such as dewatering, separation of toxic ingredients, and compaction can be used to reduce the volume of hazardous waste to be managed. However, these technologies do not reduce the toxicity or quantity of hazardous residues present. The congressional Office of Technology Assessment (1983) has suggested that source segregation is probably the simplest and least costly method of waste reduction. This approach, which prevents contamination of large volumes of waste, is often easy to implement, but is only a short-term solution. The concentrated toxic constituents must still be managed. For example, metal-finishing rinse water is rendered nonhazardous by removing the toxic metals and cyanide. The water can then be disposed of through municipal-industrial sewage systems. However, if the cost of removing the metals or cyanide is higher than treatment and disposal costs, there is no economic incentive for source segregation.

Biological, chemical, and physical treatment can also be used to remove or destroy toxic residues in hazardous industrial waste. Biological treatment, which has been used for the treatment of municipal and industrial liquid waste streams for many years, includes activated sludge and aerated lagoons. Chemical treatments use neutralization, precipitation, and oxidation reduction; physical methods are air stripping, carbon sorption, ion exchange, reverse osmosis, and filtration. Thermal technologies include incineration, fluidized bed combusters, and molten salt reactors. The following list describes volume reduction treatments (compare California Office of Appropriate Technology 1981).

Biological treatment
1. *Activated sludge*   Wastewater is mixed with recycled activated sludge to oxidize biodegradable organic waste constituents.
2. *Aerated lagoons*   Organic waste is stabilized by dispersed biological growth in tanks or ponds. Aeration is required.

Chemical treatment
3. *Oxidation reduction*   Waste streams containing reductants are converted to a less hazardous state. Chlorine is often used as the oxidizer.
4. *Precipitation*   Solid constituents are separated from an aqueous waste stream by chemical changes that convert soluble constituents to an insoluble form.

Physical treatment
5. *Air stripping*   Volatile and organic contaminants are stripped from liquid waste streams. This process is often used to remove ammonia-bearing waste.
6. *Carbon sorption*   Dissolved refractory organics are removed from waste streams. Activated carbon has been widely used to remove organics from water.

Thermal treatment
7. *Incineration*   High temperatures oxidize solid and liquid organic wastes to carbon dioxide and water in the presence of oxygen.
8. *Fluidized bed combustion*   Wastes are combusted in a bed of solid particles that behave like a fluid. Complete combustion of organic waste occurs with a minimum of excess air and heat.

The ideal treatment for hazardous waste materials would permanently reduce risks to human health and the environment by destroying the toxic character of the material or reducing it to a concentration that would not cause any adverse human health effects. Thermal treatment comes closer to this ideal than any other technology. However, elemental metals, some highly refractory organics, and products of incomplete combustion such as dioxins and dibenzofurans may be released in air emissions and ash residues. These emissions can be significantly reduced, but not totally eliminated, by proper design, operation, and monitoring of the equipment.

All of the technologies listed above produce residuals, which may contain toxic constituents. These residuals must be contained to prevent their entry into the environment.

Dilution, Containment, and Storage

Once all the management measures that are reasonably available have been used, there may still remain materials that cannot be further recycled, treated, or destroyed. Two additional control strategies remain for these materials. Those whose toxic risks are low—and especially those in which small traces of such toxicants are mixed with large volumes of water, dirt, or other nontoxic materials—may simply be released into the environment under a planned discharge regime that assures dilution to nontoxic concentrations at all times. Those materials with higher toxic risks may require containment and storage—either above ground or below ground, in tanks, landfills, vaults, or other secure facilities—for the foreseeable future.

For centuries, people have buried waste in the land. This practice has often led to the contamination of groundwater, surface water, and, to a lesser degree, the atmosphere. Even though engineered "secure" landfills are a hazardous waste disposal option under Resource Conservation and Recovery Act regulations, the U.S. Congress, many state legislatures, and the U.S. Environmental Protection Agency are considering prohibiting disposal of hazardous materials in the earth. Virtually all interested parties have acknowledged that even stringent regulatory requirements will not guarantee that toxic constituents will not migrate into the environment from these landfills (Harrison 1984). Some residuals, however, will likely continue to be disposed of in underground or aboveground facilities. These residuals include ash residues from incineration and treatment residues that have been encapsulated to prevent migration. Permanent storage appears to be the only reasonable options for the disposal of these residuals.

▌ Exposure Control

Even the best controls at the sources and in the environment cannot eliminate all risks of toxic exposure. Further control measures are sometimes necessary, therefore, to block the movement of toxic chemicals from the environment to exposed individuals. This is especially true for two groups of individuals: those who are more heavily exposed than the general population, such as people who handle toxic chemicals in their jobs, and those who are more susceptible to toxic effects of exposure.

These exposure controls are of three types. Product substitution protects individuals by exposing them to less toxic products. EPA regulations sometimes prohibit the use of especially toxic chemicals in consumer products, such as home pesticides and wood preservatives, by either banning them entirely or restricting their use to trained and licensed applicators. Personal protective measures are direct barriers to exposure, such as filter masks and protective clothing, fans and ventilation systems, and other devices that prevent or minimize exposure. The final means of exposure control is simply removal of susceptible populations. Examples include occupational screening, emergency evacuation, and personal decisions by medically sensitive individuals—when they have the option—to live and work in low-exposure areas.

▌Medical Intervention

The discussion above summarizes measures to prevent or reduce exposure to toxic chemicals. Beyond these, the only remaining options are through neutralizing or mitigating health effects: medical interventions either to block the substance's movement to a target organ or system within the body where a toxic effect can occur or to heal the effect once it has occurred. Promptly administered poison antidotes, for instance, can neutralize some acute toxic chemicals before they cause harm, and potassium iodide can block uptake of radioactive iodine by the vulnerable thyroid gland. Chelation, in contrast, mitigates the effects of lead poisoning by cleansing lead from the bloodstream, though it cannot reverse brain damage.

Choices among Controls

The choice of a control strategy depends first on the substance to be controlled. Processes for managing organic chemicals, for instance, are not necessarily appropriate for managing toxic metals (such as arsenic and lead) or radioactive materials, and vice versa. Toxic products must also be approached somewhat differently from toxic wastes, especially if their toxicity is part of the purpose of the product (pesticides, for instance); and both must be approached differently from toxic chemicals that occur from natural sources (radon, for instance).

Within the range of options that are technically suited to the substances in question, however, four principles form the basis for choice: degree of hazard, effectiveness, cost, and equity. These principles, though oversimplified, form a useful framework for analysis.

▎ Degree of Hazard

Which toxics are worth controlling? A common but unfortunate practice is simply to control those singled out for attention by particular laws or public controversies or those that are traditional priorities of the firm or agency. Some of these substances are worth controlling, but others may be less important than hazards that have received less attention.

If the purposes of toxics control are to protect human and ecological health, then control priorities should be based on degree of hazard to those aims. Three assumptions of the principle help define the degree of hazard of any substance and guide in the application of control.

De Minimis

If the amounts and concentrations released into the environment do not pose risks significant enough to be worth controlling, the only appropriate control is continuing awareness of change in the amounts or concentrations released.

Relative Risk

If the quantities or concentrations released are large but the risks are small compared to the risks of another, priority should be given to controlling the more significant hazard.

In practice, relative risk is often confounded by political and economic pressures, because some of the most significant hazards are also the most politically entrenched or most costly to control. In such cases, greater *administrative* effectiveness is often achieved by targeting the next most hazardous substances; but this should not be mistaken for *substantive* effectiveness, which is reduction of the most significant hazard.

Uncertainty

Ordinarily, controlling known risks should take precedence over controlling uncertain ones of similar magnitude. But when an uncertain (but plausible) risk would be catastrophic, prudence suggests a presumption favoring strong controls, even at substantial cost, until the risk is disproven. In less extreme cases, reasonable balancing of risk against cost might lead to more tentative measures, such as monitoring release patterns and susceptible populations, research to resolve the uncertainties, and clear liability for any effects.

▌ Effectiveness

Which control options are most effective in minimizing toxic effects? Some measures are intrinsically more effective than others, in the sense of their physical or chemical capacity to reduce toxicity; others are operationally more effective, in the sense that they are more reliable in situations where they are needed. Three assumptions of the effectiveness principle provide a guide for choosing effective toxic management measures.

Prevention Is More Effective than Cleanup

The most effective control is not to produce a toxic material in the first place; the next most effective control is to fully recycle it within the production process so that it is not released into the environment (North Carolina Department of Natural Resources and Community Development 1986). Treatment and destruction processes vary from high to low effectiveness and often leave residual waste streams requiring management; and land filling or other long-term storage of toxic chemicals is not really an effective measure at all but rather an admission of the ineffectiveness of other processes. Least effective is cleanup of toxic chemicals once they have been dispersed in the environment, which in effect requires treatment under the least favorable conditions—wide dispersal of toxic material over households, soil, or groundwater. The following list shows the hierarchy of control options from most to least effective (National Academy of Sciences 1985).

Most effective: reducing volume
1. Abatement
2. Minimization
3. Recycling
4. Reuse

Less effective: reducing hazard
5. Physical-chemical treatment
6. Biological treatment
7. Thermal treatment

Least effective: dispersing into environment
8. Landfill
9. Water cleanup

Passive Measures Are More Effective than Active Ones

Control measures built into the design of products or processes generally are more effective than measures that require conscious human choice on a case-by-case basis. This is especially true of toxic chemicals whose effects are chronic or latent, such as carcinogens. People do not read labels (some cannot); people are careless, forgetful, often unaware of their own options, and overconfident about risks they think they can understand or control; people face peer and employer pressure to not appear overcautious; and people generally make poor trade-offs between risk and convenience when risks are not obvious and personal protection measures are inconvenient (Fischhoff et al. 1981). For all these reasons, designed-in controls and ample margins of safety are generally more effective than controls that rely on proper operating procedures.

There Are Exceptions to the Preceding Two Assumptions

For instance, risk of toxic consequences may be so much higher for an identifiable subgroup than for the population as a whole, or so much higher than available technologies can reliably control, that it is more effective to limit exposure than to prevent releases or to design in safeguards.

❙ Cost

Most control measures cost money. However, the effects of these toxic substances also impose costs if they are not controlled (for instance, the cost of human health care and damage to dairy herds and fisheries); and the disposal of toxic materials as waste is an economic waste—a throwing away of potentially useful and sometimes costly materials. In choosing among control strategies, therefore, it is important to weigh all costs associated with the decision, not simply the direct costs of the technology, and to make sure that the range of options considered does not ignore important opportunities. The following three assumptions are part of the cost principle.

Pollution Prevention Pays

Prevention of toxic releases is not only the most effective control strategy but often the cheapest as well (Royston 1979; Huisingh and Bailey 1982; Huisingh and Hilger 1985). Many products can be made as cheaply with less toxic components; and if one counts the reduction of health risks and associated liabilities, cost savings may be substantial. Many waste streams can be recycled internally or diverted to by-product manufacture, saving both the cost of disposal and the value of the materials. Electroplaters, for instance, are now learning how to reclaim highly toxic but expensive trace metals from their wastewater, and to save money doing so (Kohl and Triplett 1984). Prevention of toxic wastes may be orders of magnitude less expensive than pumping out and purifying contaminated groundwater, a process that can cost millions of dollars over ten to twenty years (Andrews et al. 1986).

Costs Are Affected by Knowledge and Regulation

Why has pollution occurred in the first place, if one can save money by not doing so? First, because businesses, like people, are creatures of habit. Most of them run by standard operating procedures and take many assumptions as given. They do not constantly reexamine every aspect of their operations. This is especially true of small firms and of fixed-cost technical processes and basic capital facilities (as opposed to financial management). Most businesses reevaluate these basic processes only when some sharp change in factor prices or regulatory requirements triggers it; and when they do, they often discover unanticipated ways of saving money (compare Royston 1979).

Second, both knowledge about toxic chemicals and standards of acceptability have changed. When these substances were little regulated and liability laws lax, it was cheaper to dump waste into airstreams and rivers and landfills; but with today's tighter regulation, the calculus has shifted to favor preventive measures. When regulations differ among states or are not firmly enforced, however, control options that are more effective but also more costly than sewers and dumps may not be used, due to a lack of stable markets for their services.

Costs Serve Multiple Purposes

Economic textbooks focusing only on waste treatment often assert that costs rise geometrically as one attempts to clean up the last few percent of the waste. In reality, however, capital investments typically serve several purposes at once. A single investment in process or equipment changes to meet a toxic chemicals standard may actually achieve more treatment than the standard requires, or even remove a toxic waste stream entirely; and it may also control other substances, save energy, and produce a product more effectively. The ideal toxic chemicals control option, in fact, is one that not only is highly effective but saves costs and increases business efficiency as well; and such options are not as rare as one might initially assume.

▌ Equity

The final consideration in toxic chemicals control choices is equity: Who pays? When a direct toxic cause and effect can be proven, few would dispute that the producer of the cause should compensate the victim of the effect. But few issues are so clear-cut. Who should pay when causality is uncertain, or when several sources might be involved? And how much expense should be imposed on producers (and by implication, their customers) to prevent uncertain risks? Or to prevent risks of minor or transitory toxic effects (occasional eye irritation or bad odors, for instance), as opposed to life-threatening or carcinogenic toxic substances? The following two assumptions answer these questions.

The Costs of Preventing Toxic Chemical Risks Should Be Borne by Those Who Cause Them

A basic principle of market economics holds that all costs should be reflected in producer and consumer decisions: there should be no externalities, in which real social costs are shifted to other parties or to the public.

More recent arguments have blurred this principle, asserting instead that the cost of the harm done should be balanced against the cost of preventing it—in effect, placing the burden of proof on victims to prove health effects more costly than businesses' claims of compliance costs, rather than on businesses to prove adequate management of their toxic materials. The test of equity lies in the result, not in the cost to the producer of achieving it.

A primary cause of today's toxics problems is that the full costs of toxic contamination were not included in the business costs of producing them. Their effects on air and water and on human and ecological health were underestimated or ignored. This was especially true of toxic chemicals whose effects are hard to trace to specific causes. For instance, the effects of latent or insidious toxic chemicals such as carcinogens appear long after exposure. And the effects of some toxic chemicals are similar to those due to other causes; respiratory problems due to environmental toxins are complicated by smoking; and a lowered intelligence due to lead exposure is complicated by inherited causes.

If a substance does appear to have serious toxic effects, the producer of the substance should be given the widest possible latitude in choosing the least costly effective control measures—but must then bear responsibility for effective control.

Prevention Is More Equitable than Cleanup or Compensation

Both market economics and common law hold that individuals are entitled not to be harmed by the unilateral actions of others. When such harm occurs, payment of compensation is the least that can be demanded, but in serious cases it can never fully replace the loss of health, the stress, and the disruption of lives that result. The only truly equitable solution is to prevent toxic health effects in the first place.

Government Incentives for Implementing Controls

The control of toxic substances in the environment is important not only for individuals but also for public policy. It is not, of course, entirely new: the United States has regulated some substances, such as food and cosmetic additives, radiation, and some pesticides, for decades.

Since 1970, however, governments have enacted a complex patchwork of laws intended to more fully control the environmental release of toxic agents (Portney 1978). These laws are often thought of as the primary control mechanisms for toxic chemicals in the environment. In fact, however, they are not. They are simply implementation incentives: that is, government-sponsored rewards and punishments intended to encourage greater use of control options by others (Bower et al. 1977; Davis 1984).

Listed below, in chronological order, are thirteen major U.S. statutes controlling toxic substances in the environment. Others, and many state and local ordinances, could easily be added. In fact, many releases of toxic chemicals can be controlled effectively only at the local level (Andrews et al. 1986).

1. Food, Drug, and Cosmetics Act (1938) as amended (1958) regulates toxic additives to food and cosmetics and prohibits additive use of any known carcinogen.
2. Federal Insecticide, Fungicide, and Rodenticide Act (1947) regulates use of pesticides.
3. Clean Air Act (1970, plus amendments) regulates six major pollutants based on health effect levels, plus hazardous air pollutants more generally.
4. Occupational Safety and Health Act (1970) regulates toxic exposure in the workplace.
5. Consumer Product Safety Act (1972) regulates toxic as well as other potential hazards in consumer products.
6. Federal Water Pollution Control Act (1972, plus amendments) regulates toxic water pollutants.
7. Federal Environmental Pesticide Control Act (1972, plus amendments) tightens regulation of pesticides.
8. Safe Drinking Water Act (1974) regulates toxic substances in drinking water.
9. Toxic Substances Control Act (1976) requires premanufacture testing and control of new toxic substances.
10. Resource Conservation and Recovery Act (1976) regulates transportation, treatment, storage, and disposal of hazardous wastes, and tightens regulation of solid wastes, generally.
11. Hazardous Materials Transportation Act (1978) regulates transportation of toxic and other hazardous materials.
12. Comprehensive Environmental Response, Compensation, and Liability Act (1980) provides liability requirements and funds (superfund) for cleanup of contaminated sites.

13. Resource Conservation and Recovery Act amendments (1984) regulate toxic and other hazardous materials from "small-quantity generators," underground storage tanks, municipal landfills, and other sources not previously regulated.

Four general methods for controlling toxic substances in the environment have been available to governments. Direct regulation, such as banning particular substances, limits their uses to specified applications or sets standards limiting allowable releases of them into the environment. Economic incentives use deliberate changes in subsidies, taxes, or liability standards to make safe management less costly (or unsafe management more costly) than current practice. Educational programs—training, public information campaigns, labeling requirements—promote wider knowledge of hazards and control options (and thus, presumably, better decisions). Procedural requirements, such as record keeping, monitoring, and environmental auditing, promote greater accountability for the use of toxic substances.

Existing government regulatory programs for toxic chemicals are frequently criticized. On the one hand, only a small fraction of the toxic substances in everyday use have in fact been regulated; and some that have been restricted are arguably less hazardous than others left uncontrolled. On the other hand, these laws require substantial paperwork on the part of regulated businesses and often require costly investments in treatment technology as well. Some regulations are still in flux, posing risks that investments to comply with current requirements could prove costly mistakes once future requirements are added. Such uncertainty reduces rather than increases incentives for implementation.

Finally, while early regulations focused on large manufacturers, recent ones affect small businesses and local governments, which have less resources with which to comply. Examples include regulations covering underground storage tanks, municipal landfills, and groundwater protection.

A central issue today, therefore, is the identification of more effective implementation incentives to promote toxics control. Current proposals include risk-based regulation; economic incentives, including strict liability doctrines; and innovations in enforcement, such as environmental auditing.

Risk-Based Regulation

Current toxic chemicals control laws are a patchwork of uncoordinated mandates, involving four or more separate agencies; separate programs for air, water, pesticides, and hazardous wastes even within the same agency; disparate approaches to control, some emphasizing particular substances and others focusing on technologies and facilities; and differing criteria for control, some using absolute prohibitions and others requiring balancing of risks against the economic costs and benefits of control (cf. Doniger 1978; Lave 1981).

The U.S. Environmental Protection Agency (1986, no date) is now seeking to promote risk-based decision making to set control priorities both within and among these various programs. In this framework, control proposals must comply with statutory mandates, but priorities for implementing them are then based—insofar as possible—upon the degree of hazard involved. Hazardous waste control priorities, for instance, would be based not simply on the type of facility but also on its distance to population, hydrogeological conditions, and the toxicity, volume, transport, and likely fate of the wastes themselves.

Within each regulatory program, this approach relates decisions explicitly to the true goal of the program: to do the most to reduce toxic risks. Among programs, this approach in principle promotes a consistent decision perspective, and it also helps to assure that total risks are minimized across all environmental media, so that pollution is not simply transferred among air, water, and land.

Risk-based decision making is in principle the most logical basis for setting control priorities. Debate continues, however, as to whether, with its more extensive information needs, it is really more cost-effective than current requirements, which emphasize implementation of the best reasonably affordable control technology.

▌ Economic Incentives

The purpose of implementation incentives is to influence the behavior of people who produce or use toxic substances—businessmen, workers, consumers—so that their decisions will be appropriate to the toxicity of the substance.

A basic economic incentive for toxics control is the escalating cost of waste disposal, which is due primarily to the effects of government regulations. Customary practices of dumping many toxic chemicals in municipal landfills, sewers, and rural lands have been made illegal, and costly civil and criminal penalties have been authorized for abuses. The cost of legal disposal, meanwhile, has itself increased due to the greater cost of assuring safe management (banning liquids from hazardous waste landfills, for instance, and stringent design standards for the facilities themselves). The net effect, assuming predictable regulations and credible enforcement, is to create an economic incentive for toxic waste reduction at the source.

Additional economic incentives include subsidies for safe management. North Carolina, for instance, operates a small but well-publicized pollution prevention program, which offers technical assistance, challenge grants, and annual awards for measures to reduce toxic waste generation at the source. Many governments offer tax incentives, such as accelerated depreciation and property tax exclusions, for pollution control facilities; and some governments, especially in Europe, even provide government-subsidized waste disposal facilities. Care is required in designing such programs, however, to assure that their primary incentive is in fact for toxic waste minimization. Measures that simply reduce industrial costs through subsidized treatment and disposal may actually reduce the incentive for responsible management.

▌ Strict and Joint Liability Doctrines

Closely related to direct costs and benefits imposed by governments are changes in the doctrines of liability, which increase the economic risks of using toxic chemicals. Conventional liability doctrine requires the victim to prove a direct causal link to the source, a test that is scientifically difficult for many toxic chemicals and often impossible for those whose effects occur only after long periods of time (such as many carcinogens). It also requires that the effect be solely from that cause, not exacerbated by other sources or by the victim's behavior.

Strict liability doctrine, in contrast, holds that some substances are so intrinsically dangerous that their source must accept responsibility for any adverse effect they might have caused, regardless of other sources or the victim's actions. This doctrine has long been applied to substances such as explosives, and since 1980 has been extended to the costs of hazardous waste cleanup as well. Strict doctrines of joint and several liability extend liability to all parties that may have contributed to a toxic chemicals problem, such as all companies that may have dumped any amount of hazardous waste—however small—into a contaminated site. The purpose is to make it easier to require responsible parties to clean up their contamination, rather than leaving taxpayers stuck with the cost; but the effect is also to create a powerful economic incentive for companies to minimize their production of toxic wastes and to give close scrutiny to where they are discarded.

The doctrines of strict and joint and several liability are probably among the most powerful economic incentives available to encourage preventive management of toxic substances—far more effective than most regulatory measures, under which a government agency must prove harm and initiate enforcement on a case-by-case basis. It gets the attention of producers and users directly, and it also allows them more flexibility than many regulations in deciding how to minimize their risks.

▌ Environmental Auditing

A key element in toxic chemicals control is government enforcement, although it is often the weakest link. Government always has too few inspectors; it bears the burden of proof; and its limited resources can easily be drained down in a few costly and time-consuming lawsuits while other offenders go unchallenged. Regulations without credible enforcement, in turn, are not taken seriously and lead to cynicism and disrespect toward the laws. A basic argument for economic incentives such as strict liability, in fact, is that they decrease the need for enforcement by substituting more direct changes to the economic risks facing toxic chemicals producers.

Another current innovation is to substitute self-enforcement procedures for government inspectors. Firms have long been required to have their financial records examined regularly by independent professional auditors to certify both to government and to their investors that they have stated their financial resources honestly and managed them ethically. A similar procedure, known as environmental auditing, is already in use by some firms, and has been proposed as a general requirement for firms subject to environmental regulations (Smith 1985).

Environmental auditing typically involves inspection of each plant's operations by an independent team of professionals, who report directly to top management officials rather than through the plant manager. The procedure has three purposes. In simplest form, it is used to certify compliance with regulatory requirements and company policies. It can also be used, however, to identify and correct any liability risks, or to go even further and identify opportunities for waste minimization and cost savings. Environmental auditing is used routinely in some firms already, and in others it is used at least in corporate acquisitions, mergers, and insurance underwriting to avoid assumption of unexpected risks. As a regulatory incentive, state governments have incorporated it into some permit conditions, in order that self-enforcement may reduce the need for inspection and enforcement proceedings; and it appears to hold promise as a more general practice.

Complicating Realities

Principles for toxics control are relatively straightforward in the abstract but difficult to apply in practice. Key pieces of information may be unknown or uncertain; and human perceptions and preferences frequently do not match the logic of the principles.

Industrial processes, for instance, typically involve many substances in a series of interacting processes, emitting waste streams to air, water, and land. The optimal solution for preventing toxic emissions across all these material flows is not always readily apparent. Also, many risks from toxic substances are imperfectly understood. For many substances, few if any studies have been published, and those few typically cover only the carcinogenic effects of high doses of single substances on animal species assumed to respond similarly to humans. Data on effects on humans, data on toxic effects other than cancer, data on effects of chronic low-dose exposure, and data on complex mixtures more typical of actual environmental exposures, usually do not exist. Control decisions must therefore be based not on solid knowledge and actuarial experience but on analogies and extrapolations, assumptions, safety factors, and subjective value judgments about how much it is worth to avoid possible risks given the apparent cost of doing so.

Perceptual and organizational blinders and simple differences in human preferences also create barriers to optimal control solutions. For instance, people are more concerned about some toxic chemicals risks than others, and these preferences often are not consistent with the degree of hazard involved. Psychological factors affect whether the individual perceives the risk as familiar and controllable or not (Fischoff et al. 1981). To the extent that these factors operate, they have powerful effects not only on individual behavior but also on the political demands that shape government control priorities and regulatory programs.

Control decisions within businesses—and government agencies as well—may be influenced far more by human perceptions and preferences than by technical considerations. Environmental managers typically are trained in engineering compliance assurance and may lack both training and influence to seek toxic chemicals control through changes in factor inputs, production processes, or product formulations. Other corporate officials, conversely, often leave environmental control to engineers, without examining other options for achieving the same purposes. Similarly, government legislators as well as regulatory professionals often develop commitments to particular goals and approaches that hinder more effective integration of programs and priorities.

Toxic chemicals control is not, therefore, a matter of making a quick or easy choice among technical options. It is an ongoing management process, in which both technical and managerial innovations offer opportunities for improvement in a very imperfect patchwork. If there is a key to this process, it is to keep one's eye constantly on the basic purpose: to contribute to real reduction of human and ecological health hazards.

References

Ames, B. N. 1983. Dietary carcinogens and anticarcinogens. *Science* 221:1256–62.

Andrews, R. N. L., R. J. Burby, and A. G. Turner. 1986. *Hazardous Materials in North Carolina: A Guide for Decisionmakers in Local Government.* Chapel Hill: University of North Carolina, Institute for Environmental Studies.

Arthur D. Little, Inc. 1978. *Environmental Emergency Response: Survey of State Response Capabilities.* Washington, D.C.: U.S. Environmental Protection Agency.

Bower, B. T., C. N. Ehler, and A. V. Kneese. 1977. Incentives for managing the environment. *Environmental Science and Technology* 11:250–54.

Bryan, F. L. 1979. *Diseases Transmitted by Foods.* Publication CDC81-8237. Atlanta: U.S. Department of Health and Human Services, Center for Disease Control.

Bureau International de la Recuperation. 1980. *Handbook for the International Reclamation Bureau.* Brussels: BIR.

Caldart, C. C., and C. W. Ryan. 1985. Waste generation reduction: A first step toward developing a regulatory policy to encourage hazardous substance management through production process changes. *Hazardous Waste and Hazardous Materials* 2:309–31.

California Office of Appropriate Technology. 1981. *Alternatives to the Land Disposal of Hazardous Wastes: An Assessment for California.* Sacramento: California Publications and Information Office.

Cohen, S. Z., S. M. Creeger, R. F. Carcel, C. G. Enfield. 1984. *Potential for Pesticide Contamination of Ground Water Resulting from Agricultural Uses.* Washington, D.C.: American Chemical Society.

CONCAWE (Oil Companies European Organization for Environmental Health Protection). 1977. *Emissions and Effluents from European Refineries.* Report 6/77. The Hague: CONCAWE.

———. 1980. *The Environmental Impact of Refinery Effluents.* Report 1/80. The Hague: CONCAWE.

Council on Environmental Quality. 1982. *Environmental Quality, 1982.* 13th Annual Report. Washington, D.C.: Executive Office of the President.

Davis, G. 1984. *Measures to Promote Reduction and Recycling of Hazardous Wastes in Tennessee.* Knoxville: University of Tennessee, Energy, Environment, and Resources Center.

Doniger, D. D. 1978. *The Law and Policy of Toxic Substances Control: A Case Study of Vinyl Chloride.* Baltimore: Johns Hopkins University Press.

Elkin, H. F. 1977. Petroleum refining. In *Air Pollution,* ed. A. C. Stern. Vol. 4. New York: Academic Press.

Fischoff, B., P. Slovic, S. Lichtenstein, S. L. Derby, and R. L. Keeney. 1981. *Acceptable Risk.* Cambridge: Cambridge University Press.

Fritz, R. J., and K. M. Hanzevack. 1980. Emissions of hydrocarbons and their control. *Proceedings of the World Petroleum Congress* 10:57–64.

Harrison, D., Jr. 1984. Banning hazardous materials from land disposal facilities. *Hazardous Waste* 1:431–42.

Hess, C. T., J. Michel, T. R. Horton, H. M. Prichard, W. A. Coniglio. 1985. The occurrence of radioactivity in public drinking water supplies in the United States. *Health Physics* 48:553–86.

Huisingh, D., and V. Bailey, eds. 1982. *Making Pollution Prevention Pay.* New York: Pergamon.

Huisingh, D., and H. Hilger. 1985. *Profits of Pollution Prevention: A Compendium of North Carolina Case Studies in Resources Conservation and Waste Reduction.* Raleigh: North Carolina State University, Division of University Studies.

Kneese, A. V., and B. T. Bower. 1979. *Environmental Quality and Residuals Management.* Baltimore: Johns Hopkins University Press.

Kohl, J., P. Moses, and B. Triplett. 1984. *Managing and Recycling Solvents: North Carolina Practices, Facilities, and Regulations.* Raleigh: North Carolina State University, Industrial Extension Service.

Kohl, J., and B. Triplett. 1984. *Managing and Minimizing Hazardous Waste Metal Sludges: North Carolina Case Studies, Services, and Regulations.* Raleigh: North Carolina State University, Industrial Extension Service.

Lave, L. 1981. *The Strategy of Social Regulation.* Washington, D.C.: Brookings.

National Academy of Sciences. 1980a. *Drinking Water and Health.* Vol. 3. Washington, D.C.: National Academy Press.

———. 1980b. *Lead in the Human Environment.* Washington, D.C.: National Academy Press.

———. 1983a. *Management of Hazardous and Industrial Wastes: Research and Development Needs.* Washington, D.C.: National Academy Press.

———. 1983b. *Transportation of Hazardous Materials: Toward a National Strategy.* Transportation Research Board Special Report 197. Washington, D.C.: National Academy Press.

———. 1985. *Reducing Hazardous Waste Generation.* Washington, D.C.: National Academy Press.

North Carolina Department of Natural Resources and Community Development. 1986. *Accomplishments of N.C. Industries: Case Summaries.* Raleigh: N.C. Dept. of Natural Resources and Community Development, Pollution Prevention Program.

Patten, R. C. 1981. Aflatoxins and disease. *American Journal of Tropical Medicine and Hygiene* 30:422–25.

Patterson, L. W., and C. E. Westell, Jr. 1985. The manufacture and use of unleaded gasoline in the United States. *Industry and Environment* 8(2).

Portney, P. 1978. Toxic substance policy and the protection of human health. In *Current Issues in U.S. Environmental Policy,* ed. P. R. Portney. Baltimore: Johns Hopkins University Press.

Royston, M. G. 1979. *Pollution Prevention Pays.* New York: Pergamon.

Sarokin, D., W. R. Muir, C. G. Miller, and S. R. Sperber. 1986. *Cutting Chemical Wastes.* New York: INFORM.

Schaub, J. R. 1983. The economics of agricultural pesticide technology. In *Agricultural Chemicals of the Future,* ed. J. L. Hilton. Totowa, N.J.: Rowman and Allanheld.

Scott, E. L., and M. L. Straf. 1977. Ultraviolet radiation as a cause of cancer. In *Origins of Human Cancer.* Book A. Cold Spring Harbor, N.Y.: Cold Spring Harbor Laboratory.

Smith, M. A. 1985. *A Handbook of Environmental Auditing Practices and Perspectives in North Carolina.* Raleigh: North Carolina Department of Natural Resources and Community Development, Pollution Prevention Program.

Schwartz, J., H. Pitcher, R. Levin, B. Ostro, A. Nichols. 1985. *Costs and Benefits of Reducing Lead in Gasoline: Final Regulatory Impact Analysis.* EPA-230-05-85-006. Washington, D.C.: Environmental Protection Agency.

U.S. Congress, Office of Technology Assessment. 1983. *Technologies and Management*

Strategies for Hazardous Waste Control. Washington, D.C.: Government Printing Office.

U.S. Department of Agriculture. 1978. *The Pesticide Review.* Washington, D.C.: U.S.D.A., Agricultural Stabilization and Conservation Service.

U.S. Environmental Protection Agency. 1979. *Development Document for Effluent Limitations, Guidelines, and Standards for the Petroleum Refining Point Source Category.* Publication EPA-440-1-79-014b. Washington, D.C.: Government Printing Office.

————. 1980. *Waste Exchange: Background Information.* Publication SW-887-1. Washington, D.C.: Government Printing Office.

————. 1984. *Costs and Benefits of Reducing Lead in Gasoline.* Report EPA-230-03-84-005. Washington, D.C.: EPA, Office of Policy, Planning and Evaluation.

————. 1986. Draft hazardous waste implementation strategy. Washington, D.C.: EPA Office of Solid Wastes and Emergency Response. Unpublished.

————. No date. An overview of integrated environmental management in the Santa Clara Valley, California. San Francisco: EPA, Region IX. Unpublished.

3. Measuring Toxic Chemicals in the Environment: A Materials Balance Approach

ROBERT U. AYRES, FRANCIS C. McMICHAEL, AND
SAMUEL R. ROD

Ayres, McMichael, and Rod introduce a basic framework for thinking about toxic chemicals in the environment: the materials (mass) balance framework. Activities do not create or destroy matter, but they can transfer it chemically and change its location. For inherently toxic substances, such as the heavy metals, the total mass must be monitored, with only secondary concern given to the precise chemical form. For organic compounds, such as those involving nitrogen, the precise chemical form is more important than the mass of released nitrogen. When used by chemical engineers for a plant or process, the materials balance framework is a rigorous tool. The authors advocate its use at a more aggregate level, such as a geographical region. They explore a historical reconstruction of deposition in the New York–New Jersey region and get strong results regarding the importance of industry versus consumer sources. While the materials balance framework is more art than science at a regional level, it appears to be a valuable tool in understanding the sources of chemicals and in suggesting control strategies.

The study of toxic chemicals in the environment is complex, requiring an understanding in detail where these chemicals are found, how long they persist, and how they move about in the chemical and biological cycles of the environment. Berthouex and Rudd (1977) pointed out that there are a huge number of toxic compounds with a wide range of effects in the environment, and they made these generalizations:

> The pathways through the environment for a toxic material are so subtle and numerous that, even when man is alert to possible harmful

A portion of the work described in this chapter was supported by a grant from the Hudson River Foundation.

effects, he may not predict where in the environment the substance will reach a harmful level.

While we can use analogy and the similarity between chemical families to try and foresee troublesome environmental routes, we dare not rely on these analogies to suggest a substance is safe.

While we can make statements about the concentration of materials in a local environment or about the solubility of a substance, we must remember that the dynamic character of the environment makes all assumptions regarding the uniform distribution of materials or equilibrium conditions dangerous.

The Art and Science of Materials Balance

This chapter discusses the application to environmental problem solving of a fundamental principle of science and engineering analysis known as the conservation of mass or material. The idea is not new. Material is not created nor is it destroyed by ordinary processes, but material does change form. The materials balance method is an accounting procedure, and skill is needed to use it. The materials balance method provides a technique to describe the environment as it is today and as it might be under conditions resulting from remedial actions or from changes in the way society produces, uses, and disposes of toxic materials. Generally, the method is used in science and engineering. However, it has great utility as a tool for analyzing environmental problems as well.

The study of materials balance involves both science and art. Science provides the principle of the conservation of mass, the mathematical expressions for dealing with the flow and storage of material, and the units for expressing the mass, the mass flows, and the concentration and composition of the materials of interest. Art comes into play through the choice of particular control volumes or compartments, the selection of the shape of the boundaries for the control volumes, and the identification of the input and output flows. When the control volume has obvious physical form, such as a manufactured chemical reactor, the art is easy. When the control volume is the aluminum industry or the U.S. economy, the art is harder.

Each application of the materials balance method may be characterized by a spatial and temporal scale. Figure 3.1 shows schematically the wide range of size and time scales encountered in the application of materials balance methods. The scale for a particular problem is difficult to discuss in general terms except at the limits. At the smallest physical size are the detailed engineering balances that rigorously account for all the materials entering and leaving the process, while on the largest physical scales, such as the whole earth, the method is applied to the movement of chemi-

Figure 3.1. Time and size scales for selected applications of materials balance models.

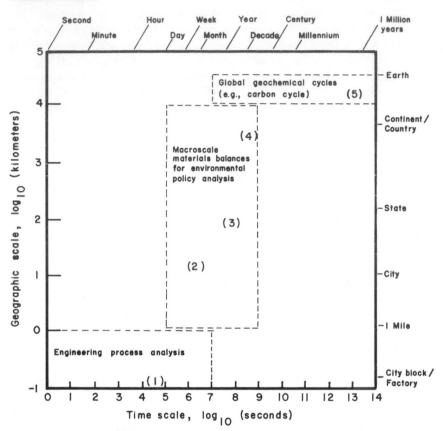

Note: Examples of (1) through (5) are discussed in text: (1) sulfur in an integrated iron and steel plant; (2) pollutants in cities; (3) lead in the Hudson-Raritan River basin, 1880–1980; (4) toxic metals end uses in the United States; (5) global carbon cycle.

cals in the geochemical and geobiological cycles (Garrels et al, 1975). At this scale, the materials balance framework is suggestive rather than rigorous. This chapter applies materials balance methods to problems between these limits—problems of a regional and national scale with time intervals measured in years and decades. Sometimes environmental problems need to be approached with a hierarchical set of materials balances. The art is often, then, in selecting the level of the detail to be included, which depends on how accurate the accounting framework can be. Of course, the selection of such a stopping rule depends on the purpose of the analysis.

In a later section, we emphasize some of the new applications of the materials balance method developed in our own research, paying attention to source or input terms for toxic substances to the environment. We identify the importance of end uses, or consumer uses, as a source of toxic substances in the U.S. environment over several decades, and we explain how indirect as well as direct data can be used to construct a materials balance. This use of indirect data is another example of the art of the method. Our strongest point is that the materials balance method is an important tool for environmental policy analysis and not simply a technical concept to be used only by engineers for process problem solving.

Materials Balance Method Applied to Toxic Chemicals

The construction of a materials balance involves several elements. First, a picture or a diagram, which engineers call a flow sheet, is drawn. The flow sheet consists of compartments and directed lines, which show the inputs and outputs. Second, a basis for describing the problem—for example, a time interval such as a day or a year—is chosen. Similarly, the size of the flows between compartments are scaled on the basis of a particular input or output. In most cases, the physical boundaries of the region over which the material balance will be made is designated. It is also possible to define boundaries in other ways (e.g., by industrial sector such as the aluminum industry, described in a following section). Since the principle of the conservation of mass applies to any and all compartments, it is best to designate boundaries that may be crossed by only a single unknown flow in order to simplify the analysis. This hierarchical manner of looking at the problem, using trial and retrial—combining fragments of information in an orderly manner to develop a complete picture of the pollution problem—is part of the art as well. Next, the nature of toxic substances is examined with a view toward using the materials balance method to address environmental regulation.

▌ Types of Toxic Chemicals

Toxic chemicals are commonly classified as (1) corrosives, (2) irritants, and (3) systemic poisons. Corrosives typically react rather indiscriminately with organic materials or with the water in human tissue. Strong acids, alkalis, and "oxidants" are examples. Irritants are mainly heavy metals and their compounds, such as arsenic, cadmium, chromium, copper, lead, mercury, nickel, silver, and zinc. These metals cause damage to all kinds of tissues. For reasons that are not entirely obvious, most of the toxic metals are likely to be found in nature in combination with sulfur. More important from the environmental perspective, they tend to be toxic in all, or nearly all, their chemical compounds. They differ in this respect from systemic poisons, which tend to be specific in their biological activity.

Systemic poisons are typically organic compounds that interfere with enzymatic reactions, oxygen metabolism, or neural functions. They do so, by and large, by virtue of chemical resemblances to organic compounds normally found in animal cells, mainly proteins. It is not accidental that most biocides—both natural and synthetic—act by combining preferentially with enzymes or other macromolecules' carriers and thereby interfering with their normal message—carrying or transport functions.[1]

Systemic toxins, therefore, are often simple variants or modifications of harmless or essential compounds. For instance, nitrogen is an essential component of all amino acids, from which protein molecules are built. Yet many nitrogenous compounds, including ammonia, cyanide, cyanates (such as MIC), nitrites and nitrates, amines, urea, and so on, are highly toxic. Nitrites are used as preservatives (e.g., of bacon) because of their bactericidal properties. Urea and ammonia are by-products of aerobic and anaerobic protein metabolism, respectively. Ptomaines are produced by anaerobic bacteria. Nitrosamines are among the most toxic and carcinogenic chemicals known. Luckily, nitrogenous materials are biodegradable and are ultimately recycled by natural processes.

Much the same holds true for organic phosphorous compounds. Phosphorus is an essential element of DNA and RNA, as well as bones and teeth, many enzymes, and adenosine triphosphate, the key to both muscular contraction and nerve function. Yet many, if not most, compounds of phosphorus are toxic. For example, phosphorylated cholinesters (including sevin, malathion, and parathion) are widely used as insecticides. Like nitrogenous toxins, toxic phosphorylated organics are biodegradable and do not persist in the environment.

Sulfur is another element essential for animal life. It is a component of three of the amino acids. Yet many organic sulfur compounds are toxic, including hydrogen sulfide, mercaptans, sulfur oxides, carbon disulfide. Copper sulfide and copper sulfate have both been used as pesticides and fungicides. The bactericidal properties of so-called sulfa drugs are well known. Organic compounds of sulfur are generally biodegradable.

The halogens (fluorine, chlorine, bromine, iodine) also tend to be toxic in most forms—although ordinary salt (NaCl) is essential to life, tiny amounts of fluorides appear to be an important ingredient in tooth enamel, chlorine is used for water disinfection, and iodine is a well-known bactericide. Virtually all chlorinated and brominated organics, such as

---

1. Carbon monoxide is toxic because it combines preferentially with hemoglobin, the blood protein that normally carries oxygen from the lungs to the tissues.

solvents, are toxic to animals.[2] Phosgene ($COCl_2$) was one of the first war gases, while DDT, endrin, dieldrin, and others were widely used as insecticides. Polychlorinated biphenyls (PCBs), used as transformer fluids and for a variety of other purposes, have also turned out to be toxic to fish and birds. Vinyl chloride monomer, the basis of PVC, is now known to be extremely carcinogenic. Among the most toxic of all known chemicals are the dioxins, particularly 2, 3, 7, 8 tetrachlorodibenzo-p-dioxin (TCDD). Dioxins are not manufactured as such but are by-products of the process of chlorinating phenols, an intermediate in the production of herbicides such as 2,4-D and 2,4,5-T (agent orange is a 50:50 mixture of these two herbicides). Unfortunately, some halogenated organics are not readily biodegradable. This is particularly true of chlorinated aromatics such as DDT and many similar compounds, PCBs, and dioxins.

It is fairly safe to classify as potentially toxic essentially *all* organic (and many inorganic) compounds of nitrogen, sulfur, phosphorus, fluorine (except the fluorocarbons), chlorine, bromine, and iodine. Similarly, the heavy metals are toxic in almost any ingestible form. While there are certainly some nontoxic compounds of these elements (as well as some toxic substances not involving these elements), the above generalization offers a useful guide. It implies, among other things, that they are likely to be hazardous in the amounts that they occur in almost any industrial waste. From an environmental health perspective, the only safe procedure is to minimize direct human contact with such chemicals. This is particularly important for metals and halogenated aromatics.

The foregoing discussion suggests an alternative classification of hazardous substances, which may be more relevant from the regulatory perspective. It would distinguish toxic chemicals in terms of persistence:

1. *Nondegradable* Substances that remain toxic (or carcinogenic) in virtually any chemical combination. The eight metals cited previously are examples. Radioisotopes also fit into this category.
2. *Semidegradable* Substances that degrade very slowly into less hazardous forms under normal conditions. PAHs and chlorinated aromatics fall into this category.
3. *Degradable* Substances that degrade fairly rapidly to volatile or harmless forms in the presence of oxygen, sunlight, or bacteria. This is true of most organic toxic substances based on nitrogen, sulfur, and phosphorus.

These three groups are not absolute. For instance, metallic forms of most of the metals are relatively harmless, as are some of the oxides and

---

2. Luckily, the chlorofluorocarbons seem to be quite inert.

other inorganic compounds. Chromium is highly toxic in only one of its two valency forms. Arsenic compounds tend to be converted by bacteria into volatile forms that disperse to harmlessly low concentrations. PCBs may be more persistent. Yet the classification is enough to suggest that the principles of accounting may be applied usefully to the first group and, within limits, the second group.

❚ Data for Materials Balance Calculations of Toxic Chemicals

Data useful in estimating toxic contaminant levels can be classified into three categories:

1. Direct data from administrative records (automobile registration, tax collection, electricity generation, water pumped, land use).
2. Direct data from technical measurements (pH readings, chemical analyses, ion concentrations, ratios of dissolved solids to suspended solids, effects on indicator species).
3. Indirect or hybrid data from models or studies done at various times for other purposes (generated often by materials balance accounting).

The direct data categories may include one or more stages of statistical massaging, like simple averaging and estimation of mean probable error. In general, direct data are preferred over indirect data whenever they are available. However, it is an awkward fact that much of the desired information regarding toxic wastes has not been measured directly and must therefore be imputed. The conventional method of estimating residual generation is not adequate for most minor residuals—including many toxic materials—for reasons briefly summarized hereafter. In some cases, a materials balance approach offers a more reasonable prospect of quantification for toxic wastes.

In brief, the conventional method determines net residual coefficients (empirically determined estimates of the residual generated per unit of energy or materials processed per dollar of sectoral output or per unit of sectoral employment). Or gross residual coefficients can be combined with degree-of-control data. If the appropriate coefficients are known and the appropriate physical or economic output measures are given, residual output can be estimated easily.

Unfortunately, for quantitatively minor residues—including most trace elements and toxic chemicals—residual coefficients are largely unavailable and would be unreliable to the point of meaninglessness. This is due primarily to variability of measuring techniques, difficulties in extrapolating from sample data to aggregates, process variability (especially for minor waste streams), and feedstock variability. By comparison, process input-output relations tend to be much more stable and reliable.

More generally, the weakness of the conventional method is that it depends ultimately on direct measurements of residuals, to the exclusion of indirect methods. This seems to be due to a somewhat excessive reliance on empirical data as opposed to "theory." However, the only theory involved in the materials balance method is the basic physical principle of conservation of mass. Chemical elements are neither created nor destroyed by ordinary processes. Hence the amount of a given chemical element that leaves any process, environmental compartment, or region (as a waste) must be exactly balanced by the amount that enters minus net accumulation within the process or compartment boundaries. This is nothing more arcane than double-entry bookkeeping (income = outgo) applied to chemical elements. However, it exploits the fact that process inputs are often easier to track than waste outputs. A formal mathematical statement of materials balance is given below.

Mathematics of Materials Balance

Materials balance, or conservation of mass, is actually a statement of the fundamental physical principle that mass cannot be created or destroyed.[3] The practical statement of mass balance may be phrased as an equation:

Mass entering the volume + change in the amount of mass stored
= mass leaving the volume.

The above statement of mass conservation holds true for total mass and for any components of the total mass that retain their chemical identities regardless of transformations in the control volume. Chemical elements are examples of such conservative substances. Many of them are toxic substances of concern (e.g., mercury, arsenic, lead) or are the key building blocks of other pollutants (e.g., sulfur, chlorine, phosphorus).

To track quantitatively the flow of specific substances that may undergo chemical or biological changes within the control volume, additional source and sink terms must be added to the mass conservation equation. The source term accounts for the creation of the specific chemical in the control volume, while the sink term accounts for its destruction. For a reactive (nonconservative) substance,

---

3. In nuclear processes, mass can be converted to energy and vice versa, but this is a special case, which for the present application can be ignored. In the realm of chemical and biological reactions, mass conservation is a strict statement of fact.

increase in mass of chemical Z in control volume = creation of Z in
control volume + inputs of Z to control volume + destruction of Z in
control volume − output of Z from control volume.

The control volume may be a section of pipe or a stretch of river or any
compartment an analyst wishes to define. By linking several control volumes together as a representative of a physical process and by imposing the
materials balance principle at every point in the network, one can rigorously account for mass flows among compartments. The mathematical expression of this procedure is shown below.

Most pollutants migrate through a complex environmental network
but are ultimately traceable to a number of primary sources. To trace their
transfer from their origins to their final fates in an ecosystem, the materials balance technique employs a materials input-output matrix with properties similar to those of the Leontiev econometric input-output model
(Herfindahl and Kneese 1974). This approach coupled with a mass conservation constraint appears to reduce uncertainties in estimating inputs of
ecosystem contaminants and to validate estimates against actual field
measurements.

The model may be applied on any scale, from a particular chemical
process in a manufacturing plant to a geographical region of any size. At
the microscale of plant processes, engineers regularly impose mass conservation constraints to analyze chemical and materials flows in the processes
and equipment they design. It is an economic necessity in a manufacturing
business to track valued materials accurately throughout a factory. This
application is well defined and can be as sensitive as is desired. The negative value of these materials, as environmental contaminants, however, was
not appreciated until the materials balance principle had been applied to
regional environmental analyses. When applied at a macrolevel, the information yield includes identification of

1.   major pollutant contributors and categories,
2.   key pathways and concentration points within a region,
3.   emissions and runoff trends over long time periods,
4.   cumulative releases and accumulations in the environment, and
5.   uncertainties in pollutant-loading estimates.

At this level, the pathways are too complicated to trace every molecule.
The many interactions and intermediate compounds are ignored when
only the total flow into and out of a sector is looked at.

The materials balance's network of compartments and the accompanying matrix can be constructed in a very formal manner for any bounded
system, from a single factory (or even a piece of equipment such as a fur-

nace or reactor) up to the earth as a whole. A general ecosystem problem is likely to require a fairly high level of aggregation. A materials balance model for the environment is essentially a formal compartmentalization, identifying stocks and flows of materials between compartments (including people). It applies mass conservation as an accounting identity to inputs, transformations, and outputs of each compartment. Figure 3.2 is a schematic of a materials balance network, showing the sources and transport routes of anthropogenic contaminants to the surface waters of a hypothetical river basin.

The next step is the quantification of mass flows, for which a matrix formulation is used to organize the network of environmental compartments. The matrix used for tracking pollutant movement in an ecosystem is adapted from the Leontiev input-output matrix used in econometrics to follow commodity flows among a nation's industries. Derivations applicable to materials balance problems exist in several texts (Herfindahl and Kneese 1974; Ayres 1978) and are not reproduced here. However, a set of definitions and assumptions pertinent to the environmental transport model are presented below.

Once the system is divided into environmental compartments such as airsheds, watersheds, land-use categories, and so on, the transfer of mass from one compartment to others is described by

$$x_i = \sum_j t_{ij} + Y_i,$$

where

x_i = the total mass output from compartment i,
t_{ij} = the mass transferred from compartment i to compartment j, and
Y_i = the mass transferred directly from compartment i to the final environmental reservoir.

An output coefficient, c_{ij}, is defined as the fraction of the total output of compartment i transferred to compartment j, while an input coefficient, a_{ij}, is the fraction of the total output of compartment j that originated in compartment i:

$c_{ij} = t_{ij}/x_i.$
$a_{ij} = t_{ij}/x_j.$

Three fundamental assumptions are made:

1. The sum of inputs to a compartment plus internal sources equals the sum of outputs plus storage (conservation of mass).

Figure 3.2. Anthropogenic emission and transport of pollutants in a hypothetical river.

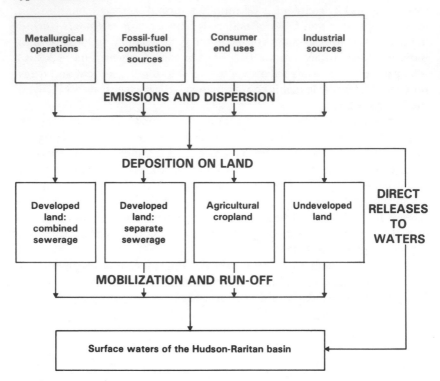

Note: Metallurgical operations include iron and steel foundries; copper, lead, zinc, and other nonferrous metal primary and secondary refiners and smelters. Fossil-fuel combustion includes all heat and power burning of coal, petroleum distillate fuels, and residual oil. Consumer end uses include all end uses by consumers, as distinguished from intermediate uses (emissions) in industrial processes. Industrial sources include all losses from industrial plants and processes other than metallurgical operations and the burning of fossil fuels for heat and power. Also, industrial emissions refer only to pollutants released from the point of production, not those embodied as trace residues in final products. Chemical uses embodied in final products ultimately are released into the environment through the consumption of the products and are therefore included in the end-use category. (*Source:* Ayres and Rod 1986; from *Environment* 28, no. 4 [May 1986]: 17. Reprinted with permission of the Helen Dwight Reid Educational Foundation. Published by Heldref Publications, 4000 Albemarle Street, N.W., Washington, D.C., 20016. Copyright 1986.)

2. Transformations that change the chemical identity of substances are defined as *removal*, and such removal has its own compartment for accounting purposes.
3. Input and output coefficients are constants for the time steps used in the analysis.

Obviously this is a simplification of a complicated structure. Different chemical forms of a substance migrate at different rates to different sinks. The path depends on ambient temperature, moisture level, and so on. The justification for these macroapplications is suggestiveness and productivity, not rigor.

By defining and ordering the compartments appropriately, a variety of information about the system can be elicited. Specifically, once the vector of pollution sources, X, and the matrix of output coefficients, C, are defined we can derive the final output vector, Y, the input coefficient matrix, A, the mass transfer matrix, T, and two other useful matrices:

D = the cumulative output matrix, in which an entry d_{ij} is the fraction of the total output from i transferred to j by all paths, direct and indirect.

B = the cumulative input matrix, in which an entry b_{ij} is the fraction of the total input to j transferred from i by all paths, direct and indirect.

Given the C matrix, calling I the identifying matrix, and defining X_{DIAG} as a matrix whose diagonal elements are the entries of the X vector ($x_{DIAGii} = x_i$) and whose off-diagonal elements are zero,

$A = (X_{DIAG})C(X_{DIAG})$,
$B = (I - A)$,
$D = (I - C)$,
$T = AX_{DIAG} = X_{DIAG}C$, and
$Y = (I - A)X$.

Materials Balance Method at Different Scales

Several studies have been performed that illustrate the use of the materials balance approach in quantifying mass flows in complex systems. The examples cover a range of scales in space and time, from a single industrial facility to the entire nation. The earliest and most frequent use of materials balance has been for engineered systems. The precision of mass flow estimates in such well-defined, manufactured systems can be within plus or minus 1 percent or smaller. For the more novel application of materials balance principles to large ecosystems, uncertainties are much larger.

The advantages and limitations of the technique in these settings are discussed below.

▌ Sulfur in an Integrated Iron and Steelmaking Plant

Materials balances of individual plants and processes are performed routinely for valuable materials and products. A similar approach to track wastes has been used less frequently, mainly since regulatory agencies have placed penalties on excessive discharges.

Figure 3.3 is taken from a study of sulfur flow in a single integrated iron and steelmaking plant. The sulfur in question is embodied in the various raw materials, intermediate substances, products, and wastes that go into the process. Nevertheless, the conservation of mass holds at all points, because elemental sulfur retains its identity through all transformations. The sulfur released into the environment (and embodied in products) from all stages of steelmaking must exactly equal the sulfur content of all the raw materials:

Sulfur in raw materials (tons per day)		Sulfur in final product and waste (tons per day)	
Blast furnace coke	38.00	Steel	1.10
Oxygen furnace scrap	0.37	Blast furnace slag	36.70
Oxygen furnace ferroalloys	0.03	Oxygen furnace slag	0.56
Total	38.40	Oxygen furnace scrap	0.04
		Total	38.40

Uncertainties do exist in these values, arising from variability of inputs, technological and operational variations in the process, and measurement errors of the concentration and mass of sulfur in the process streams. At the scale of a single plant, though, the uncertainties can be clearly identified and bounded. There are also typically several independent methods available to cross-check such estimates.

▌ Pollutants in Cities

Urban areas have received much of the attention of local, state, and federal environmental agencies with respect to quantifying pollution inventories. Up to the scale of a single city and its environs, the tasks of identifying pollution sources and transport paths, estimating emissions, and monitoring the environment seem to be managable. Also, at this scale the effect of regulations can be demonstrated. Areas much beyond the size

Figure 3.3. Flow of sulfur in a typical integrated iron and steelmaking plant.

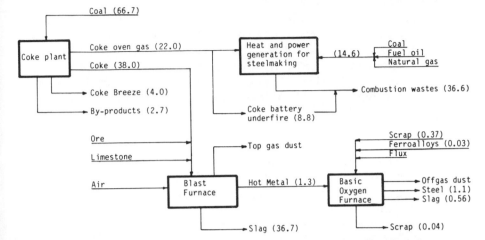

Note: Basis of calculations is 5,500 tons per day of raw steel. (*Source:* Massey 1977.)

of densely populated urban zones are subject to additional physical complexities, such as long-range versus short-range transport of pollution and the accompanying institutional (interjurisdictional) difficulties.

The materials balance principle is at the heart of an emission apportionment method known as source-receptor modeling. Its fundamentals are similar to the mathematical basis of the materials balance approach, and several references describe its theory and application (Hopke 1985; U.S. Environmental Protection Agency 1978). The materials balance technique was the organizing principle for a series of studies on the emission, transport, and deposition of heavy metals in the Los Angeles basin (Friedlander 1973; Huntzicker et al. 1975; U.S. Environmental Protection Agency 1978). Materials balance was also the basis of a retrospective study of sulfur dioxide concentrations in New York City from 1880 to 1980 (Husar and Patterson 1985). Tracing the flow of major inputs like food, water, and fuel into a city, Berthouex and Rudd (1977) constructed a flow of sewage, refuse, and air pollutants for a typical city of one-million persons. We are not aware that such a balance has been carried out in detail for any real city.

▌ Lead in the Hudson-Raritan River Basin

A simple first-order analysis of historical loadings of lead in the Hudson-Raritan River basin (Rod 1986) provided an input-output matrix for a materials balance method on the regional scale. The Hudson-Raritan basin drains much of eastern New York and northern New Jersey and has been the subject of a relative abundance of environmental measurements and modeling efforts (which have not, however, resolved the uncertainty regarding present pollution loads). Lead is a metal of long-standing ecological concern in the region. Historical records of lead production and use are good, and lead's transport properties and aquatic chemistry have been examined in some detail. The thirteen compartments of the matrix formulation are, in order,

Pure sources
1. Metallurgy (lead production)
2. Fossil fuel combustion (coal, gas, petroleum distillates)
3. Industry (losses from manufacturing processes)
4. Consumer end uses
5. Agricultural biocides
6. Nature (erosion)
Intermediate receptors
7. Developed land, combined sanitary and storm sewer systems
8. Developed land, separate sewer systems
9. Agricultural cropland
10. Undeveloped land
Retention
11. Retention on land
Final fates
12. Surface waters of the Hudson-Raritan basin
13. Loss at system boundaries (advection out)

These categories are not immutable, but for the present case they are sufficient and are the most detailed for which reliable data were obtained. Atmospheric dispersion and deposition were included implicitly in source-to-land transport, so the atmosphere is not included as a separate compartment. Also, river and harbor sediments are included as part of the final environmental reservoir, the basin's major water body.

The matrices for the benchmark year, 1980, and preceding years contain best-estimate values of transport coefficients, adapted in large part from the study of historical Hudson-Raritan basin pollution by Ayres et al. (1985) and from National Oceanic and Atmospheric Administration data (Basta et al. 1985; Basta et al. personal communication). The following list summarizes results of the 1980 lead pollution analysis. Values (in metric tons) come from cumulative input, B, and output, D, matrices (Ayres et al. 1985).

Pure sources
1. Fossil fuel combustion: 5,300 metric tons
2. Consumer end uses: 4,200 metric tons
3. Nature: 100 metric tons
4. Industry: 100 metric tons
5. Metallurgy: 50 metric tons
6. Agricultural; biocides: less than 1 metric ton

Intermediate receptors
7. Developed land, combined sewer system: 1,500 metric tons in, 1,100 out; 0.7 ratio
8. Developed land, separate sewer systems: 4,800 metric tons in, 900 out; 0.2 ratio
9. Agricultural cropland: 1,100 metric tons in, 340 out; 0.3 ratio
10. Undeveloped land: 500 metric tons in, 160 out; 0.3 ratio

Retention and final fate
11. Retention on land: 5,400 metric tons
12. Surface water: 2,500 metric tons
13. Loss at boundaries: 1,850 metric tons

The principal lead emission sources were fossil fuel burning (overwhelmingly from alkyl-lead compounds in automotive gasoline) and consumption of lead-containing products. Emissions were transported primarily to developed land, which in turn contributed the majority of the river loading of lead through urban runoff and wastewater discharges. (High combined sewer runoff fraction is due to routine storm overflow that bypasses treatment plants.) Overall, about 55 percent of the primary lead emissions in 1980 was retained on land, 20 percent flowed out to sea, and only 25 percent reached the surface waters of the Hudson-Raritan basin.

The profile of lead emissions shown in figure 3.4 provides an instructive example of changing patterns of material uses and pollution releases over time. The biggest single source of environmental lead since World War II is tetraethyl lead in gasoline. The effects of the automotive emissions regulations of the early 1970s show quite clearly that gasoline use dominated the fossil fuel combustion category. Between world wars I and II, though, lead reached the environment mainly as an ingredient in paints. The larger tonnage uses in car batteries, pipe, foil, solder, soundproofing, and radiation shielding (enclosed uses subject to commercial recycling) did not result in significant dissipative losses. Metallurgical sources of lead dominated around 1900. Two primary lead refineries in northern New Jersey accounted for 33 percent of the 222 thousand metric tons of refined lead in the United States in 1899. Other Hudson-Raritan basin facilities also refined lead and did some primary smelting, but these

Figure 3.4. Sources of lead emissions in the Hudson-Raritan River basin, 1880–1980.

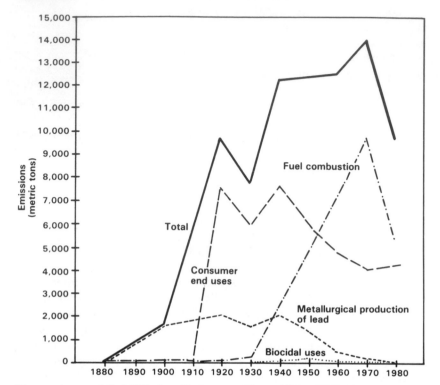

(*Source:* Ayres and Rod 1986; from *Environment* 28, no. 4 [May 1986]: 40. Reprinted with permission of the Helen Dwight Reid Educational Foundation. Published by Heldref Publications, 4000 Albemarle Street, N.W., Washington, D.C., 20016. Copyright 1986.)

operations began closing or leaving the region in the 1930s and 1940s, as reflected in figure 3.4. Secondary lead recovery is still carried out in a number of small plants in the industrial areas of northern New Jersey.

The trends revealed by this historical application of the materials balance principle are valuable for assessing the effects of past environmental interventions (e.g., leaded gasoline regulation) and for anticipating the likely effects of proposed regulation on a contaminant's sources. At the regional level, uncertainties in the best-estimate values of pollutant loadings on the order of 50 percent would be acceptable for the specific purpose of the trend analysis. Because the methodology was applied in a consistent manner over the decade time intervals, relative trends for each source category are reasonably accurate, though absolute values may have fairly large variances. A discussion of uncertainties related to the application of materials balance to pollution chronologies appears later in this chapter.

▌ Consumer End Uses of Toxic Metals in the United States

Regional-scale studies of pollution sources have in many cases revealed the end uses of products as significant sources of environmental contamination. Numerous substances embodied in products consumed by both individuals and businesses become pollutants when the products that contain them are used or disposed of. The preceding example of lead in the Hudson-Raritan basin shows that consumer end uses of lead in that region are coming to dominate lead emissions as emissions from leaded gasoline decrease through regulatory restrictions.

The recognition of the numerous distributed end uses of materials (when taken as a whole) as a major contributor to pollution has come only recently. The U.S. Environmental Protection Agency has initiated research into this area now that the more traditional industrial pollution sources have been brought under reasonably mature and comprehensive institutional controls. The EPA's National Urban Runoff Program exemplifies the basic research activities, while the attention to small quantity generators of pollutants in the 1986 reauthorization of the Resource Conservation and Recovery Act demonstrates recent regulatory concerns about the myriad small sources of pollution in the country.

This section illustrates the use of the materials balance approach to estimate environmental fluxes of eight toxic metals (from the EPA's priority pollutant list) from dissipative end uses and consumption wastes. It is important to emphasize that extraction, smelting, and refining losses and emissions are not included in the analysis (although the materials balance principle is clearly applicable to these processes). The eight examples demonstrate both the value of the technique in identifying dominant emission sources and the limitations of the current state of the science.

The emissions resulting from dissipative end uses may be radically different from one source category to another. (An obvious illustration: tetraethyl lead from automobile exhaust is rapidly dispersed into a highly mobile form, and a high proportion of it evidently appears in urban runoff; on the other hand, lead used in batteries, bullets, cable coverings, and solder is scarcely mobilized at all, and little or none appears in runoff.)

In the case of the heavy metals (silver, arsenic, cadmium, chromium, copper, mercury, lead, and zinc), ten categories of consumption are readily distinguishable in terms of degrees of dissipation in use and modes of release to the environment (table 3.1). These ten categories can be summarized as follows:

1. Metals used as alloys or amalgams (except plating, electrical equipment, catalysts, and dental work). Losses can be assumed to be due largely to wear and corrosion (primarily the latter), except for mercury, which volatilizes.

2. Plating and dip coating (e.g., galvanizing, electroplating), vacuum deposition, or chemical bath (e.g., chromic acid). These processes generally resulted in significant waterborne wastes until the 1970s. Cadmium plating processes were particularly inefficient until recently. Losses in use are mainly due to wear and abrasion (e.g., silverplate), or flaking (decorative chrome trim). In the case of mercury-tin "silver" for mirrors, the loss was largely due to volatilization.

3. Paints and pigments are lost primarily by weathering (e.g., for metal-protecting paints), by wear, or by disposal of painted dyes or pigmented objects, such as magazines. Copper-based and mercury-based paints slowly volatilize over time. A factor of 0.5 is rather arbitrarily assumed for all other paints and pigments.

4. Batteries and electronic devices include all metals and chemicals (e.g., phosphorus) in tubes and primary and secondary batteries, but excludes copper wire. Losses in manufacturing may be significant. Mercury in mercury vapor lamps can escape to the air when tubes are broken. In all other cases it is assumed that discarded equipment goes mainly to landfills. Minor amounts are volatilized in fires or incinerators or lost by corrosion; lead-acid batteries are recycled.

5. Other electrical equipment includes solders, contacts, semiconductors, and other special materials (but not copper wire) used in electrical equipment control devices, instruments, and so on. Losses to the environment are primarily through the discarding of obsolete equipment to landfills. Mercury used in instruments may be lost through breakage and volatilization or spillage.

6. Industrial chemicals and reagents include catalysts, solvents, reagents, bleaches, and so on. In some cases, a chemical is basically embodied but there are some losses in processing. Losses in chemical manufacturing per se are included here. Major examples are copper and mercury catalysts (especially in chlorine manufacturing); copper, zinc, and chromium mordants for dyes; mercury losses in felt manufacturing; chromium losses in tanning; lead losses in desulfurization of gasoline; and zinc losses in rayon spinning. In some cases, virtually all of the material is actually dissipated. Detonators, such as mercury fulminate and lead azide (and explosives), are in this category.

7. Chemical additives to consumer products include fuel additives (e.g., TEL), anticorrosion agents (e.g., zinc dithiophosphate), initiators and plasticizers for plastics (e.g., zinc oxide), and wood preservatives

Table 3.1. Emission into the environment of eight heavy metals in ten consumption categories

Metal	Metallic Uses	Plating and Coating	Paints and Pigments	Batteries and Electronic Devices	Other Electrical Equipment	Industrial Chemicals and Reagents	Chemical Additives to Consumer Products	Agricultural Biocides	Nonagricultural Biocides	Pharmaceuticals and Germicides	Other
Silver	0.001	0.02	0.5	0.01	0.01	1.0	0.40	0	0	0.5	0.05
Arsenic	0.001	0	0.5	0.01	0	0.5	0.05	0.50	0.5	0.8	0.05
Cadmium	0.001	0.15	0.5	0.02	0	1.0	0.15	0	0	0	0.05
Chromium	0.001	0.02	0.5	0	0	1.0	0.05	0	1.0	0.8	0.05
Copper	0.005	0	1.0	0	0.10	1.0	0.05	0.05	1.0	0	0.05
Mercury	0.050	0.05	0.8	0.20	0.10	1.0	0	0.80	0.9	0.2	0.50
Lead	0.005	0	0.5	0.01	0	1.0	0.75	0.05	0.1	0	0.05
Zinc	0.001	0.02	0.5	0.01	0	1.0	0.15	0.05	0.1	0.8	0.05

Source: Ayres et al. 1985.
Note: Emission coefficient is the fraction of the material released in mobile form within about a decade. Recycled waste, waste in landfills, and sludge dumped off shore are excluded.

and chromium salts embodied in leather. Losses to the environment occur when the embodying productivity is utilized; for example, gasoline containing TEL is burned and largely (0.75) dispersed into the atmosphere. However, copper, chromium, and arsenic are used as wood preservatives and dispersed only if the wood is later burned or incinerated. In the case of silver (photographic film), we assume that 60 percent is later recovered.

8. Agricultural pesticides, herbicides, and fungicides are dissipated, but heavy metals are largely immobilized by soil. Arsenic and mercury are exceptions because of their volatility.

9. Nonagricultural biocides are the same compounds as above used in industrial, commercial, or resident applications. Loss rates are higher in some cases.

10. Pharmaceuticals (including cosmetics), dental filling material, and germicides, are mostly dissipated to the environment via waste water. Silver and mercury dental fillings are likely to be buried with cadavers.

It is unfortunate (and curious) that there are almost no published data on emission coefficients for consumption activities. Obviously, most analysts have not considered such activities to be sources of pollutants.[4] In the absence of a body of literature, the choice of emission coefficients must be based on a combination of available literature, expert judgment, and educated guesswork. There remains much art in the science.

The values in table 3.1 are kept to one or two significant figures, depending on the quality of the background information, resulting in rounded values in which contributions from minor uses or emissions are effectively "lost in the noise." Nonetheless, within the limits of inherent uncertainty, the results are instructive. While many of the numerical estimates are uncertain—sometimes even by a factor of two or three—there are only a few important routes that clearly dominate for each metal. In general, only the consumption categories with large coefficients would need to be considered in greater detail in a more refined study.

To complete the example, we allocated total domestic usage of each of the eight metals over the past three decades among the input-output categories. The allocation is far from constant. Many formerly important uses have disappeared, while others have emerged as recently as the last decade. Consumption data by use is available, in general, only since World War II. For earlier periods, one must rely on a scattering of real data sup-

---

4. On the other hand, sewage treatment and waste incineration have inconsistently been so treated.

plemented by a variety of other clues. Usage of silver and lead over the last four decades for the whole United States is summarized in tables 3.2 and 3.3.

▌ Fluoride in the Primary Aluminum Industry

In each of the preceding examples, we chose physical boundaries for the regions over which the materials balance is made. It is also possible to define boundaries in other ways; for example, by industrial sector rather than by geographical region. A somewhat unconventional application of the materials balance method—to the primary aluminum industry—demonstrates its value in reducing uncertainty in the estimation of the inputs of chemical feedstocks that contain fluorine. The materials balance method was combined with empirical data in a rigorous manner to reduce inherent

Table 3.2. Silver: End uses and emissions, various years (metric tons)

Consumption category	1958	1967	1972	1980
Metallic; plating and coating				
End use	1,800	1,300	1,800	1,100
Emissions	19	14	19	12
Batteries and electronic devices				
End use	60	130	170	200
Emissions	1	1	2	2
Other electrical equipment				
End use	400	700	1,000	900
Emissions	4	7	10	9
Industrial chemicals and reagents				
End use	60	60	100	110
Emissions	60	60	100	110
Chemical additives to consumer products				
End use	700	800	1,100	1,700
Emissions	280	320	440	680
Pharmaceuticals and germicides				
End use	60	60	40	40
Emissions	30	30	20	20
Other				
End use	220	90	70	130
Emissions	11	5	4	7
Total end use	3,300	3,100	4,300	4,200
Total emissions	410	440	590	840

Source: Ayres et al. 1985.

Table 3.3. Lead: End uses and emissions, various years
(thousand metric tons)

Consumption Category	1949	1957	1972	1980
Metallic				
End use	440.0	370.0	280.0	250.0
Emissions	2.2	1.9	1.4	1.3
Paints and pigments				
End use	120.0	100.0	80.0	100.0
Emissions	60.0	50.0	40.0	50.0
Batteries and electronic devices				
End use	340.0	300.0	620.0	850.0
Emissions	3.4	3.0	6.2	8.5
Agricultural biocides				
End use	30.0	10.0	0.0	0.0
Emissions	1.5	0.5	0.0	0.0
Other				
End use	20.0	30.0	50.0	30.0
Emissions	1.0	1.5	2.5	1.5
Total end use	1,000.0	800.0	1,000.0	1,200.0
Total emissions	68.0	57.0	50.0	61.0

Source: Ayres et al. 1985.

uncertainty in quantitative predictions (including extrapolations, interpolations, forecasts, and backcasts).

Despite its conceptual simplicity, the principle of materials-energy balance is even more powerful than financial accounting, since there is not one balance condition (dollars) but as many balance conditions to be satisfied as there are atomic species involved in the process (plus one more for energy). In view of its power, it is curious that the principle has seldom been used at the macrolevel, although it is a standard tool of engineering analysis at the process level. Its potential value is illustrated by the following example, adapted from a 1978 study for EPA (Ayres et al. 1978).

Nine studies of the primary aluminum industry over the period 1968–76 revealed moderate agreement with regard to the input coefficients for alumina, petroleum coke, and pitch but surprisingly wide disagreement on inputs of fluorine-containing chemicals—synthetic cryolite, aluminum fluoride, and fluorspar (table 3.4).[5] In fact, estimates of cryolite input ranged from 5 to 50 kilograms per metric ton of aluminum, depending on the

---

5. Natural cryolite was exhausted some years ago. All cryolite used in recent years has been synthetic.

Table 3.4. Inputs in aluminum output, kilograms per metric ton, nine studies

Kilograms per Metric Ton of Aluminum Output

Input	Bureau of Mines Studies			EPA Studies			FEA Study	Balgord Study	International Research and Technology
	1	2	3	1	2	3[a]			
Alumina	1,930	1,910–1,950	1,900–1,950	2,000	1,930	1,900	1,930	1,930	1,930
Petroleum coke	...	560–600	330	500	520	450–490	550	520	500
Pitch	...	100–200	140–165	260	150	127–167	150	150	150
Synthetic cryolite	35	20–50	5–35	50	35	30–50	35	35	21
Aluminum fluoride	20–50	10–30	12.5–30	40	20	30–50	20	20	30
Fluorspar	3	...	2–4	...	...	3	...	...	...
Baked carbon	520	...	20–40	600	...	20	...	...	...

Source: Ayres et al. 1978.

Note: See source for details of the nine studies.

[a] The lower figure is for petroleum coke and soderberg, the higher figure is for prebake. For pitch, the lower figure is for prebake. For pitch, the higher figure is for prebake, the higher figure is for soderberg.

study. Estimates of aluminum fluoride input ranged from 10 to 50 kilo-grams per metric ton. The range of possible error for a median estimate is far too high for comfort.

A probably better estimate can be arrived at indirectly from the re-ported total production of aluminum fluoride, assuming it is used almost exclusively in aluminum production. In 1973 this assumed allocation ac-counted for 30 kilograms per metric ton of aluminum. This obviously con-stitutes an upper limit. It is easily verified by a materials balance calcula-tion that this level of production of aluminum fluoride would have accounted for 29 percent of reported 1973 production of hydrofluoric acid. An authoritative source, *Chemical Economics Handbook* (Stanford Re-search Institute 1973) allocated an additional 12 percent of hydrofluoric acid production to the manufacture of synthetic cryolite. Again, a materi-als balance for the chemical reactions implies a consumption level (roughly equal to production) for cryolite equivalent to 21 kilograms per metric ton of aluminum. It is noteworthy that both figures are roughly in the middle of the estimated range. Quite obviously, the range of error has been sharply reduced.

The above analysis is directly applicable to the estimation of fluorine emissions from the primary aluminum industry. The conventional ap-proach to emissions estimation for the industry is to measure the fluorine content of all effluent streams from many aluminum refineries. Such mea-surements are technically difficult and quite dependent on operating con-ditions, which are inherently variable. Typical summaries of emissions fac-tors are given in ranges, so a meaningful estimate of either average or total fluoride emissions for a given facility is almost impossible to derive from the standard tables.

With the materials balance approach, fluoride emissions equal fluo-ride inputs less any accumulation as inventory within the industry. Assum-ing no capacity growth, the calculation is straightforward: 21 kilograms of synthetic cryolite (54 percent F) plus 30 kilograms of aluminum fluoride (55 percent F) per metric ton of aluminum implies that 28 kilograms of fluorine is emitted per metric ton of aluminum. While this figure may not be exact, it is unlikely to be wrong by more than 10 percent. Moreover, the true emissions figure is much more likely to be slightly smaller rather than larger, since there may be some accumulation within the plant.

Global Balances

The study of the circulation of materials through the earth's atmo-sphere, to the land, and through the soils into the ground and surface wa-ters, then to the ocean, to the deep ocean sediments, or to the atmosphere again, is part of the geological sciences. Quantitative models based on materials balance have been constructed for major elements like carbon, nitrogen, sulfur, and phosphorus (Garrels et al. 1975). Few global models of trace element cycles have been constructed because of a general lack of environmental data. It is especially difficult to describe society's contribution to the change in the natural global cycles.

Garrels et al. described the application of the materials balance method to the synthetic organic chemical, DDT (dichlorodiphenyltrichloroethane), which is foreign to natural systems. Again, due to a lack of worldwide data, it is difficult to describe quantitatively the flows among the atmosphere, the land, the oceans, and the biota, as well as to estimate the amount of DDT stored in each compartment. The logic and organization is in the model, but the quantification is weak.

Materials Balance Estimates and Environmental Measurements

There is a paradox in the developing sciences (of which quantitative ecological research is an excellent example). How does one assess a method's predictions when that method is the first approach to a novel problem? The paradox will remain with applications of macroscale materials balance principles until comprehensive studies from the perspectives of both pollution sources and environmental receptors are completed for geographical regions of interest.

In the case of the materials balance methodology, its predictive power has been demonstrated extensively in the study of engineered systems. However, evidence in support of its practical value in ecosystem analysis is scarce because examples of separable (i.e., boundable) systems are scarce. Note that materials balance as a principle need not be validated. It is the nearest thing to an absolute law of nature that we have. In any case involving a reasonably well-defined, bounded system, if direct measurements do not agree with indirect measurements it says something about the measurements, not the method. In this section, comparisons between some materials balance estimates and relevant field measurements of an environmental system are presented. In addition to the studies of historical pollution trends in the Hudson-Raritan basin (Ayres & Rod 1986; Rod 1986; Ayres et al. 1985), there are both pollutant source estimates from materials balances and a few actual measurements of some pollutants in riverine and marine sediments.

Sediment cores taken from river beds, harbor floors, marshes, and wetlands hold the only long-term historical record of pollution in the Hudson-Raritan basin. Figure 3.5 presents a qualitative comparison of the input-output materials balance estimates of lead pollution with deposition

Figure 3.5. Lead in the Hudson-Raritan River basin: Loading and sediment concentration, 1880–1980.

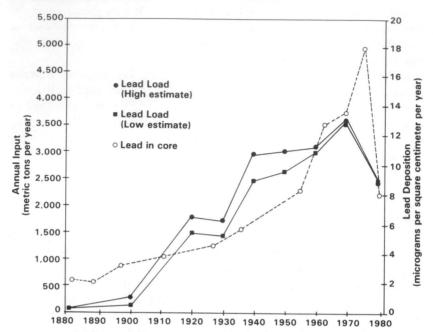

Note: Lines linking point estimates are for clarity only. They should not be used for interpolation. (*Sources:* Ayres and Rod 1986; Stevenson 1986; from *Environment* 28, no. 4 [May 1986]: 43. Reprinted with permission of the Helen Dwight Reid Educational Foundation. Published by Heldref Publications, 4000 Albemarle Street, N.W., Washington, D.C., 20016. Copyright 1986.)

data from a dated sediment core. The core was taken in the Tivoli marsh (river mile 100 on the Hudson), and dates to the early 1800s. Normalized ad hoc at the 1980 benchmark year (for want of direct theoretical links), the chronologies compare remarkably well, especially since the core could be susceptible to local effects, while lead river-loading estimates are an average for the entire basin.

No theory is yet capable of quantitatively relating river pollution inputs to sediment concentrations reliably. However, qualitative comparisons between analytical results and measurements of several pollutants in a single core and comparisons of a single pollutant in several cores are still valuable. Mercury, for instance, was also measured in the Tivoli marsh core. Figure 3.6 shows results of an input-output materials balance of mercury similar to the one for lead. The fact that the analytical method's profile matches the sediment chronology fairly well reinforces evidence of the method's applicability in this case.

Figure 3.7 compares the historical input of PCBs into the Hudson-Raritan basin, with PCB concentrations in two cores taken from the central Hudson basin at river miles 52 and 89. PCBs have been used commercially in the region since 1939. Their principal point sources were two General Electric Company capacitor plants, which opened in the mid 1950s. Until 1973 most PCBs released from the plants were trapped behind a dam upstream of the core sites. The removal of the dam in 1973 resulted in a release of PCBs so large that they appeared distinctly in both sediment cores and downstream river-loading estimates. With the 1973 peak as a normalization point, the remainder of the historical records corroborate one another, qualitatively.

Trace pesticide concentrations in another core are shown in figures 3.8 and 3.9. The figures show materials balance estimates of river loadings of the chlorinated hydrocarbon pesticides chlordane and dieldrin to concentrations of both chemicals in a dated Hudson River sediment core. Both the pesticide-loading estimates and sediment concentrations reflect the in-

Figure 3.6. Mercury in the Hudson-Raritan River basin: Loading and sediment concentration, 1880–1980.

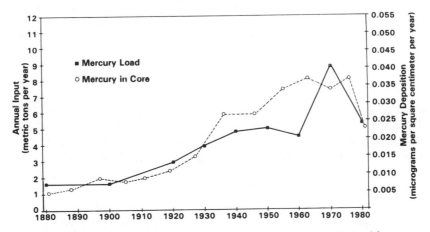

Note: Lines linking point estimates are for clarity only. They should not be used for interpolation. (*Sources:* Ayres and Rod 1986; Stevenson 1986; from *Environment* 28, no. 4 [May 1986]: 42. Reprinted with permission of the Helen Dwight Reid Educational Foundation. Published by Heldref Publications, 4000 Albemarle Street, N.W., Washington, D.C., 20016. Copyright 1986.)

Figure 3.7. PCBs in the Hudson-Raritan River basin: Loading and sediment concentration, 1940–1980.

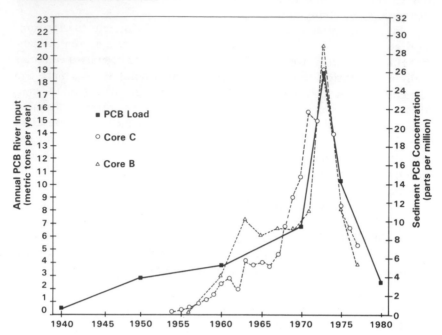

Note: Lines linking point estimates are for clarity only. They should not be used for interpolation. (*Sources:* Ayres and Rod 1986; Olsen et al. 1984; from *Environment* 28, no. 4 [May 1986]: 42. Reprinted with permission of the Helen Dwight Reid Educational Foundation. Published by Heldref Publications, 4000 Albemarle Street, N.W., Washington, D.C., 20016. Copyright 1986.)

creased usage of chlordane and dieldrin from their introductions in the 1940s to their usage peaks and their subsequent declines. However, the annual materials balance loading estimates yield a clearer picture of the river-loading chronologies for these pesticides than do the few scattered sediment measurements. Generally speaking, measurements are always imprecise to some degree, so direct and indirect measurements are likely to disagree. However, indirect measures like those that underlie the materials balance approach can be much more precise in some cases, especially where the toxic substance is a trace residual.

Comparisons between the results of analytical materials balance and sediment chronologies are encouraging. While such comparisons have so far been qualitative in the absence of mechanistic models linking river inputs to sediment concentrations, they are valuable as corroboration of the

Figure 3.8. Chlordane in the Hudson-Raritan River basin: Loading and sediment concentration, 1940–1980.

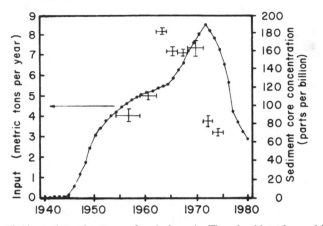

Note: Lines linking point estimates are for clarity only. They should not be used for interpolation. Error bars represent dating uncertainty due to the width of core segments and to high versus low split-sample concentration measurements. (*Sources:* Rod 1986; Bopp et al. 1982; Olsen et al. 1984.)

Figure 3.9. Dieldrin in the Hudson-Raritan River basin: Loading and sediment concentration, 1940–1980.

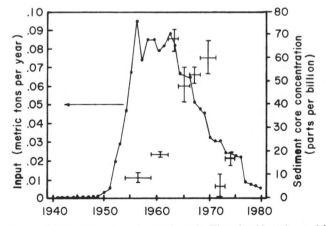

Note: Lines linking point estimates are for clarity only. They should not be used for interpolation. Error bars represent dating uncertainty due to the width of core segments and high versus low split-sample concentration measurements. (*Sources:* Rod 1986; Bopp et al. 1982; Olsen et al. 1984.)

materials balance estimate chronologies. Conversely, there are often uncertainties inherent in direct environmental measurement, which can be reduced or at least bounded by invoking materials balance principles.

Summary

The materials balance method has been used for many years to characterize the movement of chemical pollutants to different parts of our natural environment. However, the method is often viewed solely as a tool of the engineer and physical scientist, and its use in environmental planning, regulation, and management is sometimes overlooked. It is helpful for systems in which descriptive information is incomplete or in which direct measurements of residuals are impractical. It permits one to set limits on mass flows in and out of compartments and to focus attention on the data needs for environmental characterization and analysis.

The materials balance method can be applied to the analysis of environmental problems in a hierarchical fashion. One can increase the level of detail from the simple to the complex by dividing the problem into larger numbers of environmental compartments and including more transport pathways between compartments. Thus it is possible to explore problems by adding the appropriate level of detail that can be supported by the data and the appropriate level of detail to address a particular problem. At a macrolevel of analysis, this framework is necessarily a gross simplification of many complicated physical, chemical, and biological processes.

The method is not a panacea. It should be used cautiously, with attention to comparison between predictions and observations. It offers a mechanism to test knowledge of an environmental system by asking the question, How good is the materials balance? A good agreement between direct and indirect measurements indicates that the system is well bounded and the transfer functions are well understood. The major drawback of the materials balance approach is that defining clear system boundaries and determining mass flows across those boundaries are not always feasible. Cases where chemical transformations occur in the environment are particularly difficult to analyze by means of this approach. But for toxic atomic species such as heavy metals or halogens, which are quite likely to be toxic in *any* chemical form, the materials balance method is attractive.

This chapter describes the use of the materials balance at a macroscale in order to try to identify the role that consumer end use plays in the release of toxic substances, like certain heavy metals and synthetic organic chemicals, to the environment. It highlights the use of the method to construct patterns of historical chemical usage that can be related to the composition of selected environmental compartments, like river bottom sediments, which for yearly time scales act as holding reservoirs for these toxic chemicals.

Future work using the materials balance method as a policy analysis tool should address the special problems posed by chemical transformation. At the macrolevel, it should also focus on the relative importance of point sources versus distributed end-use sources. To date, our work indicates that end use is by far the dominant source of metals and of synthetic organic pesticides. There is a need to develop more detailed data bases for end-use categories in order to more completely describe the release of toxic chemicals to the environment.

References

Ayres, R. U. 1978. *Resources, Environment and Economics: Applications of the Materials/Energy Balance Principle.* New York: John Wiley and Sons.

Ayres, R. U., L. W. Ayres, J. McCurley, M. Small, J. A. Tarr, and R. C. Widgery. 1985. *A Historical Reconstruction of Major Pollutant Levels in the Hudson-Raritan Basin, 1880–1980.* Pittsburgh: Variflex Corporation.

Ayres, R. U., and S. R. Rod. 1986. Patterns of pollution in the Hudson-Raritan basin: Reconstructing an environmental history. *Environment* 28:14–20, 39–43.

Ayres, R. U., E. Weinstein, and J. Cummings-Saxton. 1978. *Assessment of Methodologies for Indirect Impact Assessment.* Final Report IRT-468-R/a. Washington, D.C.: Environmental Protection Agency.

Basta, D. J., F. D. Arnold, and D. R. Farrow. Personal communication of unpublished data from the National Coastal Pollutant Discharge Inventory, October 1985.

Basta, D. J., B. T. Bower, C. N. Ehler, F. D. Arnold, B. P. Chambers, and D. R. Farrow. 1985. The National Coastal Pollutant Discharge Inventory. In *Proceedings of the 4th Symposium on Coastal and Ocean Management.* Washington, D.C.: Department of Commerce, National Oceanic and Atmospheric Administration.

Berthouex, P. M., and D. F. Rudd. 1977. *Strategy of Pollution Control.* New York: John Wiley and Sons.

Bopp, R. F., H. J. Simpson, C. R. Olsen, R. M. Trier, and N. Kostyk. 1982. Chlorinated hydrocarbons and radionuclide chronologies in sediments of the Hudson River and estuary, New York. *Environmental Science and Technology* 16:666.

Friedlander, S. K. 1973. Chemical element balances and identification of air pollution sources. *Environmental Science and Technology* 7:235.

Garrels, R. M., F. T. Mackenzie, and C. Hunt. 1975. *Chemical Cycles in the Environment.* Los Altos, Calif.: William Kaufman, Inc.

Herfindahl, O. C., and A. V. Kneese. 1974. *Economic Theory of Natural Resources.* Columbus: Merrill.

Hopke, P. K. 1985. *Receptor Modeling in Environmental Chemistry.* New York: John Wiley and Sons.

Huntzicker, J. J., S. K. Friedlander, and C. I. Davidson. 1975. Material balance for automobile-emitted lead in the Los Angeles basin. *Environmental Science and Technology* 9:448–57.

Husar, R. B., and D. E. Patterson. 1985. *Sulfur Dioxide Concentration Estimates for*

New York City, 1880-1980. St. Louis: Washington University, Research Laboratory Report.

Massey, M. J. 1977. Environmental control of sulfur in iron and steelmaking. Ph.D. thesis. Carnegie-Mellon University.

Olsen, C. R., I. L. Larsen, R. H. Brewster, N. H. Cutshall, R. F. Bopp, and H. J. Simpson. 1984. *A Geochemical Assessment of Sedimentation and Contaminant Distributions in the Hudson-Raritan Estuary*. Technical Report NOS-OMS-2. Washington, D.C.: Department of Commerce, National Oceanic and Atmospheric Administration, Environmental Services Division.

Rod, S. R. 1986. Historical reconstruction of pollutant loadings in river basins. In Proceedings of the 17th Modelling and Simulation Conference, University of Pittsburgh. Unpublished.

Stanford Research Institute. 1973. *Chemical Economics Handbook*. Palo Alto: SRI.

Stevenson, K. Personal communication, March 12, 1986.

U.S. Environmental Protection Agency. 1978. *Mass Balance Determinations for Pollutants in Urban Regions: Methodology with Application to Lead, Zinc, Cadmium, and Arsenic*. Technical Report EPA-600/4-78-046, Environmental Monitoring Series. Washington, D.C.: EPA.

4. Environmental Monitoring of Toxic Chemicals

BERNARD E. SALTZMAN

*The previous chapters describe the release of chemicals into the environment,
their chemical transformations, and their physical movements, but detailed data
are needed to assess damage to people and the ecology. Saltzman presents the
theory and practice of environmental monitoring. Monitoring is made inherently
difficult by the enormous variation from one period to the next in the amount of
a particular compound at a particular monitoring site. Often, monitoring must
distinguish the precise chemical compound at concentrations in the parts per
million or parts per billion range. Unfortunately, the sampling process and
chemical analysis can change the chemical composition and concentration of the
substance being monitored. Great care must be taken not to contaminate
samples when the analysis is at the level of a few parts per billion. According to
the author, there is no good, general-purpose environmental monitoring
program. Rather, each monitoring program must have its own specified goals
concerning the chemical to be monitored in each medium and the desired
accuracy of measurement.*

Environmental monitoring is inherently complicated. It can involve
sampling air, water, soil, plants, animals, and materials for thousands of
chemicals in concentrations measured in parts per trillion. For example,
hundreds of toxic chemicals have been detected in water supplies, and potentially all of them might be monitored. Monitoring all the toxic chemicals in air, water, soil, and food that people might be exposed to, much less
all the toxic chemicals that could influence the ecology of a region, is an
impossible task—it would require many more resources than are available.

For this reason environmental monitoring must be designed for a specific purpose. The media, the receptor to be protected, the chemicals and
concentrations of interest, and the acceptable level of sensitivity all must
be specified. Unless all these considerations are designed into the monitor-

ing program, it is almost certain to be inconclusive and unnecessarily expensive.

The federal government has been spending many millions of dollars each year to monitor toxic chemicals in the air, water, soil, and food. However, these data often turn out to be inadequate for characterizing the state of the environment or for accomplishing legislative objectives. For example, federally supported air-monitoring stations are located in polluted, populated areas. The stations are at fixed sites (which may be changed over time) and take continuous readings of at least five pollutants. The equipment for each station costs more than $100 thousand, each requires a part-time operator, and each generates vast amounts of data. Unfortunately, these data cannot confidently tell to what degree air quality is improving in a region, or even whether air quality is improving at all. At best, these stations measure the quality of outdoor air in a particular location twenty feet off the ground. No one breathes air at that height. It would be preferable to know more about the quality of the air people breathe, both outdoors and indoors. This might call for the use of personal sampling devices, which measure the air breathed by individuals.

The point is that careful specification of the purpose of the monitoring program would permit the program to be designed to serve that particular need. If the objective were to find out the extent to which air quality in a particular city has changed over time, one would probably want to select a few sites for permanent monitors and then use mobile sampling to characterize the rest of the area. One would have to specify which pollutants were of interest and whether it was the peak concentration or some average over time that was of concern. The optimal monitoring plan would probably be quite different from anything that currently exists. If the objective were to find what humans are exposed to, one would want to use personal monitors. If the objective were to measure the amounts of pollutants being emitted from a particular facility, still a different monitoring plan would be designed.

Even beyond these considerations, the monitoring program must be designed with the characteristics of the laboratory technology in mind. The types of samples taken, storage of these samples, and analysis time all depend on the chemicals sampled and the laboratory procedures available for analysis. Finally, the monitoring plan must take account of the skills, training, and motivation of the personnel.

Environmental monitoring is technically difficult in the sense of being able to measure the chemicals of concern in a way that accurately reflects what is in the environment. For example, the monitoring procedure can transform chemicals, exclude some from collection, or be systematically biased; it can measure a chemical of no interest rather than the chemical of concern. This chapter is focused on how to monitor so that the results accurately reflect the concentration of the measured chemicals in the specified medium in the specified location. Achieving this level of accuracy and reliability means taking great pains with choosing the sampling method and the sampling instruments.

General Considerations for an Environmental Sampling Program

There may be a variety of objectives for a sampling program. The most common one is compliance with a legal standard. Detailed sampling and analytical methods are usually included in the standard, which are usually followed exactly. If different methods are used, they must be proved to be equivalent to the official method or bè accepted by the official agency.

Another common objective is to sample for a research study, for which investigators sometimes use unofficial but more suitable methods. It is important for such a study to sample all significant variables. For example, if air concentrations are to be studied, meteorological data usually should be collected. If industrial emissions or river water concentrations are to be studied, flow measurements are needed. Special sampling programs also may be conducted for public information, for the historical record, to investigate complaints, or to plan or evaluate methods of controlling an environmental hazard. Monitoring methods thus are adjusted to meet the objectives of the study.

It is important to obtain statistically representative samples. Concentrations in air may change rapidly with time. When short-term peaks are important, continuous monitoring instruments usually are used. Such data commonly are reduced to a series of one-hour averages. When such peaks need not be measured, longer-term samples may be collected or composited. Samples also should be representative of the space of interest. This may be difficult and expensive to achieve.

The sampling method used must be appropriate for the subsequent laboratory analytical procedure. Procedures generally include specifications for sampling, including the equipment and reagents to be used. Generally, blanks must be provided; the value and variability of the blank limit the sensitivity of the analysis. At least ten times the blank value of analyte should be collected, and in many cases there also is an upper limit on sample size for accurate analysis. The sampling reagents and collected samples may require preservatives or refrigeration and may have limited lifetimes. These requirements must be observed for valid results.

For legal purposes, a chain of custody must be established. Records should show complete control of the samples by each necessary participant in the sampling and analysis process, by means such as signed seals and locked storage. Finally, quality assurance procedures should be conducted by introducing replicate or known samples and by calibration and standardization checks. The choice of method is influenced by the resources available, such as the experience and skills of the staff, and the facilities, money, and time available.

Preliminary Sampling Methods

▌ Water

A preliminary study for water pollution should be conducted by traversing the drainage basin. The areas, channel dimensions and volumes, sources of contaminants, climate, biological factors, temperatures, and seasonal variations should be noted. Sampling above and below effluent outfalls should be correlated with waste loadings, industrial production, tides, and so on. Hydroelectric power stations and locks may introduce pulsations in flow, which should be noted. Sampling data are best interpreted when there is a steady state of water flow, temperature, and pollution. Then the natural self-purification process along the length of the river may be studied and the point of lowest dissolved oxygen determined. This is where many problems may occur. Good data permit calculations of reaction rates, establish causes and effects, and permit accurate future projections.

During the 1970s the EPA National Water Quality Monitoring Network was established. It was modified in the 1980s as the Basic Water Monitoring Program. These programs were designed to provide national pollution statistics and to measure progress toward achieving water quality goals. Generally, one sampling station per river is set up near an existing streamflow gauge, with little regard to sources of pollutants or the locations of bad spots with low dissolved oxygen. Analyses are conducted for standard constituents, with no modifications for local contaminants. One sample per month is collected, regardless of whether conditions are representative of a steady state or of rapid change. Some samples were from heterogeneous distributions, but normal statistics are applied. Interpretation of changes in statistical data cannot readily be related to causes. Thus, although the regulatory objectives of the monitoring are being met, the applicability of the data for study and evaluation of local pollution problems is limited. Recently, monitoring has focused on the over 100 "priority pollutants" selected as important for toxicity and carcinogenicity but whose analyses are difficult and expensive. Meanwhile, the major fraction of unknown pollutants is being ignored.

▌ Air

A preliminary study also is desirable for establishing an air pollution monitoring program. An emission inventory should be undertaken, and the locations of major sources of pollutants, the locations of the population, the topography and land use, the meteorology, and any anticipated changes should be determined. Preliminary monitoring can establish the broad relation between present concentrations and ambient air quality standards. Monitoring sites may be selected to determine the effects of major pollution sources, to determine the effects of control programs, to determine the points of maximum contamination, or to determine the exposure of the population. The monitoring is usually conducted with expensive continuous-recording instruments. Thus the site usually is air conditioned; it supplies needed utilities, provides safe storage of cylinder gases and equipment, and may have facilities for data transmission. Concentrations vary greatly in three dimensions of space and in time, and thus representative sampling is very difficult to achieve. A path of up to one kilometer may be monitored spectrophotometrically or with Lidar, but most monitoring instruments sample at one point. Mobile monitoring stations in a trailer have been used for preliminary surveys, for plume dispersal studies, for background and environmental impact studies, and for emergency episodes.

During the 1960s, the predecessor of the EPA operated the National Air Sampling Network, and since the 1970s the monitoring has been continued by state and local agencies under EPA supervision at sites selected for high pollution and population densities. A computer data bank in North Carolina stores the data and supplies requested information. Large amounts of data (hourly average values for five or more gaseous pollutants and twenty-four-hour values every sixth day for particulates) have been accumulated over many years. The objectives of obtaining national data and determining compliance with regulations are thus being achieved but at substantial expense. But the data may be of limited use for local purposes. Monitoring many sites for shorter periods of time with less accuracy might give a more representative picture and provide a means of evaluating effects of major sources and of locating all the hot spots of pollution. More intensive studies have been made in a few cities, but high costs have limited their number.

The preliminary industrial hygiene survey for monitoring workplace atmospheres also is very important. The raw materials, processes, products, byproducts, and contaminants should be determined from the management of the plant and from material safety data sheets. A walk-through survey provides information on the quality of the equipment, controls, housekeeping, and the performance of the staff. Each worker could receive a different dose of contaminants depending upon his or her location, duties, and work habits. Thus personal breathing-zone samples are collected for an entire eight-hour shift by small portable sampling pumps carried on the worker's belt. Since only a limited number of samples can be collected, there is a substantial chance that values exceeding the permissible exposure limit may be missed. Thus at 50 percent of the exposure limit, more intensive monitoring is required. Statistical methods have been applied to various sampling patterns, with allowances for the number of samples and the analytical variability. The probabilities of erroneously declaring a compliant situation as noncompliant or a noncompliant as compliant can be calculated.

Applied Sampling Methods

▌ Water

Care must be taken in collecting water samples to prevent contamination or transformation. Containers and caps must be made of suitable materials and must be carefully cleaned and stored. Allowable storage times may be as short as one day for some unstable analytes but are generally measured in weeks. Details for sampling water and wastes are available in a number of publications (Environmental Monitoring and Support Laboratory 1979a, 1979b, 1982, 1983; American Public Health Association/American Water Works Association/Water Pollution Control Federation 1985; American Society for Testing and Materials 1983; U.S. Environmental Protection Agency 1979).

Drinking Water

Drinking water is generally sampled from well-flushed consumer taps at representative points in the distribution system. Locations should be selected to represent dead ends, loops, storage facilities, pressure zones, and multiple water sources. The regulations may require monitoring of one or more of the following primary and secondary contaminants:

Primary

Arsenic	Lead	Selenium
Barium	Lindane	Silver
Cadmium	Mercury	Trihalomethanes, total
Chlorine	Methoxychlor	Toxaphene
Chromium	Nitrate	Turbidity
Coliform bacteria	Radioactivity	2,4-D
Endrin	(gross alpha and	2,4,5-TP (Silvex)
Fluoride	beta)	

Secondary

Chloride	Foaming agents	pH
Color	Iron	Solids—total, dissolved
Copper	Manganese	Sulfate
Corrosivity	Odor	Zinc

The sampling frequencies required for most components are between once a year and once every four years except for trihalomethanes (1–4 samples per quarter) and chlorine and coliform bacteria (1–500 samples per month, depending upon the population served).

Groundwater

Sampling of groundwater can be conducted for various objectives. If the objective is to determine the quality of water from a particular well, it is simple and inexpensive to collect a sample at a tap. Since groundwater moves slowly, the quality parameters change slowly. If the objective is to determine the quality of an underground aquifer or the horizontal and vertical distribution of organic pollutants, to predict their eventual fates, then soil cores, monitoring wells, and special sampling equipment may be needed, which greatly increase the required costs and efforts. If a potential contamination source is above the water table, the zone around it may have to be sampled, because it may take years before the groundwater becomes contaminated. Hydrogeological conditions must be studied when trying to intercept a pollutant plume underground. Flow patterns are complex and difficult to predict, especially in fractured rock. For monitoring groundwater near a landfill, one well up-gradient from it and a minimum of three wells down-gradient should be tested.

During the drilling of a well, sensing devices are lowered into the hole and the various layers are logged to determine the water-permeable layers. Cement grout is placed to select the desired layer and prevent intercommunication with the other layers. The hole should be as small as possible, to minimize its dead volume. The materials of construction should not contaminate the samples. A new well should be flushed; fine clays that might plug the intake screen may be removed by vigorous agitation of the water. The well then should sit idle for several days before sampling. A variety of sampling devices may be used, such as a simple bailer lowered into the hole for a grab sample, suction lift pumps when the water is less than twenty feet below the surface, submersible pumps, or air or nitrogen lift pumps. A Teflon bailer is best for sampling highly volatile organics. When high sensitivity is needed, continuous sampling through absorbents, such as macroreticular resins, activated carbon, and polyamide particles, may be used. Surface soil may be sampled by driving a porous ceramic cup into it and allowing the water to infiltrate into it.

Surface Water

There may be a variety of objectives for sampling rivers and streams, lakes, and bottom sediments. The quality may be important at locations used for domestic water supplies, recreation, or for propagation and maintenance of fish and wildlife. Locations may be sampled in areas unaffected by human activities and in areas subject to inputs of contaminants. Sampling plans may be designed to represent point discharges or the gradients in the river, based upon preliminary knowledge of the variability of the parameters. Common measurements are listed below:

Alkalinity	Organic matter and	Solids—total, dissolved,
Color	demand	suspended
Depth	Pesticides	Specific conductance
Dissolved oxygen	pH	Temperature
Heavy metals	Phosphate	Turbidity
Nitrogen series	Sediment composition	Velocity
	Silica	

Sampling may be conducted once for each season, or annually. Bottle devices or pumps may be used for obtaining water samples, and scoops or coring devices for bottom sediments. River-flow measurements may be obtained from U.S. Geological Service's gauging stations, or by recording surface elevations and measuring stream velocities with a current meter.

Wastewater

Sampling of wastewater is required under the National Pollutant Discharge Elimination System (NPDES), and the locations of sampling points, sample types, frequency, and so on, are specified in the NPDES permit. Municipal wastewaters are sampled to check on the efficiency of the treatment process and to facilitate operations. Industrial wastewaters are monitored to determine their character, variability, the performance and efficiency of process units, and to establish a sound basis for treatment. Agricultural wastewater is sampled to study and regulate runoff from feedlots and fields. Common measurements for wastewater are

Alkalinity	Fecal coliform	Organic priority
Biochemical oxygen	Fecal streptococci	pollutants
demand (5-day)	Flow	Phosphate
Chemical oxygen	Fluoride	Solids—total, dissolved,
demand	Metals	suspended, volatile
Chlorine residuals	Nitrogen series	Surfactants
Dissolved oxygen	Oil and grease	Temperature
		Total organic carbon

Grab samples may be taken to check individual unit processes and composite samples for overall monitoring. Composite samples should be proportioned according to flow rates so that they are representative of the total discharge. A variety of automatic samplers are available (U.S. Environmental Protection Agency 1979). The intake velocity should be adequate to collect suspended solids properly. Sampling frequency varies from daily to weekly. However, when a new discharge is characterized, it may be sampled hourly.

Sludge

Sludge sampling is usually conducted at municipal or industrial plants for process control and evaluation, as feed characteristics change. Common parameters are

Alkalinity	Heavy metals	Solids—total, settleable,
Biochemical	Nutrients	suspended, volatile
oxygen	Pesticides	Volatile acids
demand	pH	Temperature

Sampling locations are chosen appropriately for the unit to be studied. Since the sludge composition may be highly variable, samples from at least three locations or depths should be composited and thoroughly mixed. When possible, frequent samples should be collected and composited according to flow rates. Temperature may be monitored continuously, and other parameters should be monitored from twice daily to weekly. Automatic samplers are too readily fouled to be useful.

▌ Air

Air samples may be much more variable in time or space than water samples, and thus the problem of obtaining a representative sample is much more acute. For air pollution monitoring, the regulations require a specified number of monitoring stations depending on the population of the city. The minimum distances from traffic and local sources of pollution and the height of the sampling inlet also are specified, as they can greatly influence the result. Because of the great variability of the concentrations, instruments for continuous monitoring are generally used, and the data are reduced to hourly average values.

Since people usually spend more than 80 percent of their time indoors, outdoor measurements are not adequately representative of exposure. In industrial hygiene studies, personal sampling for an entire eight-hour shift is generally required. This is done by sampling from the worker's breathing zone with a dosimeter, or a small sampling device clipped to the worker's collar or lapel and connected to a battery-operated pump clipped to his or her belt.

Air samples may contain aerosols and gases and vapors of interest. The size of the aerosol determines how far into the lung it penetrates. Size-selective impactors are used to discard the coarse particles above $10\text{-}\mu m$ diameter when sampling "inhalable particulates" according to EPA specifications, and cyclones passing only 50 percent of $3.5\text{-}\mu m$ diameter particles for "respirable particulates" according to ACGIH specifications.

In order to sample an aerosol representatively, the sample inlet velocity should exactly match the air velocity. This is called isokinetic sampling and is difficult to achieve. In practice, different proportions of fine and coarse particles are collected and lost in the sampling inlets, and the size distribution of the collection may not be representative. The compositions of the fine and coarse fractions also may differ substantially. Thus representative sampling of aerosols is very difficult. Membrane filters are commonly used for small flows because of their high collection efficiencies and low pressure drops. Flash-fired glass fiber filters are widely used for high-volume samplers. When different size fractions are to be collected, a graduated series of impactors is frequently used.

Gases and vapors are most conveniently sampled with solid absorbents, such as carbon, Tenax, Chromosorb, Poropak, silica gel, molecular sieves, and alumina. Various types of bubblers containing liquid absorbents, evacuated bottles, and Mylar or Teflon bags also may be used. Detector tubes are simple and compact devices for rapid field surveys. These contain an indicating absorbent in a sealed glass tube. The tips are broken, and a small air sample is drawn through the tube with a calibrated syringe or rubber bulb to produce a length of stain proportional to the concentration.

The recent development of passive samplers for gases and vapors has eliminated the necessity for sampling pumps and has simplified sampling equipment. In these devices, the test substance diffuses into an absorbent at a rate proportional to its concentration, through a controlled air space or membrane. Direct-reading passive samplers produce a length of stain proportional to the concentration and thus do not require shipping the sample to a laboratory for analysis. Details of analytical procedures have been given in a number of publications (Katz 1977; Eller 1984; Environmental Monitoring Systems Laboratory 1976–77; Lioy and Lioy 1983). Lioy and Lioy have described available sampling devices and instruments.

Common measurements for air pollutants in the general environment are

Primary

Carbon monoxide	Nitrogen dioxide	Ozone
Lead	Nonmethane hydrocarbons	Particulate matter
		Sulfur dioxide

Hazardous

Arsenic	Benzene soluble particulates	Fluorides
Asbestos		Formaldehyde
Benzene	Beryllium	Halogenated organics
	Cadmium	Hydrogen sulfide

In industrial hygiene, more than a thousand compounds are of concern as air pollutants. Their threshold limit values are listed by the Chemical Substances TLV Committee (1985) of the American Conference of Governmental Industrial Hygienists. Interest shifts, but some common measurements are for

Acetone	Copper	Silica
Asbestos	Iron	Solvents
Benzene	Lead	Styrene
Benzo(a)pyrene	Manganese	Toluene
Cadmium	Naphtha	Trichloroethylene
Chromium	Nickel	Vinyl chloride
Coal tar pitch volatiles	Pesticides	Xylene

▌ Automobile and Industrial Emissions

A special problem in sampling automobile emissions is that concentrations and flow rates vary widely from minute to minute. Accordingly, a standard test cycle representative of city driving has been established by the U.S. Environmental Protection Agency (1985), in which the test vehicle is operated for a few minutes each at idle, acceleration, cruise, and deceleration, under specified loads and speeds. The exhaust gas flow, which varies up to 150 cubic feet per minute, is mixed with clean air to make a constant flow rate of 350 cubic feet per minute. The analysis of the mixture multiplied by the known constant total flow gives the total quantity of pollutant for the cycle, which is reported in grams per mile of hydrocarbons, carbon monoxide, and nitrogen oxides.

Industrial stack sampling is physically difficult and expensive because of location and because aerosol size and concentration may vary across the diameter of the stack. In order to make the sample representative, the cross section is divided into a number of equal areas, and an average gas velocity is measured in each (at the center of a rectangular area or at four equally spaced central points in an annular area). Each point is then sampled through a nozzle in sequence for the same time interval but at a flow rate to produce a nozzle velocity equal to the measured flow velocity at that point (isokinetic sampling). Heated probes are required to prevent condensation, along with a proper sampling train for the analyses desired. Sample volume must be corrected for temperature and moisture content. Details have been described by the Environmental Monitoring Systems Laboratory (1976–77) and in the regulations for emissions tabulated by Pahl (1983):

Acid mist	Opacity	Volatile organic
Carbon monoxide	Particulates	compounds
Fluorides	Sulfur dioxide	
Nitrogen oxides	Sulfur—total reduced	

▌ Hazardous Waste Sites

A major environmental concern for hazardous waste sites is the leachate resulting from percolation through the soil of the hazardous material or of infiltrating water. This may occur despite efforts to seal the fill with clay and plastic membrane liners. In some well-designed systems, drain pipes have been installed to catch the leachate for sampling or treatment. Otherwise, test wells may be drilled to trace the underground pollutant plumes described for groundwater. The methods described for wastewater may be applied to the leachate. The U.S. Environmental Agency (1984) has listed the common parameters measured:

Acidity	Nitrogen compounds	Solids—dissolved,
Alkalinity	Odor	settleable, sus-
Biochemical oxygen	Oils, greases, and	pended, volatile
demand	immiscible liquids	Temperature
Chemical oxygen	Organic carbon, total	Toxicity
demand	Oxidation reduction	Turbidity
Dissolved oxygen	potential	Volatile organic acids
Electrical	pH	Volatile solids
conductivity	Specific organic	
Heavy metals	compounds	

Atmospheric discharges also may pose a significant hazard, and sampling methods previously discussed may be applied. However, it is difficult to quantify the total emissions for a large landfill because of variable wind factors. There are a variety of hazards to the personnel working at a hazardous waste site (NIOSH/OSHA/USCG/EPA 1985). Leakage or crushing of containers may result in fires or explosions, and spills may be toxic or corrosive. Skin wipe tests may be used to evaluate penetration or permeation through protective clothing. Air sampling may be conducted, preferably with direct-reading instruments to evaluate the hazards rapidly.

▎ Radioactive Materials

Radioactive isotopes are characterized by unstable atomic nuclei, which decompose at constant rates, with the ejection of characteristic and highly energetic particles. Among these are alpha particles (helium nuclei), beta particles (electrons), and gamma particles (X ray photons). These atoms are transformed into new isotopes, which also may be unstable. This chain process continues until a stable isotope is formed. The chemical properties of radioactive and stable isotopes of the same element are identical. Thus the sampling and analytical separation procedures are similar. In some cases, the stable isotope is added to the sample as a carrier to assist in the separation processes.

Final measurements are made with instruments measuring or counting alpha, beta, or gamma particles, which can be done with extraordinary sensitivity, limited only by the background count caused by cosmic rays and natural radioactivity. When a chain process of radioactive decay occurs, the concentrations of the members of the series may vary with time but may ultimately approach an equilibrium ratio. At this time, analysis may be made for one of the members, which is taken as a proportional measure of all. Details of instruments, and sampling and analytical procedures have been given for water and wastewater (APHA/AWWA/WPCF 1985) and air (Katz 1977). Surfaces may be sampled by wipe tests with filter paper or cotton swabs and analyzed with an appropriate instrument. Direct exposure may be measured by film badges, pocket dosimeters, and survey meters. Common measurements are for

Alpha activity	Iodine-131	Radon-222
(gross)	Lead-210	Strontium-89
Beta activity (gross)	Plutonium	Strontium-90
Gamma activity	Radium	Tritium

A common survey instrument for alpha particles is the scintillation counter. It has a light-tight chamber, the outlet of which is covered with the sensitive element—a thin layer of zinc sulfide crystals covered by two thin layers of opaque plastic. Since the range of alpha particles in air is short, this film is brought as close as possible to the source. Alpha particles penetrating the plastic produce scintillations in the crystals. These scintillations are sensed by a photomultiplier tube and counted individually, or their rate is measured. Beta and gamma particles are counted at high sensitivity with a Geiger-Mueller instrument, which has a probe containing a gas-filled chamber and electrodes. Each entering particle produces a few ions, which are accelerated by the high voltages to produce an avalanche of additional ions, resulting in a current pulse, which is counted and then quenched.

In a Cutie Pie survey meter, lower potentials are used in the ionization chamber so that the pulses are proportional to the particle energy. Gamma particles are counted, and by removing a shielding cap, beta particles also are counted. A laboratory proportional counter operates on a similar principle, except that a planchet containing the sample is placed inside the chamber. At lower voltages, only the alpha particles may be counted, and at higher voltages gamma and beta particles also are counted. Laboratory gamma scintillation counters use large sodium iodide crystals as the sensitive element. The Nuclear Regulatory Commission has issued extensive regulations and specifications for controlling radioactive hazards.

Analysis Methods

❙ Atomic Spectrometry

In atomic absorption spectrometry (flame AA), a sample solution usually is atomized at a reproducible rate into a carefully controlled flame. Gaseous fuels producing successively hotter flames are propane, hydrogen, and acetylene. Emission and absorption of radiation in the flame mainly involves atoms, although the presence of molecules at high concentrations may have minor effects. Atoms of each element may exist only at a specific number of energy levels, depending upon the electronic orbitals, and may jump between these levels by absorbing or emitting photons having energies (and corresponding wavelengths) precisely equal to the energy difference. Thus each element has a characteristic spectrum of light wavelengths absorbed or emitted.

At appropriate flame temperatures, most atoms of the analyte are at the ground (low-energy) state and absorb photons from a light beam passed through the flame. The light beam originates in a hollow cathode lamp containing the test element in an emitting condition. The beam then passes through a monochromator, for selecting the appropriate specific wavelength, to a photodetector, which measures its intensity. The logarithm of the fraction of monochromatic light transmitted (with the negative sign made positive) is proportional to the concentration of the analyte in the original test solution. This method is popular because of its high sensitivity and specificity.

Various other methods also may be used to introduce the sample. By appropriate treatment with a reducing chemical, antimony, arsenic, bismuth, germanium, lead, selenium, tellurium, and tin (in the form of their hydrides) can be flushed via air out of a solution and into a flame. Introduction of these samples in this manner improves the sensitivity by one or more orders of magnitude. Mercury may be flushed out of a solution in elemental form and measured without a flame. In another flameless procedure, very small samples may be vaporized electrothermally in a hollow graphite rod, through which the light beam is passed (furnace AA).

In atomic emission spectrometry, a lamp is not required, but rather the source of the monochromatic light measured is the fraction of sample atoms existing in a high-energy state and emitting a spectrum. To increase this fraction, hotter flames are used. Samples also may be placed in a small crater in the tip of a carbon electrode and vaporized in an electric arc. More recently, samples are atomized into an argon plasma heated to ultra-high temperatures by an inductively coupled radio frequency source. This method of inductively coupled plasma (ICP) improves the sensitivity for most elements. More elaborate instruments can measure as many as thirty-five elements simultaneously by using multiple photodetectors and electronic systems for the various selected wavelengths. Metals give the greatest response, but almost all elements can be determined.

Slaven (1986) has reviewed the merits of the various methods of atomic spectrometry and has compared the detection limits for the elements commonly measured (figure 4.1). For detailed procedures, see Environmental Monitoring and Support Laboratory 1979a, 1979b, 1982, 1983; APHA/AWWA/WPCF 1985; ASTM 1983; U.S. EPA 1979; Katz 1977; Eller 1984; Environmental Monitoring Systems Laboratory 1976–77.

Gas and Liquid Chromatography and Mass Spectrometry

Specificity is a major problem in the analysis of organic contaminants in the environment because of the possible presence of thousands of compounds, many of which have almost identical chemical properties. Gas chromatography separates compounds that can be volatilized without decomposition at temperatures up to a few hundred degrees. (Over half of the industrial hygiene analyses use gas chromatography.) Liquid chromatography separates compounds that are not volatile. (About 8 percent of analyses use this method.) Mass spectrometry identifies a separated pure component by its characteristic mass spectrum.

In a gas chromatograph, a carrier gas such as helium or nitrogen from a cylinder flows continuously through a tube (column) containing a specially selected absorbent (a packing, or wall coating if the column is a capillary tube) into a detector. A small portion of sample, dissolved in a volatile solvent or in gaseous form, is injected into the carrier flow. The various sample components have differing physical and chemical affinities for the column packing and are thus retarded for different retention times. Under proper conditions, each component emerges separately from the column to

Figure 4.1. Detection limits for elements as measured by three atomic spectrometry methods.

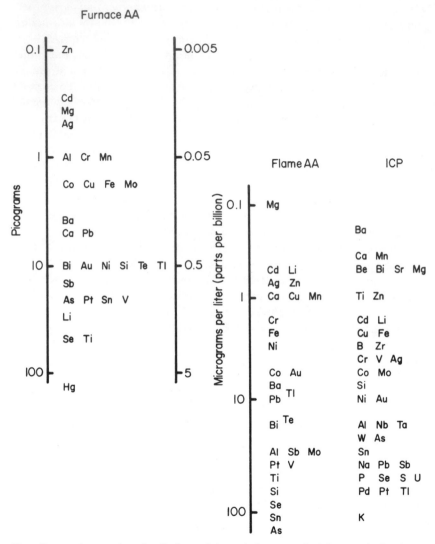

Note: Because furnace detection limits are inherently in mass units (picograms), they have been converted to concentrations by assuming a 20 μ/L sample. (*Source:* Slaven 1986.)

be sensed by the detector and to produce a peak on a recorder chart. A variety of column packings and lengths are available to accomplish the necessary separations. The temperature of the column is selected or programmed to adjust the degree of separations and retention times as desired.

A variety of detectors are available for sensing the emerging components in the carrier gas stream. This stream may be split between two detectors, or between the detector and a device, to collect part of each component. The thermal conductivity detector (TCD) is broadly applicable but relatively insensitive for trace analysis. In the widely used flame ionization detector (FID), the sample is injected into a hydrogen-air flame. Electrodes at about ninety volts measure the flame conductivity by means of an ultrasensitive electrometer circuit, giving a highly sensitive response to organic compounds containing C-H bonds. Another highly sensitive but less broadly applicable device is the electron capture detector (ECD), which detects electrophilic components such as halogens by measuring the conductivity of the gas stream. A beta source such as tritium or ^{63}Ni supplies conductive electrons, some of which are absorbed by the test component.

The quantity of each component is determined by measuring peak heights or areas and comparing each with a standard curve produced with known quantities of the pure compound. Identification is based on the retention time. However, since it is possible that other compounds may have the same retention time, confirmation may be necessary. One method is to repeat the analysis with a different column, which may change retention times for various compounds, to see if a known standard of the pure compound still has the same retention time as the component in the sample. Mass spectrometry or infrared spectroscopy of the collected component are more positive checks.

Liquid chromatographs utilize a liquid carrier stream and a high-pressure pump in a system operating on similar principles, although the detectors may not have as high a sensitivity as those for gas chromatography. Liquid chromatography is applied to high molecular weight compounds, which cannot be volatilized without decomposition. In some cases, a mixture of solvents is used as the carrier, and the proportions can be programmed to vary as the analysis proceeds. Detectors that measure ultraviolet absorption or fluorescence or the index of refraction of the emerging liquid carrier stream are commonly used. Figure 4.2 illustrates a liquid chromatogram. With some modifications, similar systems using aqueous carriers and ion exchange columns can be used for analysis of anions and cations (ion chromatography). These systems use conductivity detectors.

When positive identification is necessary, a portion of each separated component may be introduced into a mass spectrograph (MS). In this instrument, the test molecules enter an evacuated space and are fragmented and ionized by a beam of electrons. The charged fragments are deflected by electrostatic or magnetic fields and separated into a spectrum according to their mass-to-charge ratios. This spectrum is scanned by the detector and recorded as a series of peaks. Each compound produces a unique spec-

Figure 4.2. Record of polynuclear aromatic compounds measured by a liquid chromatograph.

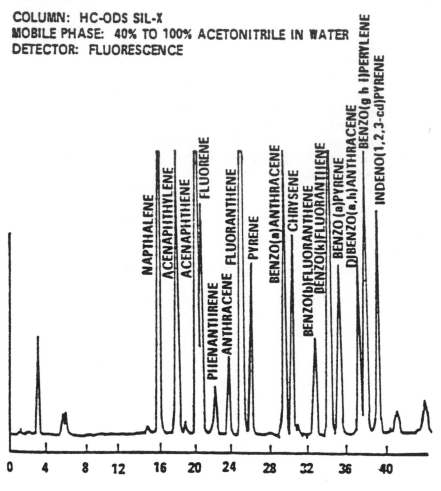

COLUMN: HC-ODS SIL-X
MOBILE PHASE: 40% TO 100% ACETONITRILE IN WATER
DETECTOR: FLUORESCENCE

RETENTION TIME-MINUTES

(*Source:* U.S. Environmental Protection Agency 1979.)

trum. Many spectra are entered into the memory of a computer and used to help identify unknown samples. Analysis by mass spectrometry may be quite expensive ($1 thousand to $2 thousand per sample) but is necessary for specific identifications in complex mixtures.

Following are some compounds or types of compounds analyzed by the methods discussed above. Those marked * are commonly analyzed by gas chromatography–mass spectrometry.

Acids*
Acrolein
Acrylonitrile
Base/neutrals*
Chlorinated
  hydrocarbons
Dioxin (TCDD)*
Haloethers
Hydrocarbons

Isophorone
Nitroaromatics
Nitrosamines
Organochlorine
  pesticides
Pesticides*
Phenols
Phthalate esters

Polychlorinated
  biphenyls
Polynuclear aromatic
  hydrocarbons
Priority pollutants*
Purgeable aromatics
Purgeable halocarbons
Purgeable organics*
Solvents

▌ Spectrophotometry, Titrimetry, Electrometry, and Other Methods

A variety of other analytical methods, mostly predating the development of the analytical systems described above, are still in use. In order to improve specificity, many are preceded by separation steps, which remove interfering substances and concentrate the test component. These separation techniques include distillation, extraction with solvents (usually after complexation with an appropriate reagent), and addition of reagents to complex and suppress interferences.

Spectrophotometric procedures generally mix the test substance with a chromogenic reagent to produce an intensely colored product. The absorption of monochromatic light of the appropriate wavelength is measured and compared with a calibration curve made with known standards. Titrimetric methods add measured amounts of a reagent of known strength to the sample to react with the test component, until a slight excess is shown by an appropriate indicator chemical or device. Electrometric methods immerse specially designed electrodes into the prepared sample solution and measure electrical potentials or currents. One electrode is designed to be permeable only to the test component. For example, special types of thin glass in a pH electrode are permeable to hydrogen ions, and certain crystals are permeable to fluoride ions. Electrometric methods have been applied to determine biochemical oxygen demand, fluoride, and pH.

In anodic stripping voltammetry, a trace metal such as lead, cadmium, copper, or zinc is concentrated by being electroplated onto an electrode and then stripped with a reverse pulse of current at controlled potential. The size of the reverse pulse is a measure of the metal concentration. X ray diffraction analysis is used to identify crystals. The pattern of scattered (diffracted) X rays after the beam strikes the sample is related to the spacing of the crystal layers. It can distinguish crystalline forms of silica (quartz, cristobolite, and tridymite) from amorphous silica, all of which are chemically identical but differ in toxic significance. Optical and electron microscopy may be used to identify and count particles and fibers, notably asbestos. Gravimetric procedures are used to weigh particulate matter in air and dissolved and suspended matter in water and wastewater.

Chemicals and characteristics tested by spectrophotometry are

Boron	Iron	Phenols
Chlorine	Nitrate	Silica
Color	Nitrite	Sulfate
Cyanide	Nitrogen dioxide	Sulfur dioxide
Fluoride	Ozone	Surfactants

Chemicals and characteristics tested by titrimetry are

Acidity	Chemical oxygen	Hardness
Alkalinity	demand	Kjeldahl nitrogen
Ammonia	Chloride	Sulfite
Biochemical oxygen	Chlorine	Sulfur dioxide
demand	Cyanide	

Monitoring Instruments

Because of the variability in the concentrations of contaminants, it is frequently necessary to collect numerous samples in order to be statistically representative. This can be laborious and expensive, especially if around-the-clock sampling is required. Automatic sampling devices can provide the necessary samples effectively. A tabulation of commercially available devices for water and wastewater has been published by the Environmental Monitoring and Support Laboratory (1983). These devices use peristaltic or piston pumps, pneumatic or vacuum systems, or dippers. Most have arrangements for a purge cycle, sample timing, and sampling proportional to total flow.

Commercially available automatic sampling devices for air sampling have been listed by Lioy and Lioy (1983). Sequential samplers for gases and vapors include a vacuum pump, flow regulating valve, flow meter, timer, and valve-switching devices to draw the sample air through a number of sampling devices in the programmed sequence for the programmed time intervals. Multiple probes may be used to sample at different points, and samples may be collected in parallel, through different absorbing reagents, for different analyses. Particles may be collected with tape samplers mounted on reels and advanced intermittently by a timer; in between these intervals, the air is drawn through the tape to produce a series of dirty gray circles. The light transmittance of these spots may be measured with a photometer. In some devices a chemically impregnated tape is employed for reacting with gases, such as hydrogen sulfide, to produce a stain. There are also automated impactors, which collect particulates on a Mylar film that is coated with adhesive. The collected samples then may be examined in a laboratory.

More powerful monitoring devices continuously complete the analysis and record the final result. These provide continuous information at greatly reduced cost and are commonly employed in air pollution studies. A comprehensive list of instruments for monitoring air contaminants (Lioy and Lioy 1983) includes a wide variety of operating principles. Specifications and test procedures for air pollution monitoring instruments have been established by the EPA (1973), together with a test laboratory in North Carolina.

Electrical conductivity analyzers that use scrubbers to collect the gas in a liquid reagent have been used for ammonia, hydrogen sulfide, and sulfur dioxide. Electrical conductivity also may be used to monitor the purity of water. More specific devices use electrolytic cells that are mainly permeable or responsive only to the test gas. Such instruments, which measure electrical potentials or currents, are used for monitoring oxygen, carbon monoxide, ozone, hydrogen sulfide, formaldehyde, and nitrogen oxides. Miniaturized versions are available as personal monitors.

Gas chromatographic detectors also are used in monitoring instruments. Process gas chromatographs use time-programmed valves and electronics to cycle through a procedure, such as a multiple analysis for total hydrocarbons, methane, and carbon monoxide. The flame ionization detector is used in monitors for hydrocarbons and organic vapors. Electron capture-and-photoionization detectors also are used as organic monitors. Some of these devices may not be specific, and all require appropriate calibrations.

Another class of monitoring instrument uses heat-of-combustion detectors. In these, the test gas passes over a catalytic surface, and the temperature rise is sensed. These instruments are used for combustible gases, methane, carbon monoxide, and hydrogen sulfide. Again, appropriate calibration is necessary, and the responses are nonspecific.

Gas phase spectrophotometric devices, using infrared measurements, are used for carbon monoxide and for a variety of organic vapors and gases, according to the wavelength selected. Ultraviolet and visible light gas phase spectrophotometers are used for ozone, mercury vapor, sulfur dioxide, and for analysis of stack gas for sulfur dioxide and nitrogen oxides. Pulsed ultraviolet fluorescence is used for monitoring sulfur dioxide. Emissions in an electric arc are used in the halide meter. Chemiluminescence after reaction with a gaseous reagent in a light-tight chamber is used for ozone and nitrogen oxides. These systems are widely used for the monitoring required by air pollution regulations. Older photometric systems using scrubbers and liquid reagents have longer response times, require troublesome maintenance of liquid-flow systems, and are no longer popular. They have been applied in the past to monitor sulfur dioxide, oxidants, and nitrogen oxides.

Direct-reading dosimeters are useful for personal monitoring. They can be clipped to a coat lapel to be near the breathing zone. These diffuse the test gas into a glass tube containing an indicating chemical absorbent; the gas produces an observable length of stain proportional to the concentration of the pollutant and the length of time the dosimeter is used. Currently available types measure acetic acid, ammonia, carbon dioxide, carbon monoxide, hydrochloric acid, hydrocyanic acid, hydrogen sulfide, nitrogen dioxide, and sulfur dioxide. New types are being developed. Dosimeters for X rays have a casing resembling a fountain pen. Inside is a highly insulated fiber electrometer charged to a high voltage. As X rays penetrate into the chamber, they produce ions, which partially discharge the fiber and cause it to move. The position of the fiber may be viewed against an optical scale through a small lens at the end of the device.

Other types of monitoring instruments are used for airborne particles. Optical devices may measure light transmission, as in measurement of opacity of stack gas. Light-scattering devices illuminate the particles with an intense beam and measure the scattered light either over a wide angle in the integrating nephelometer or through a forward angle. They use optics similar to dark-field microscopy. Some devices have used a pulsed laser as a light source. Smoke plumes can be mapped by Lidar, using a powerful pulsed laser and measuring backscattering. Special devices use flame spectrometry for elements such as sodium. Others subject particles to varying electrostatic fields to tumble and measure fibers by their varying scattered light. All of these devices respond differently to particles of different sizes and optical properties, and require careful calibrations.

Several other principles also are used for aerosol monitors. Particles may be electrically charged and their mobility measured by sensitive electronic circuits. They may be deposited on a piezoelectric quartz crystal, which is part of an oscillator circuit, and the frequency shift caused by the mass of the particles may be measured. Finally, particles may be impacted on a surface, such as a Mylar film, and their transmission of beta rays from a radioactive source may be measured. Fortuitously, the calibration for the latter device is mainly a function of mass, and chemical composition is not an important factor.

Recent developments in microelectronics and computers have revolutionized the design of monitoring instruments. New, miniaturized portable models are rapidly being developed. Some record data in an electronic memory in a form that can be read out by a computer for calculations and printing. Others provide real-time digital indications of monitored concentrations. While the electronics of these devices are sophisticated, the chemical or measurement principles in some may not be very specific or accurate. Thus the user must understand the interferences and must know what may be present in the test environment in order to properly calibrate the instrument and interpret its readings.

References

American Public Health Association/American Water Works Association/Water Pollution Control Federation. 1985. *Standard Methods for the Examination of Water and Wastewaters.* 16th ed. Washington, D.C.: APHA.

American Society for Testing and Materials. 1983. *Water and Environmental Technology, Annual Book of ASTM Standards.* Vol. 11.01 *Water I;* Vol. 11.02 *Water II;* Vol. 11.03 *Atmospheric Analysis, Occupational Health and Safety;* Vol. 11.04 *Pesticides, Resource Recovery, Hazardous Substances and Oil Spill Response, Waste Disposal, Biological Effects and Environmental Fate.* Philadelphia: ASTM.

Chemical Substances TLV Committee. 1985. *Threshold Limit Values and Biological Exposure Indices for 1985–6.* Cincinnati: American Conference of Governmental Industrial Hygienists.

Eller, P. M., ed. 1984. *NIOSH Manual of Analytical Methods.* 3d ed. Publication 84-100. Cincinnati: U.S. Department of Health and Human Services. (Revisions are issued at intervals.)

Environmental Monitoring and Support Laboratory. 1979a. *Handbook for Quality Control in Water and Wastewater Laboratories.* EPA-600/4-79-019. Cincinnati: U.S. Environmental Protection Agency.

———. 1979b. *Methods for Chemical Analysis of Water and Wastes.* EPA-600/4-79-020. Cincinnati: U.S. Environmental Protection Agency.

———. 1982. *Handbook for Sampling and Sample Preservation of Water and Wastewater.* EPA-600/4-82-029. Cincinnati: U.S. Environmental Protection Agency.

———. 1983. *Addendum to Handbook for Sampling and Sample Preservation.* EPA-600/4-83-039. Cincinnati: U.S. Environmental Protection Agency.

Environmental Monitoring Systems Laboratory. 1976–77. *Quality Assurance Handbook for Air Pollution Measurement Systems.* Vol. 1 (EPA-600/9-76-005) *Principles;* Vol. 2 (EPA-600/4-77-027a) *Ambient Air Specific Methods;* Vol. 3 (EPA-600/4-77-027b) *Stationary Source Specific Methods.* Washington, D.C.: U.S. Environmental Protection Agency. (Revisions are issued at intervals.)

Katz, M., ed. 1977. *Methods of Air Sampling and Analysis.* Washington, D.C.: American Public Health Association.

Lioy, P. J., and Lioy, M. J. Y., eds. 1983. *Air Sampling Instruments for Evaluation of Atmospheric Contaminants.* 6th ed. Cincinnati: American Conference of Governmental Industrial Hygienists.

NIOSH/OSHA/USCG/EPA. 1985. *Occupational Safety and Health Guidance Manual for Hazardous Waste Site Activities.* Publication 85-115. Atlanta: U.S. Department of Health and Human Services.

Pahl, D. 1983. EPA's program for establishing standards of performance for new stationary sources of air pollution. *Journal of the Air Pollution Control Association* 33:468-82.

Slaven, W. 1986. Flames, furnaces, and plasma: How do we choose? *Analytical Chemistry* 58:589A-97A.

U.S. Environmental Protection Agency. 1973. Ambient air monitoring equivalent and reference methods. *Federal Register* 38:28438-48.

———. 1979. Guidelines establishing test procedures for the analysis of pollutants: Proposed regulations, part 3. *Federal Register* 44:69464-574; Corrections, part 4. *Federal Register* 44:75028-52.

———. 1984. *Characterization of Hazardous Waste Sites: A Methods Manual.* Vol. 2. (EPA-600/4-84-076) *Available Sampling Methods.* 2d ed. Cincinnati: EPA.

———. 1985. Control of air pollution from new motor vehicles and new motor vehicle engines: Certification and test procedures. *Code of Federal Regulations,* title 40, pt. 86.

5. The Food Chain as a Source of Toxic Chemical Exposure

CURTIS C. TRAVIS AND ANGELA D. ARMS

Attention shifts in chapters 5 and 6 to the routes by which people are exposed to toxic chemicals in the environment. Chapter 5 examines exposure through the ingestion of food. Travis and Arms are concerned with the properties of chemicals that lead to their uptake by plants and animals and to their eventual incorporation into the food supply. Some chemicals, such as DDT, become concentrated in the food chain. DDT also accumulates in the body, as does lead and other chemicals. Still other chemicals are biologically inactive and remain in the environment. The authors focus on pesticides and develop a formula to predict how readily particular pesticides find their way into food.

Food is probably the most chemically complex part of the human environment. Foods contain hundreds of naturally occurring carcinogens and mutagens (Ames 1983). Examples can be found in herbal teas, corn, peanuts, black pepper, celery, strawberries, and many other food items (Stich 1983). The significance of these naturally occurring carcinogens and mutagens in food is unclear. However, it is known that diet is a major contributor to background cancer rates and that dietary differences throughout the world result in wide differences in the rates of many types of cancer.

Besides containing naturally occurring carcinogens and mutagens, food can be contaminated by manufactured organic chemicals. Large quantities of synthetic organic chemicals are produced in the United States each year. Production of these organic chemicals results in the annual generation of more than 2.6×10^{11} kilograms of hazardous chemical wastes (U.S. Congress, Office of Technology Assessment 1983). Only 10 percent of these wastes are disposed of in an environmentally safe manner (Fawcett 1984). During the production, use, and disposal of these chemicals, many are released to the environment, taken up by the food chain, and transferred to humans via ingestion.

Environmental contamination of food takes two forms: (1) long-term, low-level contamination, resulting from gradual diffusion of persistent chemicals throughout the environment, and (2) relatively shorter-term, higher-level contamination, stemming from direct application, accidental releases and waste disposal (U.S. Congress, Office of Technology Assessment 1979). Examples of both types of contamination abound in the literature. It is the purpose of this chapter, however, to concentrate on the former contamination because of its potential for more widespread effect on human health.

Three factors determine whether and how seriously contamination of food will affect human health: the amount of the chemical substance in the food, the amount of the contaminated food eaten, and the toxicity of the contaminant. We address the first two of these issues, attempting to characterize the nature and extent of human exposure to organic chemicals in food.

Measuring Organics in Humans and in Food

The extent of human exposure to toxic chemicals in food can be estimated in two ways: (1) determination of body burdens through examination of samples of human tissues, hair, blood, and urine, and (2) estimation of dietary intake from measured concentrations of organics in food.

▋ Human Body Burdens

The best indicators of past and present human exposure to organics are the residues of parent organic compounds and their metabolites in human tissues and fluids. Human adipose tissue is the primary repository in the body for persistent, lipophilic organic chemicals. However, it is difficult to obtain adipose tissue samples. Breast milk is an alternative medium for measuring human exposure to contaminants because it is more easily obtained for analysis.

The best quantitative data on the concentration of organics in adipose tissue come from the National Human Monitoring Program. The objective of this program is to determine on a national scale the incidence and level of exposure to pesticides of the general population (Murphy and Harvey 1985). Table 5.1 lists the frequency of detection of selected organochlorine residues in human adipose tissue. These data indicate widespread exposure of the general population to certain pesticides. The exact sources of these exposures are unknown, but the food chain is suspected as a major contributor.

Pesticide residues in breast milk also indicate that human exposure to

Table 5.1. Occurrence of selected organochlorine residues in human adipose tissue

Residue[a]	Possible Origin	Frequency of Detection (percent)
Dichlorodiphenyltrichloroethane	DDT and its analogs	100
Transnonachlor	Chlordane, heptachlor	97
Heptachlor epoxide	Chlordane, heptachlor	96
Oxychlordane	Chlordane, heptachlor	95
Dieldrin	Aldrin, dieldrin	95
β-benzene hexachloride	BHC	94
Hexachlorobenzene	Chlorinated benzene manufacture	93
Polychlorinated biphenyl	PCBs	23
λ-benzene hexachloride	Lindane	2
Other BHC isomers	BHC	<1
Mirex	Mirex	<1

Source: Murphy et al. 1983.
[a]Limits of detection: 10–20 parts per billion (10–20 µg/L).

toxic chemicals is a worldwide problem, even in remote parts of the world (Savage et al. 1981). The most frequently detected chemicals in human breast milk are dichlorodiphenyltrichloroethane (DDT), dichloro-diphenyldichloroethane (DDE), polychlorinated biphenyl (PCB), dieldrin, heptachlor epoxide, lindane, and hexachlorobenzene (Rogan et al. 1980; Savage et al. 1981; Jensen 1983; Takei et al. 1983). The concentrations of chemicals in milk fat have been correlated with that in adipose tissue (Jensen 1983).

DDT was the first toxic chemical to be detected in breast milk (Laug et al. 1951). Due to a ban on DDT in the United States, the content of DDT in the fat of human milk has declined from an average concentration of 5.5 parts per million (range of 0.8 to 16.5) in 1971 to 3 parts per million (range of 0.8 to 15.6) in 1978 (Spindler 1983). A breast milk study conducted in Hawaii showed that both the kinds and amounts of residues found in breast milk in that state are comparable to those found in the mainland states (Takei et al. 1983). The authors identified the diet of mothers as the probable means of exposure.

▍Food Chain Studies

Direct evidence of human exposure to toxic chemicals in the food chain is limited (U.S. Congress, Office of Technology Assessment 1979).

While studies have been performed to determine concentrations of chemicals in food, analysis is generally limited to a few chemicals. The best quantitative data on the extent of human exposure to chemicals in food come from Total Diet studies, through which the United States Food and Drug Administration (FDA) monitors chemical contamination in food. These studies enable investigators to measure the intake of selected pesticides, industrial chemicals, and elements (including radionuclides) in foods typical of the normal diets of infants, toddlers, and adults.

The Adult Total Diet consists of a fourteen-day supply of foods and drinking water for a sixteen- to nineteen-year-old male. This age group is assumed to have the highest dietary intake of chemical residues because of the quantities and kinds of foods consumed. More than sixty pesticides and industrial chemicals have been detected in measurable quantities in

Table 5.2. Daily intake, Adult Total Diet, ten residues, 1977–1981 (μg/kg of body weight)

Residue	1977	1978	1979	1980	1981
2-ethylhexyl diphenyl phosphate	...	...	...	1.820	0.931
Chlorpropham	0.310	0.144	0.300	0.268	0.347
Malathion	0.154	0.142	0.265	0.203	0.243
2-chloroethyl linoleate	0.078	0.228	0.079	0.197	0.140
Dieldrin	0.023	0.017	0.016	0.022	0.016
Pentachlorophenol	0.001	...	0.006	0.040	0.052
Dicloran	0.056	0.033	0.030	0.023	0.047
o-Phenylphenol	0.004	0.038	0.046	0.015	0.047
Dichlorodiphenyltrichloroethane (DDT)	0.046	0.070	0.093	0.034	0.034
Polychlorinated biphenyl (PCB)	0.016	0.027	0.014	0.008	0.003

Sources: Gartrell et al. 1985, 1986.
Note: Years are fiscal.

Table 5.3. Daily intake, Adult Total Diet, six elements, 1977–1981 (μg/day)

Element	1977	1978	1979	1980	1981
Arsenic	72	59	62	48	46
Cadmium	37	31	32	28	28
Lead	79	95	82	83	57
Mercury	6	3	5	5	3
Selenium	110	156	152	141	139
Zinc	18	17	18	18	18

Sources: Gartrell et al. 1985, 1986.
Note: Years are fiscal.

such foods (Gartrell et al. 1985; Gartrell et al. 1986). Table 5.2 shows the daily intake of ten of these residues. Table 5.3 shows the daily intake of six elements.

While data from the Total Diet studies are important, they do not provide a clear picture of the relative importance of food chain exposures to humans. What is needed is a determination of human intakes from all media: air, water, and food. We attempt to provide this perspective by considering the physicochemical properties that control the environmental fate of chemicals and their eventual partitioning into air, water, and food.

Measuring Organics in the Media

Many physical, chemical, and environmental factors affect the nature and extent of human exposure to toxic chemicals, factors often complex and inadequately understood. However, it is possible to gain a perspective on the potential for human exposure to these pollutants by considering their physicochemical properties.

Basically, chemicals are found in the media in which they are most soluble. Trichloroethylene (TCE) and tetrachloroethylene (two volatile organics) are most soluble in air; thus they tend to be found in air, and inhalation is the principal means of human exposure. DDT and PCB are most soluble in organic matter; thus they tend to bioconcentrate in biota and transfer to humans through the food chain.

Chemicals released to the environment partition between air, water, soil, and biota. Henry's Law Constant (H) and the octanol-water partition coefficient (K_{ow}) are two of the fundamental physicochemical parameters that control the partitioning of chemicals among these four media.

▎ Henry's Law Constant

Henry's Law Constant relates the equilibrium concentration of a compound in air to its equilibrium concentration in water. Henry's Law Constant can be expressed as

$$H = P/S,$$

where P is the vapor pressure of the contaminant, and S is the water solubility of the contaminant.

Thus H provides a relative measure of a chemical's solubility in air (its vapor pressure) to its solubility in water. When vapor pressure is large relative to solubility, Henry's Law Constant is large, and the chemical dissolves mainly into the air. When water solubility is large relative to vapor pressure, the chemical dissolves mainly into water.

Octanol-Water Partition Coefficient

Assessment of the environmental fate of toxic chemicals depends largely on predicting the extent they bioaccumulate in living organisms (such as fish). Their concentrations in such organisms may be greater than their concentrations in the medium (such as water). A convenient characterization of this potential is the bioconcentration factor, which is the dimensionless ratio of the concentration of the chemical in the organism to that in the media.

In living organisms, chemicals tend to bioaccumulate in the lipid component. Thus one measure of the potential for bioconcentration in the organism is the concentration of the chemical in the organism's lipid component. However, since to directly measure this concentration would require a controlled experiment with a living organism, the equilibrium partitioning between the liquid chemical octanol (a good surrogate for fat) and water is measured instead.

The K_{ow} is defined as the ratio of a chemical's concentration in the octanol phase to its concentration in the aqueous phase of a two-phase octanol-water system (Lyman et al. 1982). That is

$$K_{ow} = Co/Cw,$$

where Co is the concentration of the chemical in octanol, and Cw is the concentration of the chemical in water.

The K_{ow} is directly related to a chemical's potential to bioaccumulate in biota. It can be used to calculate the bioaccumulation factor in fish (Mackay 1982), the soil-plant bioconcentration factor (Baes 1982), and the fractional transfer to beef and milk of a chemical in forage and grains ingested by cattle and milk cows (Kenaga 1980). The K_{ow} is also correlated to two other physicochemical properties. It is inversely correlated with water solubility (Kenaga and Goring 1980; Chiou and Schmedding 1982), and directly correlated with the soil-water partition coefficient, K_{oc} (Lyman et al. 1982). Taken together, these correlations indicate that a chemical with a large K_{ow} tends to accumulate in soil and biota and not in water. Conversely, a chemical with a low K_{ow} tends to accumulate in water and not in soil and biota.

Equilibrium Partitioning Model

The environmental fate of chemicals can also be studied using the level III fugacity model proposed by Mackay et al. (1985). This model partitions the environment into six compartments: air, water, soil, sediment, suspended solids (in water), and biota (in water). Although this model contains many simplifying assumptions, given our current knowledge concerning environmental transport of chemicals, the model is adequate for predicting the equilibrium partitioning of nonparticulate pollutants (Mackay et al. 1985; Mackay and Paterson, 1982; Cohen and Ryan 1985).

Applications of the Equilibrium Partitioning Model

Mackay et al. (1985) applied the equilibrium partitioning model to fourteen benchmark chemicals for which suitable physicochemical and reactivity data are available. The application of the partitioning model to one of these chemicals, trichloroethylene (TCE), indicates the reasonableness of the results using this approach.

TCE is a widely used organic solvent. It has a large Henry's Law Constant (log H = 3.1) and a medium range octanol-water partition coefficient (log K_{ow} = 2.3). The high log H indicates a rapid loss from water to air and, together with the medium range K_{ow}, indicates a rapid loss from soil to air. Thus one would expect TCE to dissolve mainly into air.

Assuming environmental releases of TCE are 90 percent into air, 5 percent into water, and 5 percent into soil (a close approximation to actual releases), model predictions of the mass distribution of TCE under equilibrium conditions are as follows:

Media	Percent
Air	92.4
Water	7.2
Soil	0.3

Multimedia environmental measurements of TCE have been reported for the La Jolla, California, region (Su and Goldberg 1976) and for the

Table 5.4. Concentrations of trichloroethylene in partitioning model, Liverpool and La Jolla

Compartment	Partitioning Model	Liverpool	La Jolla
Air	1.4×10^3	6.4×10^3	7.1×10^3
Sea water	9.4×10^4	3.0×10^5	1.0×10^4
Fresh water	9.4×10^4	6.0×10^6 (max)	...
Soil	5.7×10^5	...	...
Sediment	4.5×10^5	1.0×10^5	...
Fish	8.8×10^5	1.0×10^7 (max)	...

Sources: Mackay et al. 1985; Cohen and Ryan 1985; Pearson and McConnel 1975; Su and Goldberg 1976.

Liverpool area (Pearson and McConnel 1975). The model results and the *in situ* concentrations at the above two sites are shown in table 5.4. The predicted concentrations agree well with the reported *in situ* measurements (that is, the predicted concentrations are generally within the same order of magnitude as the environmental measurements).

Cross-Media Partition Profiles

We are now interested in answering the question, Once released into the environment, where do chemicals go? Cross-media partition profiles are designed to answer this question.

Air

Figure 5.1 presents the cross-media partition profiles of a chemical chronically released into air. As can be seen, when log H is greater than about 0.3, a significant amount of the chemical remains in air. TCE is an industrial solvent, and aldicarb is a pesticide used on potatoes, cotton, sugar beets, and other farm produce. TCE has a log H of 3.1 and a log K_{ow} of 2.3, while aldicarb has a log H of minus 3.4 and a log K_{ow} of 0.7. As shown in figure 5.1, 99 percent of TCE would remain in the air, 0.06 percent would end up in water, and a little over 0.002 percent in the soil. Seventy percent of aldicarb would end up in water, 31 percent would remain in the air, and only 0.02 percent would enter the soil.

Figure 5.1d summarizes the partition profiles. Regions are identified where greater than 50 percent of the chemical mass would be in air, water, or soil. TCE would partition more than 50 percent into air, while aldicarb would partition more than 50 percent into water. It is interesting to note that aldicarb was used for years in the United States with no consideration given to its potential effect on groundwater. It has now been widely detected in groundwater and banned for agricultural use in several states (Harris and Davids 1982; Gruson 1983).

Water

Figure 5.2 presents the cross-media partition profiles of a chemical chronically released into water. As can be seen, a significant amount remains in the water for nearly all values of the physicochemical parameters H and K_{ow}. The air never contains more than 43 percent of the chemical mass, with the result that figure 5.2d contains no region marked as air. Soil contains more than 50 percent of the chemical mass only with very high values of K_{ow}.

It should be pointed out that the profiles in figure 5.2 describe environmental partitioning of a chemical when released in water with no fur-

Figure 5.1. Cross-media partition profiles of a chemical released into the air as a function of H and K_{ow}.

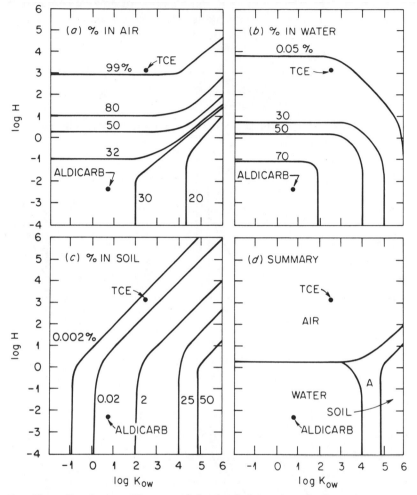

Note: No medium has over 50 percent of the chemical mass in region A, section d.

ther human intervention. For example, when TCE is discharged from an industrial plant directly into a stream or lake, one might expect about 40 percent of the discharge to eventually volatilize to the atmosphere (figure 5.2a and 5.2b). However, if the liquid discharge is subsequently treated at a wastewater treatment plant, aeration could result in almost all of the

TCE being released to the atmosphere. In a study of the Philadelphia metropolitan area on human exposure to toxic substances through air and drinking water, the EPA found that volatilization of organic compounds from the largest sewage treatment plant accounted for almost half of the estimated cancer risks to the population from breathing measured carcinogens in air (Haemisegger et al. 1985).

Figure 5.2. Cross-media partition profiles of a chemical released into water as a function of H and K_{ow}.

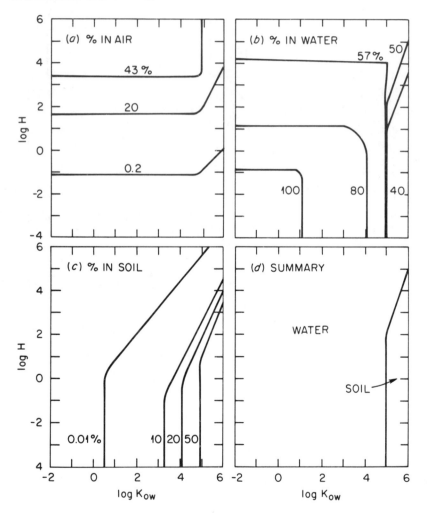

Soil

Figure 5.3 presents the cross-media partition profiles of a chemical chronically released into soil. As can be seen, partitioning into air is controlled by a trade-off between H and K_{ow}. When log K_{ow} is less than 1 and log H greater than 2, over 97 percent of the chemical enters the air. As the chemical's ability to adsorb to soil increases (i.e., increasing K_{ow}), the vola-

Figure 5.3. Cross-media partition profiles of a chemical released into soil as a function of H and K_{ow}.

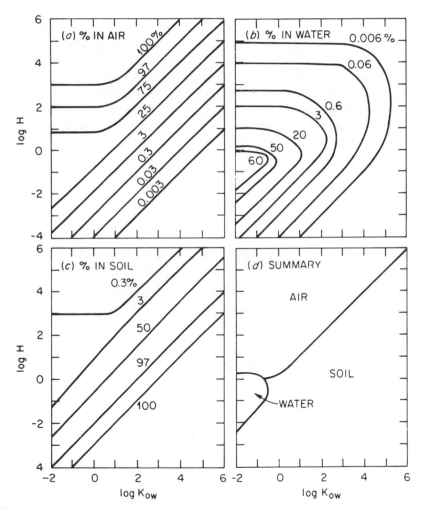

tility of the chemical must increase (i.e., increasing H) if the fraction of the chemical ending up in the air is to remain high.

▌ Uptake of Toxic Chemicals by the Food Chain

The equilibrium partitioning model can be extended for prediction of the uptake of toxic chemicals in vegetation, beef, and milk. Plant uptake of chemicals from soil is a complex process, involving not only root uptake but also subsequent translocation into shoots. Root uptake has been shown to be correlated with the octanol-water partition coefficient (Briggs et al. 1982; Baes 1982). Translocation from roots to shoots is poorly understood but is known to be most efficient for compounds with a log K_{ow} equal to 1.8 (Shone and Wood 1974). Plant leaves can take up vapors from surrounding air (Gaggi et al. 1985; Vaughan 1984), and for some chemicals this pathway contributes more than roots do to total plant uptakes (Nash and Beall 1970).

Root uptake of chemicals distributed in soil is described by the parameter B_v, representing soil-to-plant transfer coefficients for the vegetative portion of food crops. The parameter B_v is unitless, as it represents the ratio of the pollutant concentration in plants to the concentration in soil at harvest. Baes (1982) has related B_v to K_{ow} and has derived the following regression equation:

$$\text{Log } B_v = 2.71 - 0.62 \, (\log K_{ow}).$$

Kenaga (1980) has shown a positive correlation between the K_{ow} and the bioconcentration factor in beef fat (the ratio of the quantity of a chemical found in beef fat to the quantity in the diet). Based on the average fat content of various commonly ingested beef cuts and milk and the average consumption of feed per head of cattle, Baes (1982) derived the following regression equations:

$$\text{Log } F_f = -5.15 + 0.50 \, (\log K_{ow}).$$
$$\text{Log } F_m = -6.13 + 0.50 \, (\log K_{ow}).$$

The terrestrial food chain model is applied below to three chemicals: DDT, PCB, and dieldrin. These applications indicate the reasonableness of the results of the partitioning model approach.

DDT

DDT is a synthetic, fat-soluble insecticide that is highly persistent in the environment. It was used extensively in the United States until undesirable reductions in bird populations were attributed to the chemical and prompted its ban by the EPA in 1972. DDT is still used in many tropical countries to combat malaria.

Human exposure to DDT and its more persistent metabolite, DDE, (dichlorodiphenyldichloroethane) is primarily through the food chain. In 1965 food intake accounted for 0.087 milligrams of DDT per person per day (Spindler 1983). By 1970 the daily food intake of DDT was reduced to 0.029 milligrams. The Total Diet study of 1981/82 gave an average daily intake of 0.002 milligrams (Gartrell et al. 1986). Despite the decline in DDT intakes, however, DDT residues can still be detected in virtually every person in the United States (see table 5.1). Application of the equilibrium partitioning model to DDT results in the following estimates of human daily intakes:

Media	Daily intake ($\mu g/d$)
Air	0.00057
Water	0.00030
Food	5.70000

Intake of DDT via the food chain predicted by the model compares well with measured values (2.4 to 6.5 $\mu g/d$; see table 5.2). Thus virtually 100 percent of human intake of DDT is the result of contamination of the food chain (Spindler 1983).

PCB

PCBs are synthetic chlorinated compounds, which have a wide number of industrial applications. The Monsanto Company voluntarily restricted PCB production following highly publicized incidents of accidental food contamination in 1971. Later reports of PCB contamination in fish in the Hudson River again focused national attention on the problem. Manufacture of PCB was banned in 1979 (Cordle 1983).

PCBs have a low Henry's Law Constant and a high octanol-water partition coefficient. Analysis with the equilibrium partitioning model shows that 99 percent of PCB mass is expected to be found in soil. Thus one might not expect PCB to be a multimedia problem. However, evaporation of PCB from spills, landfills, road oils, and so on results in small but measurable atmospheric emissions (Weaver 1984; Lewis and Martin 1985), and atmospheric transport is now recognized as the primary mode of its global distribution. The large bioaccumulation potential of PCB (its bioaccumulation factor in fish and shellfish is 40 thousand) results in uptake in biota and thus in an environmental problem of significant proportions.

Human exposure to PCB has come primarily via low-level food contamination. A single incident of food contamination can have widespread repercussions, as illustrated by the following example. In 1979, a single transformer used at a hog-processing plant in Montana leaked more than 200 gallons of PCB-contaminated oil into a nearby underground storage bin containing meat waste products (Drotman et al. 1983). The contaminated meat was used to make animal feed, which was sold to feed manufacturers and farmers. This led to contamination of poultry and egg products in seventeen states and in countries as far away as Japan. It is clear from this incident that our food supply is vulnerable to even a single mishap.

Application of the equilibrium partitioning model to PCB results in the following estimates of human daily intake:

Media	Daily intake (µg/d)
Air	0.15000
Water	0.00002
Food	0.31000

Measured values of the daily intake of PCB from the food chain range from 0.2 to 1.9 µg/d (see table 5.2). Thus the model predicts that at least 67 percent of the daily intake of PCB is the result of food chain contamination, with the remainder contributed through inhalation. This conclusion is substantiated by environmental measurements (Murphy et al. 1983; Eisenreich et al. 1981; Nisbet and Sarofin 1972).

Dieldrin

Dieldrin is a highly persistent, synthetic compound with a higher acute toxicity than DDT. Manufactured by the Shell Chemical Company in the United States, dieldrin was primarily used for the control of corn pests. The EPA banned the manufacture of dieldrin in 1974 (Sittig 1981). Shell then began its manufacture in Holland. Dieldrin is still used in many of the industrial countries.

Food ingestion is the primary route of human exposure to dieldrin. From 1977 to 1982, the average daily intake in the United States was estimated to be less than 0.002 milligrams per day (Gartrell et al. 1986). In the late 1960s, intakes in many countries averaged about ten times higher (Hunter et al. 1969). Dieldrin is detectable in adipose tissue samples of 96 percent of the United States population (Murphy et al. 1983). It is difficult to detect dieldrin in human blood serum, since serum levels of dieldrin are about 150 times lower on the average than adipose tissue levels (Hunter et al. 1969). Nevertheless, dieldrin has been detected in blood serum lipid specimens of 8.6 percent of the general population, ages twelve to seventy four years (Murphy and Harvey 1985).

Another example of the potential for human exposure through accidental contamination of the food chain comes from an incident involving dieldrin in Scotland (Bell and MacLeod 1983). Approximately 350 hens died during a six-week period at a chicken farm in West Lothian. The deaths were attributed to dieldrin-contaminated wood litter used in nesting boxes. Humans were exposed through consumption of contaminated eggs. Blood tests revealed that farm workers and members of their families had blood dieldrin levels between four and thirty-two times the background level. If excessive mortality of the poultry had not alerted veterinary officers, human exposure from this incident could have been much wider.

Application of the equilibrium partitioning model to dieldrin results in the following estimates of human daily intake:

Media	Daily intake (µg/d)
Air	0.00100
Water	0.00004
Food	1.10000

The daily dieldrin intake from food predicted by the model compares well with measured values (1.1 to 1.6 µg/d; see table 5.2). Virtually 100 percent of human dieldrin intake occurs via the food chain.

❚ The Food Chain in Cross-Media Partition Profiles

The equilibrium partitioning model, modified to account for the terrestrial food chain, can be applied to determine the relative importance of the food chain to total human exposure to toxic chemicals. We are trying to answer the question, Under what conditions is the food chain the dominant source of human exposure to toxic chemicals? Since cross-media par-

Figure 5.4. Cross-media partition profile of a chemical released into air.

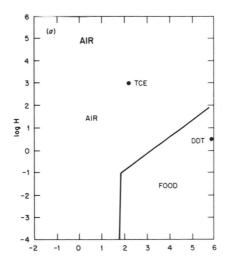

titioning is dependent on the medium into which a chemical is released, each medium is considered separately.

Figures 5.4, 5.5, and 5.6 present profiles for a chemical chronically released into the air, the water, and the soil. Parameter spaces where human exposure to a chemical is predominantly (greater than 50 percent of

Figure 5.5. Cross-media partition profile of a chemical released into water.

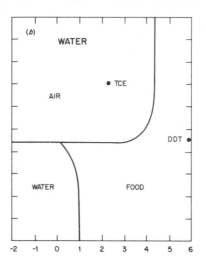

Figure 5.6. Cross-media partition profile of a chemical released into soil.

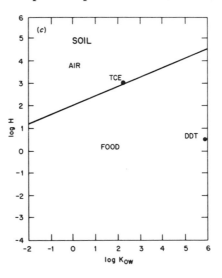

total exposure) from air, water, or food are identified. Figure 5.4 shows that in an atmospheric release more than 50 percent of the human daily intake of TCE would result from inhalation, while the majority of human exposure to DDT would result from ingestion of food.

Taken as a whole, the figures indicate that for light-weight, volatile chemicals, inhalation is likely to be the dominant human exposure pathway. For chemicals with large octanol-water partition coefficients, the food chain is the dominant human exposure pathway.

Summary

Toxic chemicals end up in media in which they are most soluble. Trichloroethylene and tetrachloroethylene are most soluble in air; thus they tend to be found in air; and thus inhalation is the principal means of human exposure to these organics. DDT and PCB are most soluble in organic matter; thus they tend to bioconcentrate in biota and vegetation and transfer to humans through the food chain. The above analysis shows that, for a large class of organics, the food chain is the dominant source of human exposure.

References

Ames, B. N. 1983. Dietary carcinogens and anticarcinogens, oxygen radicals and degenerative diseases. *Science* 222:1256-64.

Baes III, C. F. 1982. Prediction of radionuclide K_d values from soil-plant concentration ratios. *Transactions of the American Nuclear Society* 41:53-54.

Bell, D., and A. F. MacLeod. 1983. Dieldrin pollution of a human food chain. *Human Toxicology* 2:75-82.

Briggs, G. G., R. H. Bromilow, and A. A. Evans. 1982. Relationships between lipophilicity and root uptake and translocation of non-ionized chemicals by barley. *Pesticide Science* 13:495-504.

Chiou, C. T., and D. W. Schmedding. 1982. Partitioning of organic compounds in octanol-water systems. *Environmental Science and Technology* 16:4-10.

Cohen, Y., and P. A. Ryan. 1985. Multimedia modeling of environmental transport: Trichloroethylene test case. *Environmental Science and Technology* 19:413-17.

Cordle, F. 1983. Use of epidemiology and clinical toxicology to determine human risk in regulating polychlorinated biphenyls in the food supply. *Regulatory Toxicology and Pharmacology* 3:252-74.

Drotman, D. P., P. J. Baxter, J. A. Liddle, C. D. Brokopp, and M. D. Skinner. 1983. Contamination of the food chain polychlorinated biphenyls from a broken transformer. *American Journal of Public Health* 73:290-92.

Eisenreich, S. J., B. B. Looney, and J. D. Thornton. 1981. Airborne organic contaminants in the Great Lakes ecosystem. *Environmental Science and Technology* 15:30-38.

Fawcett, H. H. 1984. *Hazardous and Toxic Materials: Safe Handling and Disposal.* New York: Wiley-Interscience.

Gaggi, C., E. Bacci, D. Calamari, and R. Fanelli. 1985. Chlorinated hydrocarbons in plant foliage: An indication of the tropospheric contamination level. *Chemosphere* 14:1673–86.

Gartrell, M. J., J. C. Craun, D. S. Podrebarac, and E. L. Gunderson. 1985. Pesticides, selected elements, and other chemicals in Adult Total Diet samples, October 1978–September 1979. *Journal—Association of Official Analytical Chemists* 68:862–75.

———. 1986. Pesticides, selected elements, and other chemicals in Adult Total Diet samples, October 1980–March 1982. *Journal—Association of Official Analytical Chemists* 69:146–61.

Gruson, K. 1983. A pesticide too good to be true? *New York Times,* April 24.

Haemisegger, E. R., A. D. Jones, and F. L. Reinhardt. 1985. EPA's experience with assessment of site-specific environmental problems: A review of IEMD's geographic study of Philadelphia. *Journal of Air Pollution Control* 35:809–15.

Harris, D., and H. W. Davids. 1982. *Report on the Occurrence and Movement of Agricultural Chemicals in Groundwater: South Fork of Suffolk County.* Long Island, N.Y.: Suffolk County Department of Health Services, Bureau of Water Services.

Hunter, C. G., J. Robinson, and M. Roberts. 1969. Pharmacokinetics of dieldrin (HEOD): Ingestion by human subjects for 18 to 24 months, and postexposure for eight months. *Archives of Environmental Health* 18:12–21.

Jensen, A. A. 1983. Chemical contaminants in human milk. *Residue Reviews* 89:1–128.

Kenaga, E. E. 1980. Correlation of bioconcentration factors of chemicals in aquatic and terrestrial organisms with their physical and chemical properties. *Environmental Science and Technology* 14:553–56.

Kenaga, E. E., and C. A. I. Goring. 1980. Relationship between water solubility, soil sorption, octanol-water partitioning and concentration of chemicals in biota. In *Aquatic Toxicology,* ed. J. E. Eaton, P. R. Parrish, and A. C. Hendricks. Philadelphia: American Society for Testing Materials.

Laug, E. P., F. M. Kunze, and C. S. Prickett. 1951. Occurrence of DDT in human fat and milk. *Archives of Industrial Hygiene and Occupational Medicine* 3:245.

Lewis, R. L., and B. E. Martin. 1985. Measurement of fugitive atmospheric emissions of polychlorinated biphenyls from hazardous waste landfills. *Environmental Science and Technology* 19:986–91.

Lyman, W. J., W. F. Reehl, and D. H. Rosenblatt. 1982. *Handbook of Chemical Property Estimation Methods.* New York: McGraw-Hill.

Mackay, D. 1982. Correlation of bioconcentration factors. *Environmental Science and Technology* 16:274–78.

Mackay, D., and S. Paterson. 1982. Fugacity revisited. *Environmental Science and Technology* 16:654A–60A.

Mackay, D., S. Paterson, B. Cheug, and W. B. Neely. 1985. Evaluating the environmental behavior of chemicals with a level III fugacity model. *Chemosphere* 14:335–74.

Murphy, R., and C. Harvey. 1985. Residues and metabolites of selected persistent halogenated hydrocarbons in blood specimens from a general population survey. *Environmental Health Perspectives* 60:115–20.

Murphy, R., F. W. Kutz, and S. C. Strassman. 1983. Selected pesticide residues or metabolites in blood and urine specimens from a general population survey. *Environmental Health Perspectives* 48:81–86.

Nash, R. G., and M. L. Beall, Jr. 1970. Chlorinated hydrocarbon insecticides: Root uptake versus vapor contamination of soybean foliage. *Science* 168:1109-11.

Nisbet, C. T., and A. F. Sarofin. 1972. Rates and routes of transport of PCBs in the environment. *Environmental Health Perspectives* 1:21-38.

Pearson, C. R., and G. McConnel. 1975. *Proceedings of the Royal Society of London* 13:189.

Rogan, W. J., A. Bagniewska, and T. Damstra. 1980. Pollutants in breast milk. *New England Journal of Medicine* 302:1450-53.

Savage, E. P., T. J. Keefe, J. D. Tessari, H. W. Wheeler, F. M. Applehans, E. A. Goes, and S. A. Ford. 1981. National study of chlorinated hydrocarbon insecticide residues, USA. *American Journal of Epidemiology* 113:413-22.

Shone, M. G. T., and A. V. Wood. 1974. A comparison of the uptake and translocation of some organic herbicides and a systemic fungicide by barley. *Journal of Experimental Botany* 25:390-400.

Sittig, M. 1981. *Handbook of Toxic and Hazardous Chemicals.* Park Ridge, N.J.: Noyes Publications.

Spindler, M. 1983. DDT: Health aspects in relation to man and risk/benefit assessment based thereupon. *Residue Reviews* 90:1-34.

Stich, H. F. 1983. *Carcinogens and Mutagens in the Environment.* Vol. 1. *Food Products.* Boca Raton, Fla.: CRC Press.

Su, C., and E. D. Goldberg. 1976. In *Strategies for Marine Pollution Monitoring,* ed. E. D. Goldberg. New York: John Wiley & Sons.

Takei, G. H., S. M. Kauahikaua, and G. H. Leong. 1983. Analyses of human milk samples collected in Hawaii for residues of organo-chlorine pesticides and polychlorobiphenyls. *Bulletin of Environmental Contamination and Toxicology* 30:606-13.

U.S. Congress, Office of Technology Assessment. 1979. *Environmental Contaminants in Food.* Washington, D.C.: Government Printing Office.

———. 1983. *Technologies and Management Strategies for Hazardous Waste Control.* Washington, D.C.: Government Printing Office.

Vaughan, B. E. 1984. State of research: Environmental pathways and food chain transfer. *Environmental Health Perspectives* 54:353-71.

Weaver, G. 1984. PCB contamination in and around New Bedford, Mass. *Environmental Science and Technology* 18:22A-27A.

6. Toxic Chemical Exposure and Dose to Target Tissues

MORTON LIPPMANN

Chapter 6 examines various pathways by which toxic chemicals in the environment enter the human body. Lippmann surveys exposure from food, from water used for drinking and washing, from skin contact, and from breathing. The body has defense mechanisms to keep out chemicals and to limit exposure once chemicals have entered the body. For example, the upper airways are designed to remove large particles and water-soluble gases; those small particles that reach the lower airway are removed by the ciliar escalator or by macrophages. To cause damage, chemicals must cross membrane barriers to the target organ, while avoiding detoxification.

Toxic chemicals in the environment that reach sensitive tissues in the human body can cause discomfort, loss of function, and changes in structure leading to disease. This chapter addresses the pathways and transport rates between chemicals in environmental media and critical tissue sites, as well as retention times at those sites. It is designed to provide a conceptual framework, as well as brief discussions of (1) the mechanisms for—and some quantitative data on—uptake from the environment; (2) translocation within the body, retention at target sites, and the influence of the physicochemical properties of the chemicals on these factors; (3) the patterns and pathways for exposure of humans to chemicals in environmental media; and (4) the influence of age, sex, size, habits, health status, and so on.

An agreed upon terminology is critically important when discussing the relationships between toxic chemicals in the environment and human health. The terms used in this chapter are defined below:

Exposure   Contact with external environmental media containing the chemical of interest. For fluid media in contact with the skin or respiratory tract, both concentration and contact time are critical. For ingested material, concentration and amount consumed are important.

Deposition   Capture of the chemical at a body surface site on skin, respiratory tract, or gastrointestinal tract.

Clearance   Translocation from a deposition site to a storage site or depot within the body or elimination from the body.

Retention   Presence of residual material at a deposition site or along a clearance pathway.

Dose   Amount of chemical deposited on or translocated to a site on or within the body where toxic effects take place.

Target tissue   A site within the body where toxic effects lead to damage or disease. Depending on the toxic effects of concern, a target tissue can extend from whole organs down to specific cells to subcellular constituents within cells.

Exposure surrogates or indices   Indirect measures of exposure, such as (1) concentrations in environmental media at times or places other than those directly encountered; (2) concentrations of the chemical of interest, a metabolite of the chemical, or an enzyme induced by the chemical in circulating or excreted body fluids; (3) elevations in body burden as measured by external probes.

In summary, exposure represents contact between a concentration of a chemical agent in air, water, food, or other materials and the person or population of interest. The agent is the source of an internal dose to a critical organ or tissue. The magnitude of the dose depends on a number of factors: (1) the volumes inhaled or ingested; (2) the fractions of the inhaled or ingested material transferred across epithelial membranes of the skin, the respiratory tract, and the gastrointestinal tract; (3) the fractions transported via circulating fluids to target tissues; and (4) the fractional uptake by the target tissues. Each of these factors can have considerable intersubject variability. Sources of variability include activity level, age, sex, and health status, as well as such inherent variabilities as race and size.

With chronic or repetitive exposures, other factors affect the dose of interest. When the chemical's retention at, or its effects on, the target tissue are cumulative, and clearance or recovery is slow, the dose of interest can be represented by cumulative uptake. However, when the agent is rapidly eliminated, or when its effects are rapidly and completely reversible upon removal from exposure, rate of delivery may be the dose parameter of primary interest.

Concentration of Toxic Chemicals in Human Microenvironments

The technology for sampling air, water, and food is relatively well developed, as are the technologies for sample separation from copollutants, media, and interferences, and the technologies for quantitative analyses of the components of interest. However, knowing when, where, how long, and at what rate and frequency to collect data relevant to the exposures of interest is difficult, requiring knowledge of temporal and spatial variability of exposure concentrations. Unfortunately, one seldom has enough information of these kinds to guide sample collections. Many of these factors relating to inhalation exposures are discussed in detail in chapter 4 and Lioy (1983), while those for food are discussed in chapter 5.

▌ Water

Concentrations of environmental chemicals in food and drinking water are extremely variable, and there are further variations in the amounts consumed due to the extreme variability in dietary preferences and food sources. The number of foods for which up-to-date concentration data for specific chemicals are available is extremely limited. Relevant human dietary exposure data are sometimes available in terms of market basket survey analyses. In this approach, food for a mixed diet is purchased, cleaned, processed, and prepared as for consumption, and one set of specific chemical analyses is done for the composite mixture. Temporal trends for dichlorodiphenyltrichloroethane (DDT), dieldrin, and polychlorinated biphenyls (PCBs) from such surveys are illustrated in figure 6.1.

The concentrations of chemicals in potable piped water supplies depend greatly on the source of the water and its treatment history. Surface waters from protected watersheds generally have low concentrations of both dissolved minerals and environmental chemicals. Well waters usually have low concentrations of bacteria and environmental chemicals, but often have high mineral concentrations. Poor waste disposal practices may contribute to groundwater contamination, especially in areas of high population density. Some survey data on groundwater contamination by volatile organics are illustrated in figure 6.2 Treated surface waters from lakes and rivers in densely populated or industrialized areas usually contain a variety of dissolved organics and trace metals, the concentrations of which vary greatly with season (due to variable surface runoff), with proximity to pollutant sources, with upstream usage, and with treatment efficacy.

Uptake of environmental chemicals in bathing water by intact skin is usually minimal in comparison to uptake via inhalation or ingestion. It depends on both the concentration in the fluid surrounding the skin surface and the polarity of the chemical, with more polar chemicals having

Figure 6.1. Time trends in levels of PCB, DDT, and dieldrin in foods.

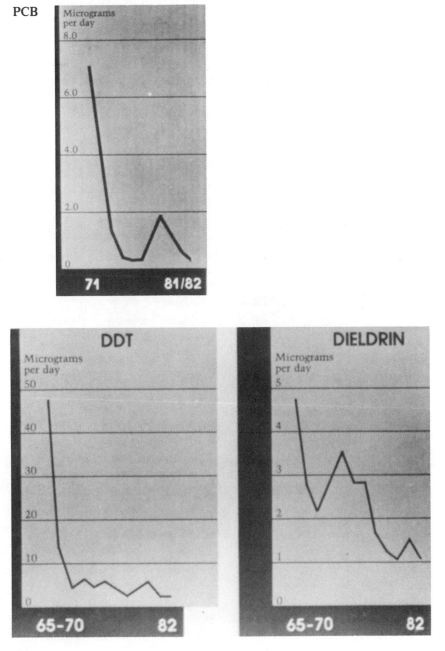

(*Source:* U.S. Environmental Protection Agency 1965–82.)

less ability to penetrate the intact skin. Uptake via skin can be significant for occupational exposures to concentrated liquids or solids.

▌ Air

While chemical uptake through ingestion and the skin surface is generally intermittent, inhalation provides a continuous means of exposure.

Figure 6.2. Groundwater contamination by volatile chemicals.

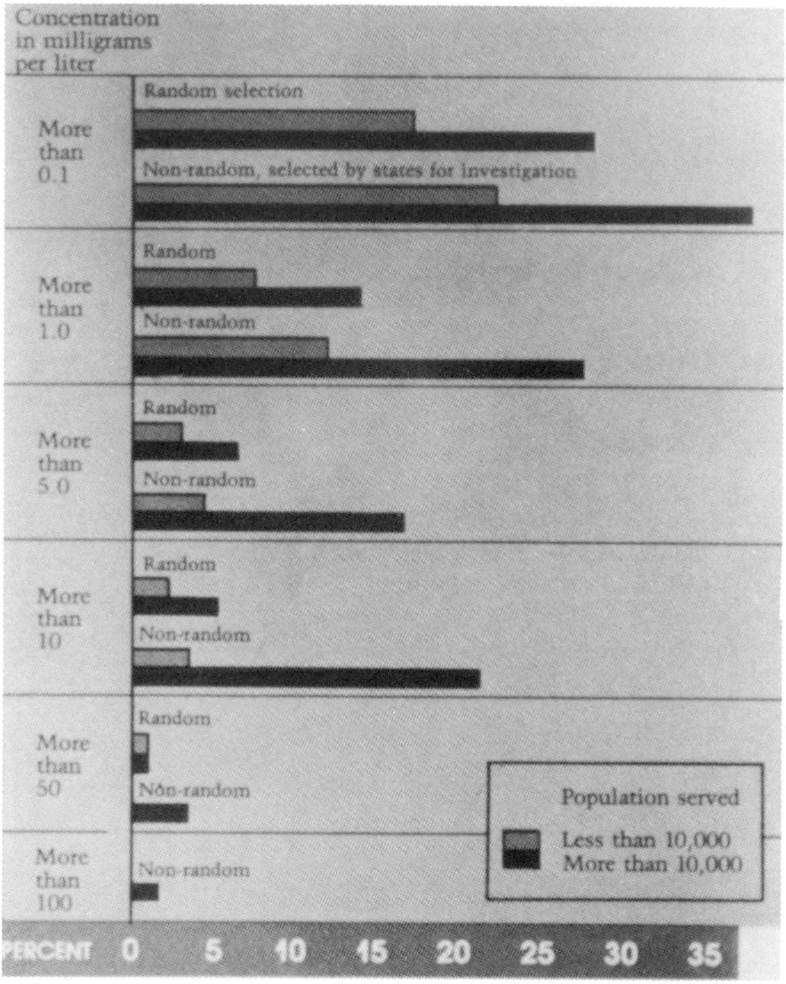

(*Source:* U.S. Environmental Protection Agency 1984.)

The important variables affecting the uptake of inhaled chemicals are the depth and frequency of inhalation and the concentration and physico-chemical properties of the chemicals in the air.

Exposures to airborne chemicals vary widely among inhalation micro-environments, the categories of which include workplace, residence, out-door ambient air, transportation, recreation, and public spaces. There are also wide variations in exposure within each category, depending on the number and strength of the sources of the airborne chemicals, the volume and mixing characteristics of the air within the defined microenvironment, the rate of air exchange with the outdoor air, and the rate of loss to surfaces within the microenvironment.

Workplace

Exposures to airborne chemicals at work are extremely variable in composition and concentration, depending on the material handled, the process design and its operation, the engineering controls applied to mini-mize chemical release to the air, the work practices followed, and the per-sonal protection provided. Workplace air monitoring often involves breathing-zone sampling—generally with passive samplers for gases and vapors and, for both gases and particles with personal battery-powered extraction samplers, which operate over periods of one to eight hours. These samplers can provide accurate measures of individual exposures to specific air contaminants.

Workplace air is also frequently monitored with fixed-site samplers or direct reading instruments. However, air concentrations at fixed sites may differ substantially from those in the breathing zones of individual work-ers. The fixed-site data may be relatable to the breathing zone when ap-propriate comparisons can be made, but otherwise they are crude surro-gates of exposure. The characteristics of equipment used for air sampling in industry are described in detail in Lioy (1983).

Residence

Airborne chemicals in residential microenvironments are attributed to their presence in the air infiltrating from out-of-doors and to their re-lease from indoor sources. The latter include unvented cooking stoves and space heaters, cigarettes, consumer products, and volatile emissions from wallboard, textiles, carpets, and so on. Personal exposures to chloroform, largely from indoor residential sources, are illustrated in figure 6.3, while the influence of smoking in the home on indoor exposures to respirable particulate matter is illustrated in figure 6.4. Indoor sources can release enough nitrogen dioxide, fine particle mass, and formaldehyde to make their indoor concentrations much higher than those in ambient outdoor air. Furthermore, the contributions of these chemicals to the total human exposure are usually even greater, since people usually spend much more time indoors than in the outdoor ambient air.

Outdoor Ambient Air

For pollutants having national ambient air quality standards (particulate matter, SO_2, CO, NO_2, O_3, and Pb) there is an extensive network of fixed-site monitors, generally on rooftops. Although these devices generate

Figure 6.3. Chloroform: Estimated frequency distributions of personal air exposures, outdoor air concentrations, and exhaled breath values, Elizabeth-Bayonne, N.J., area.

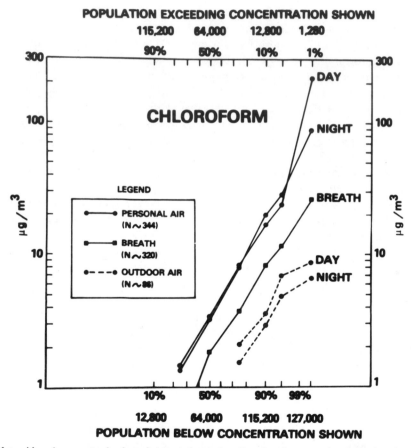

Note: Air values are twelve-hour integrated samples. Breath value was taken following the daytime air sample (6:00 A.M. to 6:00 P.M.). Outdoor air samples were taken near participants' homes. (*Source:* Wallace et al. 1985.)

Figure 6.4. Respirable particle concentrations, six U.S. cities, November 1976 to April 1978.

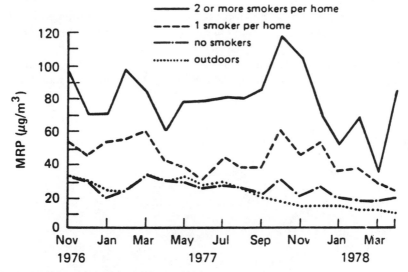

(*Source:* National Academy of Science 1981.)

large volumes of data, the concentrations at these sites may differ substantially from the concentrations that people breathe, especially tailpipe pollutants such as CO and Pb. Data for other toxic pollutants in the outdoor ambient air are not generally collected on a routine basis. Ambient concentrations of the criteria air pollutants have decreased in recent years, as shown in figure 6.5.

Transportation

Many people spend from a half hour to three hours each day in automobiles or buses going to work, to school, or shopping. Inhalation exposures to carbon monoxide (CO) in vehicles and garages can represent a significant fraction of total CO exposure.

Recreation and Public Spaces

Recreational exposure while exercising may be important to total daily exposure, because the increased respiratory ventilation associated with exercise can produce much more than proportional increases in delivered dose and functional responses. Spectators and athletes in closed arenas can be exposed to high concentration of pollutants. Spengler et al. (1978) has documented high exposures to CO at ice skating rinks from exhaust discharges by the ice scraping machinery.

Inhalation Exposures and Respiratory Tract Effects

❙ Deposition and Absorption

The surface and systemic uptake of chemicals from inhaled air depends both on the physical and chemical properties of the chemicals and on the person's anatomy and pattern of respiration. The structure of the respiratory tract is illustrated in figure 6.6. The following discussion outlines some of the primary factors affecting the deposition and retention of

Figure 6.5. Time trends in ambient levels of criteria air pollutants, 1975–82.

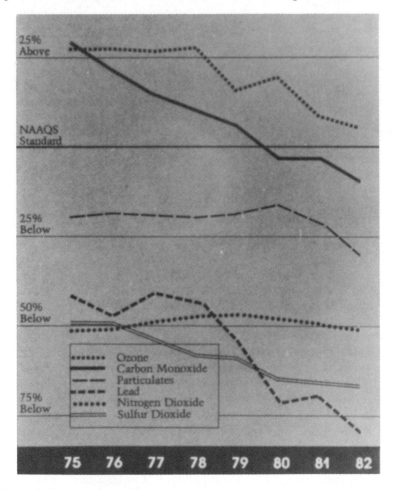

(*Source:* U.S. Environmental Protection Agency 1984.)

Figure 6.6. Structure of the respiratory tract. (Reproduced from National Research Council 1979.)

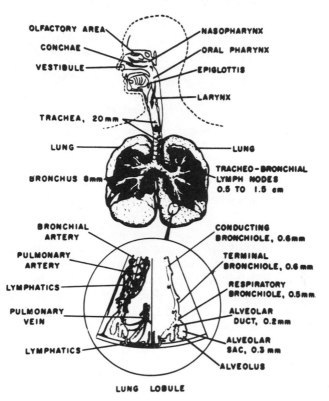

inhaled chemicals. More comprehensive discussions are available in review papers (Lippmann and Schlesinger 1984; Overton 1984).

Gases and vapors rapidly contact airway surfaces by molecular diffusion. Surface uptake is limited for compounds that are relatively insoluble in water, such as ozone. For such chemicals, the greatest uptake can be in the lung periphery, where the residence time and surface areas are the greatest. For more water-soluble gases, dissolution or reaction with surface fluids on the airways facilitates removal from the airstream. Vapors that are highly water soluble, such as sulfur dioxide, are almost completely removed in the airways of the head and very little vapor penetrates into lung airways.

For airborne particles, the most critical parameter affecting patterns and efficiencies of surface deposition is particle size. The mechanisms for particle deposition within respiratory airways are illustrated in figure 6.7.

Figure 6.7. Schematic of mechanism for particle deposition in respiratory airways.

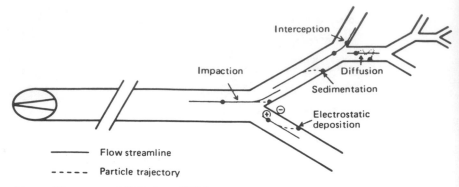

(*Source:* Lippmann and Schlesinger 1984.)

Almost all of the mass of airborne particulate matter is found in particles with diameters greater than 0.1 μm. Such particles have diffusional displacements many orders of magnitude smaller than those of gas molecules, and they are small in relation to the sizes of the airways in which they are suspended. Thus the penetration of airborne particles into the lung airways is determined primarily by convective flow—that is, the motion of the air in which the particles are suspended.

Some deposition by diffusion does occur for particles smaller than 0.5 μm in small airways, where it is favored by the small size of the airways and the low flow velocities in such airways. For particles larger than 0.5 μm, deposition by sedimentation occurs in small to mid-sized airways. For particles with aerodynamic diameters larger than 2 μm, particle inertia is sufficient to cause particle motion to deviate from the flow streamlines, resulting in deposition by impaction on surfaces downstream of changes in flow direction, primarily in mid- to large-sized airways, which have the highest flow velocities. The concentration of deposition on limited surface areas within the large airways is of special interest with respect to dosimetry and the pathogenesis of chronic lung diseases, such as bronchial cancer and bronchitis.

While particle inertia accounts for much of the "hot-spot" deposition on the trachea below the laryngeal jet and at the bifurcations of large lung airways, some of it is attributable to inertial airflow, which directs a disproportionately large fraction of the flow volume toward such surfaces and, at the same time, lessens the boundary layer thickness. Thus, to a lesser but still important extent, there is preferential deposition of submicrometer-sized particles and gas molecules at airway bifurcations.

Quantitative aspects of particle deposition are summarized in figures 6.8 through 6.11. It can be seen that deposition efficiencies in the major structural-functional regions of the human respiratory tract are both strongly dependent on particle size and highly variable among healthy humans. Additional variability results from structural changes in the airways associated with disease processes. Generally, these involve airway narrowing or localized constrictions, which act to increase deposition and concentrate it on limited surface areas.

All of the preceding was based on the assumption that each particle has a specific size. Hygroscopic particles grow considerably as they take up water vapor in the airways. Some hygroscopic growth curves for acidic and ambient aerosols are illustrated in figure 6.12.

Materials that dissolve the mucus of the conductive airways or the surfactant layer of the alveolar region can rapidly diffuse into the underlying epithelia and the circulating blood, thereby gaining access to tissues throughout the body. Chemical reactions and metabolic processes may occur within the lung fluids and cells, limiting access of the inhaled material to the bloodstream and creating reaction products with either greater or lesser solubility and biological activity. Few generalizations about absorption rates are possible.

▌ Translocation and Retention

Particles that do not dissolve at deposition sites can be translocated to remote retention sites by passive and active clearance processes. Passive transport depends on movement on or in surface fluids lining the airways. There is a continual proximal flow of surfactant to and onto the mucociliary escalator, which begins at the terminal bronchioles where it mixes with secretions from Clara and goblet cells. Within midsized and larger airways there are additional secretions from goblet cells and mucous glands, producing a thicker mucous layer having a serous subphase and an overlying, more viscous gel layer. The gel layer, lying above the tips of the synchronously beating cilia, is found in discrete plaques in smaller airways and becomes more of a continuous layer in the larger airways. The mucus reaching the larynx, and the particles carried by it, is swallowed and enters the gastrointestinal tract.

The total transit time for particles depositing on terminal bronchioles varies from about two to twenty-four hours in healthy humans, accounting for the relatively rapid bronchial clearance phase. Macrophage-mediated particle clearance via the bronchial tree takes place over a period of several weeks. The particles deposited in alveolar airways are ingested by alveolar macrophages within about six hours, but the movement of the particle-laden macrophages depends on the several weeks that it takes for the nor-

Figure 6.8. Deposition of monodisperse aerosols in the extrathoracic region for nose breathing in humans.

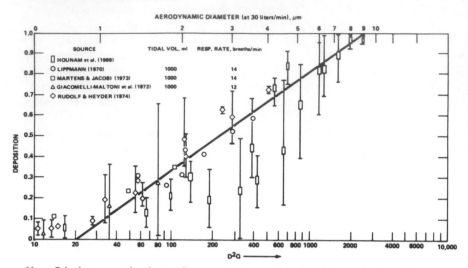

Note: Q is the average inspiratory flow rate in liters per minute. Solid line is deposition model of the International Commission on Radiological Protection. Other data show the median and range of other studies cited by the EPA. (*Source:* U.S. Environmental Protection Agency 1982.)

Figure 6.9. Deposition of monodisperse aerosols in the extrathoracic region for mouth breathing in humans.

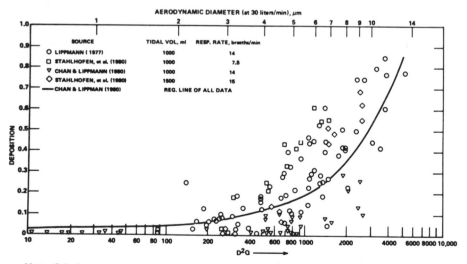

Note: Q is the average inspiratory flow rate in liters per minute. Solid line is overall regression. Other data are individual observations of investigators cited by the EPA. (*Source:* U.S. Environmental Protection Agency 1982.)

126

Figure 6.10. Deposition of monodisperse aerosols in the tracheobronchial region for mouth breathing in humans (percentage of aerosols entering the trachea).

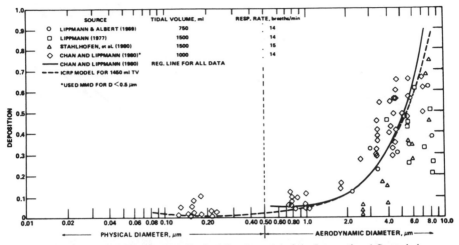

Note: Solid line is deposition model. Dashed line is model of the International Commission on Radiological Protection. Below 0.5 μm, deposition is plotted versus physical diameter by other studies cited by the EPA. (*Source:* U.S. Environmental Protection Agency 1982.)

Figure 6.11. Deposition of monodisperse aerosols in the pulmonary region for mouth breathing in humans.

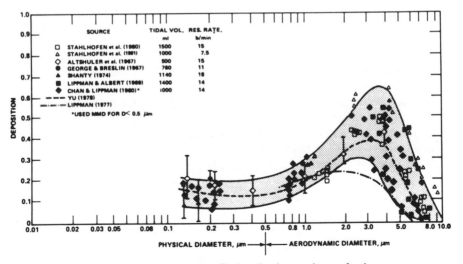

Note: Dashed line is the deposition model. Broken line is an estimate of pulmonary deposition for nose breathing. The eye-fit band envelops data from other studies cited by the EPA. (*Source:* U.S. Environmental Protection Agency 1982.)

127

Figure 6.12. Hygroscopic growth for acidic and ambient aerosols.

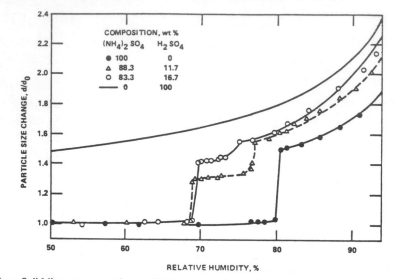

Note: Solid lines represent theory. Points are experimental observations. (*Source:* U.S. Environmental Protection Agency 1982.)

mal turnover of the resident macrophage population. At the end of several weeks, the particles not cleared to the bronchial tree via macrophages have been incorporated into epithelial and interstitial cells from which they are slowly cleared by dissolution or as particles via lymphatic drainage pathways, passing through pleural and, eventually, hilar and tracheal lymph nodes. Clearance times for these later phases depend strongly on the chemical nature of the particles and their sizes, with half times ranging from about thirty to a thousand days, or more.

All of the characteristic clearance times cited refer to inert, nontoxic particles in healthy lungs. Toxicants can drastically alter clearance times. Inhaled materials affecting mucociliary clearance rates include cigarette smoke (Albert et al. 1974, 1975), sulfuric acid (Lippmann et al. 1982; Schlesinger et al. 1983), ozone (Phalen et al. 1980), sulfur dioxide (Wolff et al. 1977), and formaldehyde (Morgan et al. 1984). Macrophage-mediated alveolar clearance is affected by sulfur dioxide (Ferin and Leach 1973), nitrogen dioxide and sulfuric acid (Schlesinger et al. in press), ozone (Phalen et al. 1980; Schlesinger et al. in press), and silica dust (Jammet et al. 1970). Cigarette smoke is known to affect the later phases of alveolar zone clearance in a dose-dependent manner (Bohning et al. 1982). Clearance pathways as well as rates can be affected by these toxic chemicals, affecting the distribution of retained particles and their dosimetry.

Ingestion Exposures and Gastrointestinal Tract Effects

Chemical contaminants in drinking water or food reach human tissues via the gastrointestinal tract. Ingestion may also contribute to uptake of chemicals that were initially inhaled, since material deposited on or dissolved in the bronchial mucous blanket is eventually swallowed.

The gastrointestinal tract may be considered as a tube running through the body, the contents of which are actually external to the body (figure 6.13). Unless the ingested material affects the tract itself, any systemic response depends upon absorption through the mucosal cells lining the lumen. Although absorption may occur anywhere along the length of the gastrointestinal tract, the main region for effective translocation is the small intestine. The enormous absorptive capacity of this organ is due to

Figure 6.13. The gastrointestinal tract.

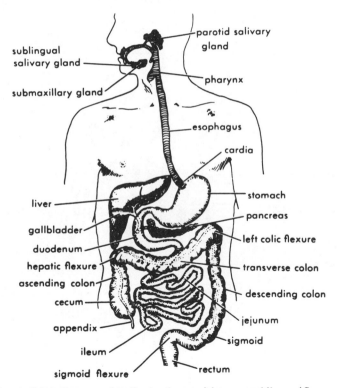

Note: The small intestine comprises the duodenum, jejunum, and ileum. (*Source:* McGraw-Hill 1960.)

the presence in the intestinal mucosa of projections, termed villi, each of which contains a network of capillaries; the villi result in a large effective total surface area for absorption (figure 6.14).

Although passive diffusion is the main absorptive process, active transport systems also allow essential lipid-insoluble nutrients and inorganic ions to cross the intestinal epithelium, and are responsible for uptake of some toxic chemicals. For example, lead may be absorbed via the system that normally transports calcium ions (Sabel et al. 1938). Small quantities of particulate material and certain large macromolecules, such as intact proteins, may be absorbed directly by the intestinal epithelium.

Materials absorbed from the gastrointestinal tract enter either the lymphatic system or the portal blood circulation; the latter carries material to the liver, from which it may be actively excreted into the bile or diffused into the bile from the blood. The bile is subsequently secreted into the intestines. Thus a cycle of translocation of a chemical from the intestine to

Figure 6.14. Longitudinal section of the small intestine.

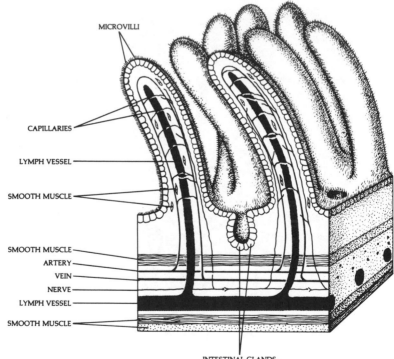

MICROVILLI

CAPILLARIES

LYMPH VESSEL

SMOOTH MUSCLE

SMOOTH MUSCLE
ARTERY
VEIN
NERVE
LYMPH VESSEL
SMOOTH MUSCLE

INTESTINAL GLANDS

Note: The absorptive area of the small intestine is increased by numerous fingerlike projections called villi, which cover the entire internal surface. (*Source:* Curtis 1983.)

the liver to the bile and back to the intestines (known as the enterohepatic circulation) may be established. Enterohepatic circulation usually involves contaminants that undergo metabolic degradation in the liver. For example, DDT undergoes enterohepatic circulation; a product of its metabolism in the liver is excreted into the bile, at least in experimental animals (Hayes 1965).

Various factors modify absorption from the gastrointestinal tract, enhancing or depressing its barrier function. A decrease in gastrointestinal mobility generally favors increased absorption. Specific stomach contents and secretions may react with the contaminant, possibly changing it to a form with different physicochemical properties—for example, solubility—or they may absorb it, altering the available chemical and changing translocation rates. The size of ingested particulates also affects absorption. Since the rate of dissolution is inversely proportional to particle size, large particles are absorbed to a lesser degree, especially if they are of a fairly insoluble material in the first place. For example, arsenic trioxide is more hazardous when ingested as a finely divided powder than as a coarse powder (Schwartz 1923). Certain chemicals—for example, chelating agents such as EDTA—also cause a nonspecific increase in absorption of many materials.

As a defense, spastic contractions in the stomach and intestine may serve to eliminate noxious agents via vomiting or by acceleration of the transit of feces through the gastrointestinal tract.

Skin Exposure and Dermal Effects

The skin is generally an effective barrier against the entry of environmental chemicals. In order to be absorbed via this route (percutaneous absorption), an agent must traverse a number of cellular layers before gaining access to the general circulation (figure 6.15). The skin consists of two structural regions, the epidermis and the dermis, which rest upon connective tissue. The epidermis consists of many layers of cells and has varying thickness depending upon the region of the body; the outermost layer is composed of keratinized cells. The dermis contains blood vessels, hair follicles, sebaceous and sweat glands, and nerve endings. The epidermis represents the primary barrier to percutaneous absorption, the dermis being freely permeable to many materials. Passage through the epidermis occurs by passive diffusion.

The main factors that affect percutaneous absorption are degree of lipid solubility of the chemicals, site on the body, local blood flow, and skin temperature. Some environmental chemicals readily absorbed through the skin are phenol, carbon tetrachloride, tetraethyl lead, and or-

Figure 6.15. Idealized section of skin.

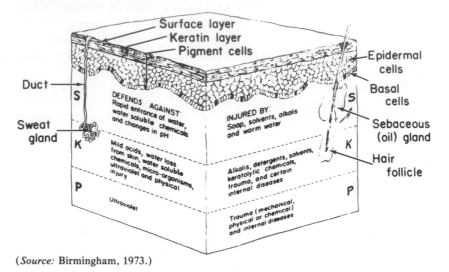

(*Source:* Birmingham, 1973.)

ganophosphate pesticides. Chemicals such as dimethyl sulfoxide and formic acid, alter the integrity of skin and facilitate penetration of other materials by increasing the permeability of the stratum corneum (the outer, horny layer of the epidermis). Moderate changes in permeability may also result following topical applications of acetone, methyl alcohol, and ethyl alcohol. In addition, cutaneous injury may enhance percutaneous absorption.

Interspecies differences in percutaneous absorption are responsible for the selective toxicity of many insecticides. For example, DDT is about equally hazardous to both insects and mammals if ingested but is much less hazardous to mammals when applied to the skin. This is due to the poor absorption through mammalian skin compared to its ready passage through the insect exoskeleton. Although the main route of percutaneous absorption is through the epidermal cells, some chemicals may follow an appendageal route—that is, entering through hair follicles, sweat glands, or sebaceous glands. Cuts and abrasions of the skin provide additional pathways for penetration.

Absorption through Membranes and Systemic Circulation

Depending upon its specific nature, a toxic chemical may exert its toxic action at various sites in the body. At a portal of entry—the respiratory tract, gastrointestinal tract, or skin—the chemical may have a topical effect. However, for actions at sites other than a portal, the chemical must be absorbed through one or more body membranes and enter the general circulation, from which it may affect internal tissues (including the blood itself). The ultimate distribution of any chemical in the body is, therefore, highly dependent upon its ability to traverse biological membranes. There are two main processes by which this occurs: passive transport and active transport.

Passive transport is absorption according to purely physical processes, such as osmosis; the cell has no active role in transfer across the membrane. Since biological membranes contain lipids, they are highly permeable to lipid-soluble, nonpolar, or nonionized agents, and less so to lipid-insoluble, polar, or ionized materials. Many chemicals may exist in both lipid-soluble and lipid-insoluble forms; the former is the prime determinant of the passive permeability properties for the specific agent.

Active transport involves specialized mechanisms, with cells actively participating in transfer across membranes. These mechanisms include carrier systems within the membrane and active processes of cellular ingestion, that is, phagocytosis and pinocytosis. Phagocytosis is the ingestion of solid particles, while pinocytosis refers to the ingestion of fluid containing no visible solid material. Lipid-insoluble materials are often taken up by active transport processes. Although some of these mechanisms are highly specific, if the chemical structure of a contaminant is similar to that of an endogeneous substrate, the former may be transported as well.

In addition to lipid solubility, affinity for specific tissues or tissue components affects the distribution of a chemical contaminant. Internal distribution may vary with time after exposure. For example, immediately following absorption into the blood, inorganic lead is found to localize in the liver, the kidney, and in red blood cells. Two hours later, about 50 percent is in the liver. A month later, approximately 90 percent of the remaining lead is localized in bone (Hammond 1969).

Once in the general circulation, a chemical may be translocated throughout the body. In this process it may (1) become bound to macromolecules, (2) undergo metabolic transformation (biotransformation), (3) be deposited for storage in depots, which may or may not be the sites of its toxic action, or (4) be excreted. Toxic effects may occur at any of several sites.

The biological action of a chemical may be terminated by storage, metabolic transformation, or excretion, the latter being the most permanent form of removal.

Accumulation in Target Tissues and Dosimetric Models

Some chemicals tend to concentrate in specific tissues due to physicochemical properties, such as selective solubility, or to selectively absorb or combine with macromolecules, such as proteins. Storage of a chemical often occurs when the rate of exposure is greater than the rate of metabolism or excretion. Storage or binding sites may not be the sites of toxic action. For example, carbon monoxide produces its effects by binding with hemoglobin in red blood cells; on the other hand, inorganic lead is stored primarily in bone but acts mainly on the soft tissues of the body.

If the storage site is not the site of toxic action, selective sequestration may be a protective mechanism, since only the freely circulating form of the contaminant produces harmful effects. Until the storage sites are saturated, a buildup of free chemical may be prevented. On the other hand, selective storage limits the amount of contaminant excreted. Since a bound or stored chemical is in equilibrium with their free form, as it is excreted or metabolized it is released from the storage site. Contaminants that are stored may remain in the body for years without effect (e.g., DDT). However, accumulation may produce illnesses that develop slowly, such as chronic cadmium poisoning.

A number of descriptive and mathematical models have been developed to permit estimation from both knowledge of exposure and one or more of the following factors: translocation, metabolism, and effects at the site of toxic action.

The use of these models for airborne particulate matter generally requires a knowledge of the concentration within specific particle-size intervals or of the particle-size distribution of the compounds of interest. Simple deposition models break the respiratory tract into regions (summarized by Phalen et al. 1986):

Head airways, nasopharynx, extra-thoracic
Nose
Mouth
Nasopharynx
Oropharynx
Laryngopharynx

Table 6.1. Gastrointestinal retention of ingested chemicals

Gastrointestinal Tract	Mass of Walls (grams)	Mass of Contents (grams)	Mean residence Time (hours a day)	λ Day^{-1}
Stomach	150	250	1	24.0
Small intestine	640	400	4	6.0
Upper large intestine	210	220	13	1.8
Lower large intestine	160	135	24	1.0

Source: International Commission on Radiological Protection 1979.

Table 6.2. Respiratory tract deposition and clearance of inhaled chemicals

Respiratory Tract Region and Compartment[a]	Day		Week		Year	
	Day	Fraction	Day	Fraction	Day	Fraction
Nasopharynx						
Compartment a	0.01	0.50	0.01	0.10	0.01	0.01
Compartment b	0.01	0.50	0.40	0.90	0.40	0.99
Tracheobronchial						
Compartment c	0.01	0.95	0.01	0.50	0.01	0.01
Compartment d	0.20	0.05	0.20	0.50	0.20	0.99
Pulmonary						
Compartment e	0.50	0.80	50.00	0.15	500.00	0.05
Compartment f	...	...	1.00	0.40	1.00	0.40
Compartment g	...	...	50.00	0.40	500.00	0.40
Compartment h	0.50	0.20	50.00	0.05	500.00	0.15
Lymphatic						
Compartment i	0.50	1.00	50.00	1.00	1,000.00	0.90
Compartment j	...	...	...	...	0	0.10

Source: International Commission on Radiological Protection 1981.
[a]Compartments are shown in figure 6.18.

Tracheobronchial
Larynx
Trachea
Bronchi
Bronchioles (to terminal bronchioles)
Gas exchange, pulmonary, alveolar
Respiratory bronchioles
Alveolar ducts
Alveolar sacs
Alveoli

These regions permit size-selective aerosol sampling, so that collection is limited to the size fraction that affects the potential for disease.

More complex models requiring data on translocation and metabolism have been developed for inhaled and ingested radionuclides by the International Commission on Radiological Protection (1966, 1979, 1981). Table 6.1 shows the ICRP model for gastrointestinal retention of ingested chemicals, while table 6.2 and figures 6.16 through 6.18 show respiratory tract deposition and clearance of inhaled chemicals.

Figure 6.16. Respiratory tract deposition model.

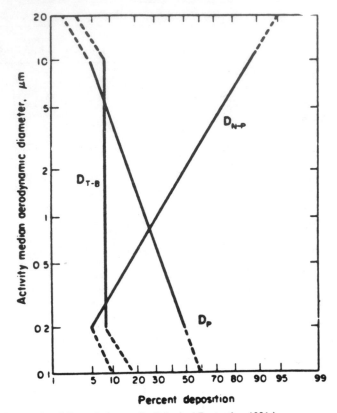

(*Source:* International Commission on Radiological Protection 1981.)

Indirect Measures of Past Exposures

Documented effects of environmental chemicals on humans seldom contain quantitative exposure data and only occasionally include more than crude exposure rankings based on known contact with or proximity to the materials believed to have caused the effects. Reasonable interpretation of available data on human experience requires some appreciation of its uses and limitations in estimating the exposure side of the exposure-response relationship. The discussion that follows is an attempt to provide background for interpreting data and for specifying the data needed.

Both direct and indirect exposure data can be used to rank exposed individuals by exposure intensity. External exposure can be measured di-

Figure 6.17. Schematic of gastrointestinal tract.

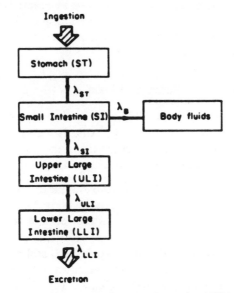

(*Source:* International Commission on Radiological Protection 1979.)

Figure 6.18. Schematic of gastrointestinal and respiratory tracts.

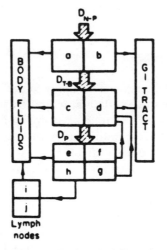

(*Source:* International Commission on Radiological Protection 1981.)

rectly by collection and analysis of biological fluids on *in vivo* retention. Indirect measures generally rely on work or residential histories, using knowledge of exposure intensity at each exposure site or some enumeration of the frequency of process upsets or effluent discharges that result in high-intensity, short-term exposures.

Concentrations in Air, Water, and Food

Historic data may occasionally be available on the concentrations of materials of interest in environmental media. However, they may or may not relate to the exposures of interest. Among the more important questions to be addressed in attempts to use such data are

1. How accurate and reliable were the sampling and analytical techniques used in the collection of the data? Were they subjected to quality assurance protocols? Were standardized and reliable techniques used?
2. When and where were the samples collected, and how did they relate to exposures at other sites? Air concentrations measured at fixed (area) sites in industry may be much lower than those occurring in the breathing zone of workers close to the contaminant sources. At fixed (generally elevated) community air-sampling sites chemical concentrations can be either much higher or much lower than those at street level and indoors, due to strong gradients in source and sink strengths in indoor and outdoor air.
3. What is known or assumed about the ingestion of food or water containing the measured concentrations of the contaminants of interest? Time at home and dietary patterns are highly variable among populations at risk.

Biological Sampling Data

Many of the same questions that apply to the interpretation of environmental media concentration data also apply to biological samples, especially quality assurance. The time of sampling is especially critical in relation to the times of the exposures and to the metabolic rates and pathways. In most cases, it is quite difficult to separate the contributions of recent exposures from the contributions of long-term reservoirs.

Exposure Histories

Exposure histories per se are generally unavailable, except in the sense that work histories or residential histories can be interpreted in terms of exposure histories. Job histories are often available in company or union records and can be converted into relative rankings of exposure groups with the aid of long-term employees and managers familiar with the work processes, history of process changes, material handled, tasks performed, and the engineering controls of exposure.

Routine, steady-state exposures may be the most important and dominant exposures of interest in many cases. On the other hand, for some health effects, the occasional or intermittent peak exposures may be of primary importance. In assessing or accumulating exposure histories or estimates, it is important to collect evidence for the frequency and magnitude of the occasional or intermittent releases associated with process upsets.

Research toward Effective Assessment of Exposure and Dose

The greatest needs in environmental exposure and dose assessment are to assemble and verify sufficient data bases on (1) concentrations of chemicals in environmental media and their temporal and spatial variability; (2) activity patterns of humans, to permit determinations of their contact with the environmental media; and (3) interindividual variability in uptake of chemicals. All of these data bases are currently inadequate for most assessments. The only situations for which substantial data bases are currently available pertain to some of the criteria air pollutants (e.g., O_3, SO_2, CO), some drinking water contaminants (e.g., As, Pb, Cr, NO_3), and pesticide residues in food. In addition, knowledge about mechanisms for transmedia transport and for deposition, translocation, and retention in the body is relatively complete.

The adequacy of mathematical models for exposure and dosimetry is largely unknown, at least in terms of the relevant coefficients. Few definitive tests have been run for these models, primarily because of the expense of testing. The use of unverified exposure models by the regulatory agencies results in a selection of coefficients that lead to either overly restrictive regulations or too lenient regulations.

References

Albert, R. E., J. Berger, K. Sanborn, and M. Lippmann. 1974. Effects of cigarette smoke components on bronchial clearance in the donkey. *Archives of Environmental Health* 29:99–106.

Albert, R. E., H. T. Peterson, Jr., D. E. Bohning, and M. Lippmann. 1975. Short-term effects of cigarette smoking on bronchial clearance in humans. *Archives of Environmental Health* 30:361–67.

Birmingham, D. J. 1973. Occupational dermatoses: Their recognition and control. In *The Industrial Environment: Its Evaluation and Control.* Washington, D.C.: U.S. Department of Health, Education, and Welfare.

Bohning, D. E., H. L. Atkins, and S. H. Cohn. 1982. Long-term particle clearance in man: Normal and impaired. *Annals of Occupational Hygiene* 26:259–71.

Curtis, H. 1968. *Biology.* New York: Worth.

Ferin, J., and L. J. Leach. 1973. The effect of SO_2 on lung clearance of TiO_2 particles in rats. *American Industrial Hygiene Association Journal* 34:260–63.

Hammond, P. B. 1969. Lead poisoning: An old problem with a new dimension. In *Essays in Toxicology,* ed. F. R. Blood. New York: Academic Press.

Hayes, W. J., Jr. 1965. Review of metabolism of chlorinated hydrocarbon insecticides especially in mammals. *Annual Review of Pharmacology* 5:27–52.

International Commission on Radiological Protection. 1966. Task Group on Lung Dynamics. Deposition and retention models for internal dosimetry of the human respiratory tract. *Health Physics* 12:173.

———. 1979. *Limits for Intakes of Radionuclides by Workers.* Part 1. New York: Pergamon.

———. 1981. Ibid., Part 3.

Jammet, H., J. LaFuma, J. C. Nenot, M. Chameaud, M. Perreau, M. LeBouffant, M. Lefevre, and M. Martin. 1970. Lung clearance: Silicosis and anthacosis. In *Pneumoconiosis: Proceedings of the International Conference, Johannesburg 1969,* ed. H. A. Shapiro. Capetown: Oxford Press.

Lioy, P. J., ed. 1983. *Air Sampling Instruments.* 6th ed. Cincinnati: American Conference of Governmental Industrial Hygienists.

Lippmann, M., and R. E. Albert. 1979. Effects of inhaled particles on humans and animals: Deposition, retention, and clearance. In *Airborne Particles,* Report of the National Academy of Sciences Subcommittee on Airborne Particles. Baltimore: University Park Press.

Lippmann, M., and R. B. Schlesinger. 1984. Interspecies comparison of particle deposition and mucociliary clearance in tracheobronchial airways. *Journal of Toxicology and Environmental Health* 13:441–69.

Lippmann, M., R. B. Schlesinger, G. Leikauf, D. Spektor, and R. E. Albert. 1982. Effects of sulphuric acid aerosols on the respiratory tract airways. *Annals of Occupational Hygiene* 26:677–90.

McGraw-Hill. 1960. *McGraw-Hill Encyclopedia of Science and Technology.* Vol. 4. New York: McGraw-Hill.

Morgan, K. T., D. L. Patterson, and E. A. Gross. 1984. Frog palate mucociliary apparatus: Structure, function, and response to formaldehyde gas. *Fundamental and Applied Toxicology* 4:58–68.

National Academy of Science. 1981. *Indoor Pollutants.* Washington, D.C.: National Academy Press.

National Research Council. 1979. *Airborne Particles.* Baltimore: University Park Press.

Overton, J. H., Jr. 1984. Physicochemical processes and the formulation of dosimetry models. *Journal of Toxicology and Environmental Health* 13:273–94.

Phalen, R. F., W. C. Hinds, W. John, P. J. Lioy, M. Lippmann, M. A. McCawley, O. G. Raabe, S. C. Soderholm, and B. O. Stuart. 1986. Rationale and recommendations for particle size-selective sampling in the workplace. *Applied Industrial Hygiene* 1:3–14.

Phalen, R. F., J. L. Kenoyer, T. T. Crocker, and T. R. McClure. 1980. Effects of sulfate aerosols in combination with ozone on elimination of tracer particles inhaled by rats. *Journal of Toxicology and Environmental Health* 6:797–810.

Schlesinger, R. B., K. E. Driscoll, B. D. Naumann, and T. A. Vollmuth. In press. Particle clearance from the lungs: Assessment of effects due to inhaled irritants. *Annals of Occupational Hygiene.*

Schlesinger, R. B., B. D. Naumann, and L. C. Chen. 1983. Physiological and histological alterations in the bronchial mucociliary clearance system of rabbits following intermittent oral or nasal inhalation of sulfuric acid mist. *Journal of Toxicology and Environmental Health* 12:441–65.

Schwartz, E. W. 1923. The so-called habituation to "arsenic": Variation in the toxicity of arsenious oxide. *Journal of Pharmacology and Experimental Therapeutics* 20:181–203.

Sobel, A. E., O. Gawron, and B. Kramer. 1938. Influence of vitamin D in experimental lead poisoning. *Proceedings of the Society of Experimental Biology and Medicine* 38:433–37.

Spengler, J. D., K. R. Stone, and F. W. Lilley. 1978. High carbon monoxide levels measured in enclosed skating rinks. *Journal of Air Pollution Control Association* 28:776–79.

U.S. Environmental Protection Agency. 1975–1982. *National Air Quality and Emissions Trend Report.* Washington, D.C.: EPA.

———. 1982. *Air Quality Criteria for Particulate Matter and Sulfur Oxides.* Vol. 3. Springfield, Va.: NTIS.

———. 1984. *Environmental Progress and Challenges: An EPA Perspective.* Washington, D.C.: EPA.

U.S. Food and Drug Administration. 1965–1982. *Dietary Studies.* Washington, D.C.: FDA.

Wallace, L. A., E. D. Pellizzari, and S. M. Gordon. 1985. Organic chemicals in indoor air: A review of human exposure studies and indoor air quality studies. In *Indoor Air and Human Health,* ed. R. B. Gamonage and S. V. Kaye. Chelsea, Mich.: Lewis.

Wolff, R. K., M. Dolovich, G. Obminski, and M. T. Newhouse. 1977. Effect of sulfur dioxide on tracheobronchial clearance at rest and during exercise. In *Inhaled Particles IV,* ed. W. H. Walton. Oxford: Pergamon.

7. Biological Monitoring of Environmental Toxic Chemicals

GERALD N. WOGAN AND STEVEN R. TANNENBAUM

> After the toxic chemicals enter the human body, the issue of interest is the resulting health effects. In this first of two chapters on health effects, Wogan and Tannenbaum examine the biological monitoring of genotoxins to discover precursors to disease. They focus on genotoxins because of concerns with cancer and genetic effects. Environmental monitoring measures concentrations of toxic chemicals seldom ingested by people; and even direct measurements of ingested chemicals do not account for the proportions of chemicals excreted or detoxified. Therefore, biological monitoring is used to measure the biologically effective dose. The authors examine DNA and protein adducts as dosimeters, as well as cytogenetic, pulmonary, and reproductive markers. They believe that biological markers will play an increasingly important role in characterizing human exposure to environmental chemicals.

Biological monitoring of exposure to chemicals has the objective of estimating the level of specific chemicals at critical target sites where their toxic effects are initiated. This level has been referred to as the *biologically effective dose* or the *internal exposure level,* and efforts to estimate it have been made by a variety of experimental approaches. Two categorical types of measurement can be made for this purpose: (1) measurement of concentrations of chemicals, or derivatives of them, in body fluids or excreta; and (2) measurement of toxicological effects such as mutations, chromosomal aberrations, or sister chromatid exchanges induced by chemicals in cells and tissues of exposed individuals.

In this chapter, we review the main avenues of research that are currently being pursued in addressing the objective stated above, and in doing so, we have selected examples to illustrate major points rather than attempting comprehensive coverage of a large and complex literature. Various aspects of biological monitoring have been the subjects of major sympósia held in the recent past, and the proceedings of these meetings provide an excellent source of information about the field. The following publications provide a relatively comprehensive coverage, and are recommended to those interested in further details: Berlin et al. 1979, 1984; Bridges et al. 1982; Omenn and Gelboin 1984; and Sorsa and Norppa 1986.

Methods and Objectives of Exposure Monitoring

Quantification of chemicals in body fluids (e.g., blood, milk, saliva, semen) or in excreta can be measured by direct chemical analysis and immunologic analysis and can be inferred from the results of a bioassay for mutagenicity. Most of the existing chemical methods and available data relate to occupational exposure, since such measurements have been used in occupational hygiene programs for many years. Immunoassays and bioassays are more recent developments, which have as yet found only limited application. With the recognition that most genotoxic chemicals require metabolic activation to electrophilic forms in order to exert their effects, an additional strategy for chemical dosimetry has been developed based upon the detection and quantification of covalently bound derivatives formed between activated chemicals and cellular macromolecules such as nucleic acids and proteins. Immunologic and chemical analytical methods have been developed that are sufficiently sensitive to detect evidence of ambient exposure in the general environment as well as in the workplace.

Prevention of excessive exposure to chemicals in industry has been approached traditionally by setting standards for the concentration of compounds in ambient air. Air monitoring has therefore constituted the principal means of assessing exposure, an approach that obviously takes into account only exposure via the pulmonary route and thus underestimates total exposure. Over the past two decades, analytical methods have been developed for many compounds, representing a variety of chemical classes, to which people are exposed in the workplace. Lauwerys (1983) summarized these methods from the perspective of their usefulness in biological monitoring programs and identified a total of sixty-nine chemicals for which analytical methodology was considered to be sufficiently well validated for application in worker surveillance programs. Lauwerys, as well as Baselt (1980) and Linch (1974), summarized the analytical methodology, together with additional pertinent information, including representative values for each of the chemicals in body fluids.

In addition to their use in monitoring programs in the workplace, a few of these methods have also been applied to population studies involving large numbers of subjects. For example, chlorinated hydrocarbons have been extensively studied with respect to their storage and accumulation in adipose tissue and other body compartments. Hayes (1975) summarized the literature concerning levels of DDT and its derivatives in adipose tissue and other body compartments in large numbers of people studied over a period of two decades. More recently, levels of chlorinated pesticides and PCBs have been quantified through analysis of human milk samples.

With reference specifically to environmental carcinogens and mutagens, the monitoring field is in a more primitive state of development. The main focus of research has been on the development of analytical methods for detection of carcinogens that can occur as contaminants of foods, and consequently most of the existing methods were intended for the purpose of food analysis. Methods have been published for some N-nitroso compounds, polycyclic aromatic hydrocarbons, aromatic amines, vinyl chloride, and mycotoxins. The suitability of these methods for analysis of media other than foods has not usually been evaluated, and in many instances they are impractical for analysis of large numbers of samples. More analytical methods are available for aflatoxins, a group of mycotoxins that frequently occur as food contaminants, than for any other class of environmental carcinogens. In this case, some methods originally developed for food analysis have been adapted to measure aflatoxins and metabolites in tissues of exposed people. Aflatoxins have been extensively studied with respect to exposure and cancer risk, and some of the information available on them is summarized later for illustrative purposes.

Some further general comments are appropriate before specific methodologies are considered. Biological monitoring of exposure to chemicals may have several objectives, which may in turn require specific methodological adaptations for different situations. Chemical dosimetry, for example, can be used to insure that current or past exposure does not entail an unacceptable health risk or to detect potentially excessive exposure before adverse health effects occur. The results of a biological monitoring program can be interpreted on an individual basis, and thus can be used to estimate for an individual the amount of chemical(s) absorbed during a specific time interval or the amount retained or bound to critical sites. Results for groups of individuals within the general population may also be used to characterize community exposure conditions. In this respect, biological monitoring is complementary to environmental monitoring, but has certain advantages in evaluating internal dose and estimating health risks (Lauwerys 1983). The greatest advantage of biological monitoring is that the data are more directly related to adverse effects than any environmental measurement and thus provide a better estimate of risk than ambient monitoring. Biological monitoring takes into account absorption by all routes, integrates exposure from all sources, and therefore can be used as a basis for estimating total risk from single or multiple chemicals.

Over the past decade, awareness of the large number of carcinogens and mutagens in the environment and concern over the potential health risks posed by their presence have greatly increased. Consequently, there has been a heavy emphasis in research dealing with studies of the mechanisms of action of chemical carcinogens and mutagens, and this in turn has led to the development of methods for evaluating the genotoxic chemicals (carcinogens and mutagens) and for detecting them in the environment.

Biochemical Markers

The majority of chemical carcinogens and mutagens exert their effects only after metabolic conversion to chemically reactive forms, which bind covalently to cellular macromolecules, including the nucleic acids (DNA and RNA) and proteins, to form addition products called adducts. Certain low-molecular-weight chemicals important in cellular function, such as water and glutathione, are also readily attacked. In some cases, formation of these adducts may be catalyzed by enzymes such as glutathione-S-transferase. The overall process whereby electrophiles react with nucleophiles forms a central theorem in carcinogenesis, and particular emphasis has been placed on DNA adducts, since these are thought to represent the initiating events leading ultimately to mutation or malignant transformation. It has been empirically established that the carcinogenic potency of a large number of chemicals bears a proportionality to their ability to bind to DNA—the so-called covalent binding index—when reacted *in vivo* with DNA (Lutz 1979). Covalent adducts formed in RNA and proteins have no putative mechanistic roles in carcinogenesis but are expected to relate quantitatively to total exposure and activation, and therefore they represent dosimeters for both exposure and activating capability. The proportionality of response among different target molecules in different tissues and cells forms the basis of an approach to biological monitoring in which the goal is to determine the size of the accumulated dose of the ultimate carcinogenic form of a chemical to the critical target that leads to the undesired biological response. We approach this discussion through a description of general principles and then give specific examples of well-studied chemical carcinogens.

▌ A General Working Model

A practical approach to the problem of monitoring the critical target dose can be described through a general working model outlined in figure 7.1. This figure summarizes, in a simplistic way, the relations among

Figure 7.1. Monitoring critical target doses of environmental carcinogens and mutagens: A working model.

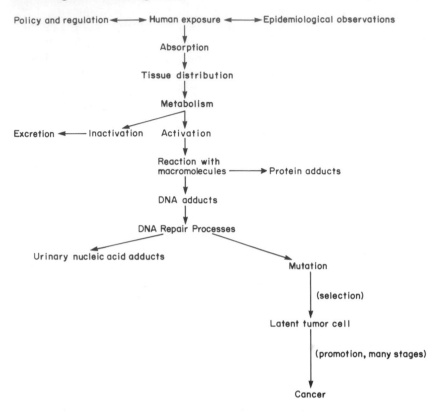

stages of exposure, metabolic and physiological processing, and the ultimate biological effects of genotoxic chemicals. Any measure of exposure or target dose should reflect the capacity of the individual for absorption, metabolism, and excretion of the particular carcinogen, to give a more accurate and relevant index than the simple measurement of the concentration of the compound in air, water, or food. The measurement of DNA adducts and of mutation or some other genetic defect has been the conventional approach to biological monitoring, rather than the measurement of protein adducts. However, having information on both types of adducts would greatly aid the interpretation of results and provide important and useful information on the target dose integrated over a time frame of weeks or months. DNA adducts might be more biologically meaningful than protein adducts, but their toxic levels may reflect exposure over only days or weeks because of the process of DNA repair. Again, it is difficult to generalize, and a clearer picture will emerge in the specific examples given below.

▌ DNA Adducts as Dosimeters

The use of DNA adducts to determine the critical tissue dose may be approached in two ways. First, measurements can be made of the levels of DNA adducts derived from a chemical of interest in cells of an accessible tissue, such as white blood cells or biopsy or autopsy material. If the chemical nature and stability of the DNA adducts for the compound of interest have been fully characterized, qualitative as well as quantitative identification of adduct levels can, in principle, provide an indication of exposure history as well as individual capability to activate the carcinogen to DNA-binding forms.

A second approach takes advantage of the fact that some adducts are known to be removed from cellular DNA (and also from RNA) and excreted in urine. Detection and measurement of their excretion rates can, in principle, provide information on the recent exposure history of the subject, and possibly also indications of that individual's capability for DNA repair. Thus studies of urinary excretion of adducts may provide data complementary to measurement of adduct levels in cellular DNA in the same individual.

Although, in principle, DNA adducts offer the most direct biological monitor for a carcinogen in which DNA is clearly the ultimate target, interpretation of data derived from DNA adduct measurements is in fact highly complex. It is well established that carcinogens—varying in structural complexity from simple alkylating agents to complex molecules that require multiple steps of activation—react to form covalent bonds at a variety of nucleophilic sites on all four DNA bases as well as on the phosphate backbone of DNA. Thus, from a qualitative viewpoint, detection of all DNA adducts derived from even a single carcinogen is a complex analytical problem. From a quantitative point of view, the problem is complicated even further by the fact that adducts are removed from DNA by chemical or enzymatic processes at different rates. The rates may vary for each adduct, for each tissue, or even for the same adduct in different types of cells in the same tissue. Singer and Grunberger (1983) gave a comprehensive review of the types of DNA adducts formed by different carcinogens and mutagens, as well as their repair characteristics.

In the past few years, analytical methods of several types have been devised for the detection and the quantitative analysis of carcinogen-DNA adducts at levels reflective of exposure to ambient concentrations of the agents (see Wogan and Gorelick 1985 for review). Most of the information concerning DNA adducts in experimental systems has been obtained through physicochemical or radiochemical detection. The usefulness of these two methods is limited by their relative insensitivity and inapplicability, respectively. In a few instances (e.g., benzo(a)pyrene and aflatoxins), ultrasensitive physicochemical methods based on the inherent property of fluorescence have been successfully applied to the detection of carcinogen-DNA adducts in human material. A postlabeling method, in which modified DNA bases are detected by ^{32}P-labeling of mononucleotides produced by enzymatic hydrolysis of DNA, has been devised and shown to be effective in detecting adducts of a large number of carcinogens of differing chemical structures (Randerath et al. 1985). Immunoassays have been developed with a sensitivity that approaches the levels required for the detection of modified DNA in exposed populations (Poirier 1981; Montesano et al. 1982). These methods are currently being validated in pilot studies of workers and others known to be exposed to polycyclic aromatic hydrocarbons and other environmental carcinogens.

The precise mechanism that yields mutations from DNA adducts is unknown for human cells, but the concept that adduct persistence is related to target cell risk has been widely accepted (see Wogan and Gorelick 1985 for review). Although a positive correlation has often been observed between adduct persistence and sensitivity to tumor induction for different species, differences in this parameter do not correlate well with the carcinogenic potency of the same compound in different strains of the same species. It is difficult to draw firm conclusions from these data, however, because the experimental data have not always been obtained under comparable conditions. Additional information suggests that, in some experimental systems, the relative rates of removal of specific adducts rather than their persistence may be related to susceptibility to tumor formation.

Collectively, this information emphasizes the uncertainties involved in the interpretation of data concerning DNA adduct levels, especially to estimate cancer risk. At this time, such data must be viewed as of unknown relevance to ultimate cancer risk in the exposed individual.

▌ Protein Adducts as Dosimeters

The chemical modification of proteins is a well-established phenomenon. Indeed, clinical application of a hemoglobin dosimeter has already been successfully used in monitoring the excessive exposure of diabetics to blood glucose. Circulating glucose reacts via a carbonylamine condensation to form a Schiff's base, predominantly with the N-terminal amino groups of the globin chains, to yield a glycosylated hemoglobin named hemoglobin A_{1c}. Levels of this modified hemoglobin are significantly elevated in diabetics, and its level in a given person is reflective of the degree of diabetic control. This approach has been regarded as being more useful than measurement of glucose levels in blood or urine, because it gives an integrated picture of exposure. The projected use of hemoglobin alkylation products, formed as a result of exposure to environmental carcinogens, is based on the same principles.

The main nucleophilic centers in proteins are the sulfur atoms of cysteine and methionine, nitrogens of amino groups, guanido groups, ring systems, and oxygen atoms. The chemical reactivity of the nucleophilic sites of proteins is determined by several factors, such as polarizability, protonation state, and pK_a, among others. Experience has shown that the simple concept of an electrophile reacting with a nucleophile is not sufficient to predict the nature of the site participating in protein-carcinogen adduct formation. The type of adduct formed is frequently unpredictable and may involve the affinity of the carcinogen for induced binding sites on the protein, which steer the proximal reactive form of the carcinogen to a particular nucleophilic site on the protein.

Ehrenberg and his colleagues conducted the pioneering work on the use of protein adducts as dosimeters and have made many contributions to the field, only the main points of which can be mentioned here. Ehrenberg and Osterman-Golkar (1980) reviewed the rationale and technical requirements for the use of protein alkylation for detecting mutagenic agents. Important among the requirements is that exposure must result in the formation of stable covalent derivatives of amino acids for which assay methods of adequate sensitivity and specificity can be devised. Further, the target protein should be found in easily accessible fluids (e.g., blood) and should be present in concentrations adequate to provide sufficient material for analysis. Although any protein could, in principle, be used to monitor alkylated derivatives, hemoglobin was suggested by Osterman-Golkar et al. (1976) as a suitable dose-monitoring protein, and the majority of the relevant literature concerns studies of hemoglobin alkylation. More recently, albumin has been recognized as a potentially useful dose monitor, since it is abundant and reactive, has a long half-life, and is synthesized in the hepatocyte—a cell in which many carcinogens are metabolized to their most reactive forms. Also, since albumin is a component of the interstitial fluid that bathes all cells, it may capture carcinogen metabolites from any tissue.

In an extensive series of studies, Ehrenberg and his colleagues characterized the essential attributes of hemoglobin as a dosimeter, which can be summarized as follows. The stability of alkylated residues in hemoglobin modified by ethylene oxide or dimethylnitrosamine was established, and the half-life of alkylation levels produced by a single dose of either agent was found to be equivalent to the life-span of the erythrocyte in the mouse. The validity of the steady-state level of alkyl residues in hemoglobin as a measure of chronic repeated exposure was subsequently established in mice dosed repeatedly with methylmethane sulfonate. Calleman (1982) reviewed studies of hemoglobin alkylation in people occupationally exposed to ethylene oxide. Blood samples were obtained from workers exposed to known levels of ethylene oxide (established by analysis of air samples), and hemoglobin was analyzed for the presence of N-3-(2 hydroxyethyl) histidine by mass spectrometry and by ion-exchange amino acid analysis. The authors concluded that the hemoglobin alkylation values accurately reflected exposure and were in good agreement with earlier data derived for ethylene oxide in the mouse.

Pereira and Chang (1981) surveyed the ability of carcinogens and mutagens (representing a broad spectrum of chemical classes) to bind covalently to hemoglobin in rats. Animals were dosed with ^{14}C-labeled carcinogens, and blood was collected twenty-four hours later. Covalent binding was determined by analysis of purified hemoglobin for ^{14}C bound to the protein. All the carcinogens studied were found to form covalent hemoglobin adducts in a dose-related manner, but the absolute binding level was *not* related to known carcinogenic potency.

In order for protein alkylation to be useful as a monitoring procedure, reliable dose-response relationships between exposure dose and production of alkylated amino acids must be established. This requirement has been satisfied for the exposures studied to date, all of the observations having been made in experimental animals dosed with various known carcinogens. Thus GC-MS determination of the levels of S-methylcysteine in hemoglobin of rats following injection of methylmethane sulfonate showed that the level of alkylated amino acid was linearly related to dose. For ethylene oxide, a virtually linear relationship was observed between dose and production of N-3-(2-hydroxyethyl)-histidine in hemoglobin, in experiments in which the alkylating agent was administered by inhalation at doses of 0 to 100 parts per million in air, thirty hours a week for two years. Other agents for which dose-response relationships have been established include trans-4-dimethylaminostilbene, chloroform, dimethylnitrosamine, and 4-aminobiphenyl, which are discussed in more detail subsequently.

On this basis, it can be concluded that the amount of alkylated hemoglobin is directly related to the erythrocyte dose, and that erythrocyte dose and exposure dose are almost always linearly related to each other. Thus many of the requirements to validate hemoglobin adducts as exposure dosimeters have been met. It is important to consider whether this parameter could also be used as an estimator of carcinogenic risk. The observation of hemoglobin alkylation per se can be taken as an indicator of genotoxic risk only when it has been shown that such alkylation correlates with reactions at the target DNA site, that is, that the erythrocyte dose is directly related to the target dose. This relationship has been studied in only a few experimental systems, in which the amounts of DNA and hemoglobin-binding products have been compared following dosing with carcinogens. Observed levels of alkylation of guanine in liver DNA and testis DNA by ethylene oxide deviated no more than twofold from the amount expected from hemoglobin alkylation. Thus the degree of alkylation of DNA could be estimated approximately from the erythrocyte dose for this compound. Similar relationships have also been shown for trans-4-dimethylaminostilbene and 2-acetylaminofluorene. Thus, in at least *some* instances, it seems possible to predict DNA binding by measuring protein binding, and therefore the latter may in some cases be taken as an indication of genotoxic risk.

One of the most important questions remaining is how cancer risk is *quantitatively* related to DNA binding. Our current studies on protein adducts focus on carcinogens that extend aromatic structures and that represent some of the most important classes of potential human environmental carcinogens. These include the aromatic amines, aflatoxins, and polycyclic aromatic hydrocarbons. Efforts have been made to determine what types and quantities of adducts are formed with hemoglobin and serum albumin, their stability, and whether methods can be devised for their routine assay in human populations. The current status of work on a carcinogen in each of the three groups is briefly summarized below:

1. 4-Aminobiphenyl is a typical aromatic amine. Briefly, it interacts through its hydroxylamine with hemoglobin and through its hydroxamic acid with albumin. For purposes of measuring exposure, hemoglobin gives an overwhelmingly higher yield of adduct than albumin. The adduct with hemoglobin is biologically stable and follows the kinetics predicted by the earlier work of Ehrenberg. (4-aminobiphenyl is discussed more extensively in the following section.)

2. Aflatoxin B_1 is a potent liver carcinogen whose metabolism has been extensively characterized. Binding to DNA occurs *via* a very reactive epoxide, and binding to proteins has generally been suggested to proceed either through the epoxide or through a dialdehyde generated by hydrolysis of the epoxide. There is a much higher level of binding to albumin than to hemoglobin, suggesting that this reaction may take place predominantly in the liver, the site of albumin synthesis. (A more detailed discussion of this carcinogen follows.)

3. Fluoranthene is a typical polycyclic aromatic hydrocarbon and is both a mutagen and carcinogen. It is widely distributed in the environment, since it is universally produced during the combustion of fossil fuels. The structure of its principal DNA adduct has been identified, and activation takes place through a diolepoxide intermediate. Although binding to albumin and hemoglobin are quantitatively similar, preliminary studies have shown that different types of adducts are

formed on the two types of proteins. A scheme showing the metabolism and potential routes of binding of this compound to DNA and proteins is given in figure 7.2.

It is clear from the work done to date that the nature of the binding of carcinogens to proteins is not readily predictable from simple *a priori* considerations. In the case of small alkylating agents, the tendency is to form reaction products with the most nucleophilic sites on the protein, but it is well known that the reactivity of individual side chains is strongly influenced by the tertiary structure of the protein. For large hydrophobic molecules, site selectivity is of even greater importance, and the ability of the carcinogen to bind to the protein in the region of a reactive site on the protein determines where and how the activated carcinogen will react.

An impressive example of this type of selectivity is given in the nature of the *in vivo* binding of 4-aminobiphenyl to serum albumin (Skipper et al. 1985). The binding takes place almost exclusively on the sole tryptophan

Figure 7.2. Metabolism of fluoranthene and potential routes of binding to DNA and proteins.

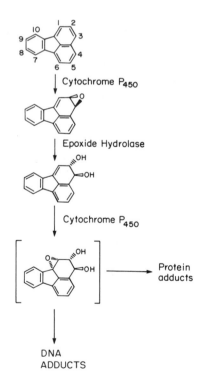

residue in albumin, *via* an ester of the hydroxamate. This residue is apparently not on the surface of the protein but is buried adjacent to a high-affinity, fatty acid binding site. This result can be explained at present only by assuming that the reactive form of the carcinogen penetrates and binds hydrophobically to the protein before reacting with tryptophan.

An important general goal for the use of proteins in molecular epidemiology is to devise methods for the detection of undisclosed or cryptic exposure to carcinogens. Törnqvist et al. (1986) proposed using the N-terminal valine of hemoglobin as a general trap for alkylating agents and devised a method of selectively cleaving N-terminal alkylated valines from hemoglobin, using an Edman degradation procedure, which yields derivatives suitable for highly sensitive mass spectrometric analysis. In its present form, the method is suited for the identification and determination of alkyl adducts of low molecular weight, as has been demonstrated with methyl, hydroxyethyl, hydroxypropyl, and hydroxyphenylethyl adducts.

An important finding from the work of Ehrenberg and his collaborators is the great extent of alkylation of hemoglobin side chains, particularly with methyl and hydroxyethyl residues of unknown origin. Perhaps their approach holds even more surprises as its reliability and sophistication improve.

Biochemical Monitoring of Two Carcinogens

We have selected two environmental carcinogens to illustrate the kinds of research approaches currently used, the results being obtained, and the status of the field—an aromatic amine, 4-aminobiphenyl, and the mold metabolites, aflatoxins. Both are subjects of active research programs, both are widely disseminated, and both are of different origins and chemical structures. Furthermore, for both, extensive human exposure is known to occur, whose quantitative estimates are extremely useful in risk assessment. Exposure to 4-aminobiphenyl takes place through cigarette smoke, among other sources. Exposure to aflatoxins takes place through food contaminants.

4-Aminobiphenyl

The aromatic amines are generally recognized to be an important class of human carcinogens and have been implicated in particular in the etiology of bladder cancer (International Agency for Research on Cancer 1982). A variety of other species of animals are also susceptible to aromatic amines, but it is the dog that most closely resembles the human in response to these chemicals. Thus extensive investigation of the dog has finally led to elucidation of the various mechanisms and factors influencing the course of arylamine-induced bladder cancer in humans (Beland et al.

1983). Although carcinogenic arylamines have been withdrawn from commercial production, they still enter the environment from their use as synthetic intermediates, as contaminants of industrial products, and from cigarette smoke (Patrianakos and Hoffmann 1979). A key compound of this type is 4-aminobiphenyl, the focus of the following discussion.

The mechanism of bladder cancer induction by 4-aminobiphenyl involves a series of steps that is shown diagrammatically in figure 7.3. In this scheme, the amine is oxidized to the hydroxylamine in the liver. This intermediate is then conjugated with glucuronic acid in the liver, transported *via* the blood to the kidney, and eventually excreted in the urine. Under neutral physiological conditions, the glucuronide is stable, but in the acidic pH found in the urine of dogs and humans, the glucuronide is hydrolyzed to the free hydroxylamine. The hydroxylamine is a neutral species, which can diffuse through the bladder mucosa into the capillary bed, where it can react with hemoglobin. This reaction sequence involves several steps, in which the hydroxylamine is first oxidized to a nitrosoaryl compound, which subsequently reacts with a cysteine sulfhydryl group to yield the biologically stable sulfinamide adduct of the original arylamine (Green et al. 1984). In fact, the adduct forms exclusively on the beta-93 cysteine of human hemoglobin.

In parallel with the process described above, the arylhydroxylamine can also undergo an acid-catalyzed reaction with bladder DNA through the very reactive nitrenium ion. Kadlubar and colleagues (Beland et al. 1983) identified the DNA lesions that form in dog bladder epithelium following administration of 4-aminobiphenyl. The modified bases were characterized by comparison with the adducts that form after treatment of either calf thymus DNA or intact cells of *S. typhimurium* with the hydroxylamine (table 7.1). The structures of the three principal adducts are shown in figure 7.4 for the several types of DNA. In an *in vivo* experiment in dogs, the same three adducts were isolated in approximately the

Table 7.1. Radioactivity in DNA (percent)

DNA Adduct[a]	Calf Thymus	S. typhimurium Cells	Dog Bladder
N-(deoxyguanosin-8-yl)-4-aminobiphenyl	70	71	72
N-(deoxyguanosin-N^2-yl)-4-aminobiphenyl	5	5	13
N-(deoxyadenosin-8-yl)-4-aminobiphenyl	17	6	6

Source: Beland et al. 1983.
[a]See figure 7.4 for structure.

Figure 7.3. Bladder cancer induction by 4-aminobiphenyl.

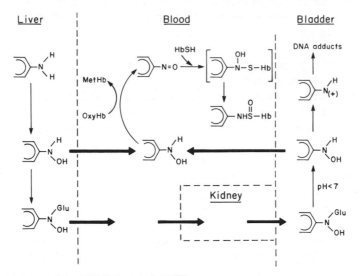

(*Source:* Adapted from Kadlubar et al. 1977.)

Figure 7.4. 4-Aminobiphenyl DNA adduct structures.

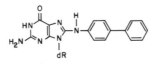

N-(deoxyguanosin-8-yl)-4-aminobiphenyl

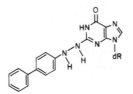

N-(deoxyguanosin-N^2-yl)-4-aminobiphenyl

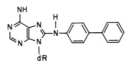

N-(deoxyadenosin-8-yl)-4-aminobiphenyl

same proportions from both liver and bladder DNA, and the adduct levels in both tissues remained close to the same value for seven days. Since liver tumors have not been observed in dogs exposed to 4-aminobiphenyl (but nearly *all* such animals develop bladder tumors), the nature and quantity of the DNA adducts formed is clearly not a sole predictor for the later appearance of tumors.

The model presented in figure 7.3 proposes a parallel process for formation of hemoglobin adducts and bladder DNA adducts, so the level of hemoglobin adducts should give an estimate of the exposure of an individual to a particular aromatic amine (Neumann 1981, 1984). The characteristics of hemoglobin as a dosimeter for 4-aminobiphenyl have been demonstrated in rat studies (Green et al. 1984). The binding is proportional to dose down to doses of tens of nanograms per kilogram body weight. Experiments with multiple doses over periods of several months confirm the stability of the adduct, and its rates of accumulation and decline conform to the kinetics predicted by Ehrenberg's calculations discussed earlier.

To extend these studies to human populations, a mass spectrometric method was developed for the analysis of small (10 ml) blood samples (Bryant et al. in press). In this method, the adduct is hydrolyzed from the globin to yield the original aromatic amine and derivatized to a perfluorinated amide suitable for gas chromatography. Using a technique called single-ion monitoring, the mass spectrometer is capable of detecting quantities down to one picogram of 4-aminobiphenyl. When this method was applied to blood samples collected from smokers and nonsmokers, several interesting observations were made. The mean adduct level for smokers was about five times that of nonsmokers, but the distribution of adduct levels in smokers was quite broad (figure 7.5). Whether this represents individual variations in smoking behavior, metabolic individuality, or a combination of variables remains to be explored. Studies of smokers who quit substantiated this biochemical dosimeter, since adduct levels declined slowly over a period of weeks to the level of nonsmokers.

Future studies in both dogs and humans will be necessary to establish the relationships between exposure to 4-aminobiphenyl, the steady-state amount of hemoglobin adduct, and the nature and modification of bladder DNA.

Aflatoxins

Aflatoxins are highly carcinogenic chemicals, consistently found as contaminants in the human diet in many areas of the world. Exposure to them has been linked epidemiologically to increased incidence of human liver cancer in Asia and Africa (see Busby and Wogan 1984 for review). The toxic and carcinogenic properties of aflatoxins are dependent upon their metabolism to chemically reactive forms (in common with many

Figure 7.5. Protein adduct levels in smokers and nonsmokers.

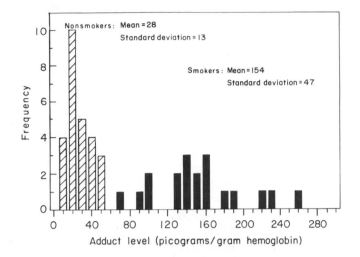

other carcinogens, as discussed above). The metabolism of aflatoxins has been extensively studied and, among other pathways, the spectrum of DNA adducts formed has been rather completely characterized (see Busby and Wogan 1984). An important generalization that can be drawn from this literature is that the same pattern of DNA adducts form in all experimental systems in which mutations or tumors are induced by these carcinogens. It is particularly noteworthy that human cells and tissues activate aflatoxins to form the same DNA adducts and, as is discussed below, evidence has recently been obtained that people exposed to these compounds in their diet excrete in their urine the major adduct as well as other metabolites.

Early attempts to identify and measure aflatoxin derivatives in human tissues or excreta involved techniques such as thin-layer chromatography, HPLC, or immunoassays, and investigators using them reported a number of derivatives in urine and serum. A major disadvantage of all of these approaches is lengthy preparation time and complex analytical methodology, which limits their application to relatively small-scale studies. Using a monoclonal antibody, our group devised a procedure that substantially simplifies the analysis of human samples through affinity purification of the aflatoxin derivatives before quantification (Groopman et al. 1984). Through this approach, we showed that individuals in a defined population in the Guangxi Province of China, with independently determined aflatoxin exposure, excrete several aflatoxin metabolites in their urine (Groopman et al. 1985). We are currently characterizing the quantitative relationships between aflatoxin intake and excretion of these products. By comparing these findings with similar information from experimental animals dosed with aflatoxins, in which the dose-response relationships between the formation and excretion of DNA adducts and tumor induction have been well established, we hope to evaluate adduct measurement as an exposure dosimeter and, possibly, to add to an understanding of aflatoxins as risk factors for liver cancer in humans.

Aflatoxins have long been known to bind to proteins as well as to nucleic acids, but little work had been done until recently to develop a protein dosimeter for aflatoxins in a manner comparable to that described above for aromatic amines and other carcinogens. We therefore have begun a program of research with that objective in mind, in order to be able to measure DNA and protein adducts in the same individuals. In the scheme shown for aflatoxin metabolism in figure 7.6, the same metabolic routes that lead to DNA binding produce metabolites capable of reacting with proteins. These would include either the 2,3-oxide, or the dihydrodiol and its equilibrium forms. Although any readily accessible protein should react with these aflatoxin metabolites, in fact the covalent binding is rather specific. Hemoglobin binds in very low yield, and of all the serum proteins, only albumin binds aflatoxin to any significant extent (Skipper et al. 1985). In the case of albumin, however, the yields are quite high, reaching 3 percent of a single dose bound to total intravascular serum albumin after twenty-four hours in rat experiments. The potential utility of this system as a biological dosimeter is further supported by the extensive experiments of

Figure 7.6. Pathways of metabolism of aflatoxin B₁.

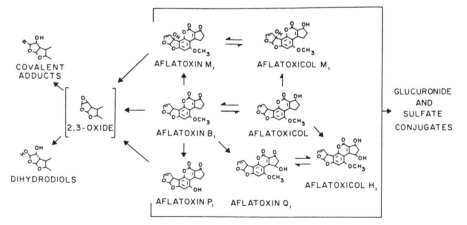

(*Source:* Essigman et al. 1982.)

Campbell and coworkers (Appleton et al. 1982), in which doses down to ten nanograms per kilogram of body weight were shown to bind in linear proportion to DNA, RNA, and liver protein.

Recent work has shown that there is probably a single major covalently bound adduct formed *in vivo* between aflatoxin B_1 and one or more lysine residues of serum albumin (Sabbioni et al. 1986). This adduct is formed by interaction of the aldehyde form of the dihydrodiol to form a Schiff base, which ultimately rearranges to an aflatoxin derivative with a terminal pyrolidine ring.

As explained in an earlier section, the kinetics of albumin turnover are different from those for hemoglobin. The utility of albumin as a dosimeter has therefore been evaluated through studies of clearance in the rat over a 14-day period and by studies of chronic dosing. Both types of study indicate that the adduct lifetime is equivalent to that of albumin (i.e., in the rat it has a half-life of 2.5 to 3 days).

Since excreted RNA and DNA adducts probably reflect only the previous twenty-four- to forty-eight-hour exposure (Essigmann et al. 1982), a protein-based dosimeter that reflects weeks of exposure history could add greatly to the interpretation of epidemiological data. If, as seems likely, aflatoxin adducts of albumin form within the liver, they also may serve as a dosimeter for the putative target organ in humans.

Mutagens in Body Fluid

The availability of well-characterized bioassay systems for the detection of chemical mutagens has made it feasible to detect and quantify the presence and amounts of mutagenic substances present in body fluids as indicators of exposure to mutagens or promutagens. Determination of requirements for metabolic activation, customarily evaluated as a component of routine mutagenicity assays, can provide further information concerning the nature of unidentified mutagenic substances.

Application of bacterial mutagenicity assays has revealed high levels of mutagens in the urine of people exposed to genotoxic agents under a variety of circumstances, including patients treated with cytostatic drugs, cigarette smokers, and workers employed in the manufacture of rubber or exposed to epichlorhydrin. In contrast, no evidence of this kind of exposure was found in workers engaged in styrene production or in coke manufacturing (Bloom 1981).

A number of bacterial mutagenicity assays carried out on nurses and pharmacists handling cytotoxic drugs have given conflicting results. In most of these studies, urine (concentrated to partially purify solutes) was subjected to either the Ames test or a more sensitive bacterial fluctuation test. The usual purification process has been found to produce some spurious positive results, but even when another process was used, Gibson et al. (1984) concluded that it is doubtful whether the available bacterial mutagenicity assays are sufficiently sensitive to be useful in screening personnel handling cytotoxic drugs. Thus, although these assays have proven valuable in documenting exposure to genotoxic agents, in demonstrating the existence of presumptive genetic hazards, and in tracing the origin of suspected agents, quantitative measurements of excreted mutagens have not been of value in assessing an individual's risk of toxic effects or development of tumors. Camus et al. (1984) addressed this problem by comparing the metabolism and urinary excretion of mutagenic metabolites of benzo(a)pyrene in two strains of mice differing greatly in susceptibility to its carcinogenicity and found general agreement between ability to activate the compound to mutagenic forms and susceptibility to tumor induction. Further studies of this kind will be required to evaluate fully the usefulness of this approach as a quantitative indicator of genetic hazard.

Although it is not valid to equate mutagenicity of body fluids with actual mutation in the exposed individual, it is reasonable to assume that persons with such mutagenicity are at elevated risk. An important advantage of this approach is that interpretable data can be obtained in single individuals, making the test especially valuable is assessing the exposure of small groups of subjects. However, a number of disadvantages must also be taken into account in further development of methodology. Body fluid samples contain potential confounding sources of mutagenic activity, such as drugs, food, beverages, cigarettes, and cosmetics. In some cases, mutagens are excreted in conjugated form, which may require hydrolysis before assay. Certain chemical classes of mutagens, such as nitrosamines, have short half-lives in blood and excreta and may therefore be undetectable.

Further developmental work is required to determine which classes of chemical hazard can be detected by mutagenesis assays on body fluids. An important avenue for technical improvement involves the manner in which samples are processed before testing. Organic compounds can be extracted or concentrated by a variety of techniques, and enzyme treatment will liberate conjugated chemical species. These and other technical modifications are under current study, and may enhance the value of this screening method for biological monitoring.

Cytogenetic Markers

Structural changes in chromosomes were among the earliest manifestations of genetic injury in persons exposed to ionizing radiation. The linear interdependence of dose of ionizing radiation and the number of structural chromosome aberrations in circulating lymphocytes has made it possible for the method to be used for biological dosimetry, even at low radiation levels (Evans et al. 1979). Cytogenetic monitoring based on the detection of chromosomal damage in somatic cells is finding increasing application, especially in the occupational setting (Vainio et al. 1983).

Damage to chromosomes can take various forms: structural aberrations, sister chromatid exchanges, and numerical abnormalities (Bloom 1981; Evans 1983). The types of alteration produced depend on the lesions induced in the chromosomes and, therefore, on the nature of the genotoxic injury in question. Structural chromosome aberrations result from the breakage and rearrangement of whole chromosomes and are most efficiently induced by those substances that directly break the backbone of DNA (e.g., ionizing radiation and radiomimetic chemicals) or significantly distort the DNA helix (such as intercalating agents). Sister chromatid exchanges result from the breakage and rejoining of DNA strands without observable morphological distortion of chromosome structure. They are efficiently induced by genotoxic agents that form covalent adducts with DNA or interfere with DNA synthesis or repair. Numerical alterations (aneuploidy) represent gains or losses of whole chromosomes or parts thereof. It is believed that aneuploidy arises following exposure of the cell to substances that interfere with the apparatus of cell division. Because the three types of cytogenetic endpoints respond to different cellular lesions, information about them is complementary, and all should be taken into account in assessing the possible genotoxicity of environmental chemicals.

▌ Chromosomal Aberrations

The system used most frequently in monitoring exposure to clastogenic agents involves the study of mitogen-stimulated lymphocytes in short-term cultures of blood samples. Because of the long life span of lymphocytes, detection of aberrations in mitogen-stimulated cells offers some possibility of detecting both short-term and accumulated damage, although the kinetics of damage of this type are poorly understood. Structural aberrations can be classified as either unstable or stable, depending on whether they are able to persist in dividing cell populations. Unstable aberrations (dicentrics, rings, deletions, and other asymmetrical rearrangements) lead to cell death. Stable alterations consist of balanced translocations, inversions, and other symmetrical rearrangements and are transmitted to progeny at cell division. The biological relevance of these stable rearrangements in somatic cells is not well defined, but recent evidence suggests that certain of them, such as stable translocations, can persist and may confer a growth advantage in dividing cell populations. For example, translocation of an oncogene, the c-*myc* gene, to a site in which its transcription is placed under control of regulatory elements of the immunoglobulin genes has been observed in patients with Burkitt's lymphoma, and the abnormal expression of these genes in such patients may be causally related to the rearrangement. An oncogene has also been mapped to the site of the rearrangement in chronic myelogenous leukemia, and other rearrangements in malignancy may be related to the translocation of other oncogenes.

❙ Sister Chromatid Exchanges

Recent developments in chromatin staining methods have made possible the detection of intrachromosomal exchanges between sister chromatids. Although the molecular mechanisms underlying these changes have not been fully characterized, it is clear that measurement of sister chromatid exchanges (SCEs) offers a sensitive indicator of exposure to DNA-damaging agents. While the biological consequences of SCE formation are poorly understood, formation of this lesion in a chromosome represents, at the very least, the breakage and rejoining of four DNA strands. It has been amply demonstrated that the frequency of SCE formation is dramatically increased when cells, animals, or people are exposed to known carcinogens or mutagens (Latt 1981).

The assay methods are quantitative and sensitive, and the occurrence of SCEs has been linearly and positively correlated with specific locus mutations *in vitro*, with transformation *in vitro*, and with lung tumor induction in mice. Experiments in rats, mice, and rabbits have demonstrated that it is possible to measure an increase in SCEs in peripheral blood lymphocytes for several days following *in vivo* exposure. Increased SCEs have been observed in the lymphocytes of cigarette smokers, workers exposed occupationally to ethylene oxide, individuals undergoing cancer chemotherapy, and those exposed to certain drugs. As a result of these findings, the SCE techniques are considered a valuable adjunct to measurement of chromosomal aberrations in cytogenetic monitoring.

Nonetheless, controversy has developed over the cytogenetic examination of human populations occupationally or otherwise exposed to putative genotoxic hazards. The major criticism of such studies is that chromosomal damage measured in the lymphocytes of peripheral blood has not predicted specific adverse health effects. One can justifiably question, therefore, the legitimacy of using this technology in routine surveillance or monitoring programs, given the fact that lack of clear understanding of the health significance of increased chromosomal damage makes interpretation of the results difficult. Consequently, a great deal of additional research is required to clarify the relationships between cytogenetic evidence of exposure and health effects.

Pulmonary Markers

The preceding discussion focuses on the use of biochemical and biological markers to detect exposure to genotoxic agents and their effects.
Similar approaches have been used to study the same parameters in the
case of nonneoplastic diseases, in particular those affecting the respiratory
system. This section focuses on biochemical and cellular markers that may
indicate exposure to toxic gases and particles, increased susceptibility to
these agents, or evidence of lung injury or pulmonary disease.

▋ Bronchoalveolar Lavage

The technique of bronchoalveolar lavage (BAL) consists of filling all
or part of the lungs with saline through the airways, then withdrawing the
fluid, which will then contain cells and dissolved or suspended material
from the internal surfaces of the lungs. BAL is therefore, in essence, a
method for biopsy of the extensive internal surface lining the respiratory
tree. By virtue of the fact that the entire surface is sampled, the method
obtains evidence of effects averaged over the entire lung, but by its nature
it cannot detect highly localized effects. In recent years, BAL has been
used increasingly in inhalation toxicology to assess lung injury and disease
mechanisms in both experimental animals and humans (see, for example,
Beck et al. 1983; and Davis et al. 1982). An extensive literature has developed concerning the use of the technique as an animal bioassay system as
well as a tool for detecting lung damage in humans. Only some main points
can be touched upon here.

The components of fluid generated by BAL include both cellular elements and dissolved and suspended materials. The cells include macrophages, polymorphonuclear leukocytes (PMN), and lymphocytes. Alveolar
macrophages are important, since their migratory patterns and phagocytic
behavior significantly affect the outcome of the interactions between toxic
particles from the environment and the lung (Brain 1984). Macrophages
influence the residence time of inhaled toxic and carcinogenic particles in
the respiratory tract and therefore are important determinants of the dose
to the target tissues affected by them. The number and migratory properties of macrophages in BAL fluid are therefore important markers of pulmonary exposure. PMN usually represent less than 5 percent of the total
cells in BAL fluid, but they increase dramatically following exposure to
toxic particles and play an important role in antimicrobial defenses and
wound healing. However, there is increasing evidence that they may also
have adverse affects, having been implicated in certain disease processes.
Under normal conditions, lymphocytes compose 15 percent or less of the
total cells in BAL fluid, and increases in their numbers may reflect immu-

nological alterations, which may be involved in hypersensitivity reactions.

Many studies of lung injury have described changes in the types and amounts of various proteins in BAL fluid. The following are some frequently used protein indicators, their sources, and their putative relevance to disease processes.

1. Albumin, derived from blood serum, can appear in the fluid as a result of its passage across endothelial and epithelial barriers. Thus elevation in the albumin level can be used as an indicator of pulmonary edema, a common manifestation of acute pulmonary injury.
2. The immunoglobulins IgG and IgA are usually present in the BAL fluid of humans and animals. Under normal conditions, IgG is of serum origin, whereas IgA is secreted by the cells of the respiratory airways. Changes in these proteins can therefore be used as indices of the integrity of the epithelial barrier and its functional status.
3. As in other organs and tissues, release of cytoplasmic or membrane-bound enzymes into the extracellular space can be indicative of cell damage or death in the respiratory tract.
4. Elevated levels of lactic dehydrogenase, alkaline phosphatase, and acid hydrolase in BAL fluid have been found to reflect acute cell injury and cell death resulting from various types of toxic exposure.
5. The balance between proteases and antiproteases in the lung is of critical importance. Uncontrolled proteolytic activity may lead to the development of emphysema, as has been shown in experimental animal systems as well as in man.
6. Degradation of elastin is a key event in the enlargement of alveolar spaces and the loss of lung elasticity. Thus elastase levels in BAL fluid can provide an index of elevated risk of emphysema.
7. Normal lung tissue contains an effective antiprotease system, an important component of which is alpha-1-antiprotease derived from serum. Reduced levels of this protein, which occurs in cigarette smokers as well as in some genetically deficient individuals, are signs of increased risk for emphysema.

Some changes in the numbers and types of cells recovered in BAL can be correlated with similar alterations in human lung tissue obtained by biopsy. Such correlations include increased PMN and macrophages in smokers, increased lymphocytes in sarcoid tissue, and increased PMN in idiopathic pulmonary fibrosis.

▌ Serum and Urine Analyses

A variety of methods are needed to monitor the development of non-neoplastic pulmonary diseases. Individuals who are affected may be highly susceptible or have had a high toxic dose. In addition to classic approaches, such as radiographic examination and pulmonary function tests, new techniques such as BAL and biochemical markers in blood and urine may be useful. Recent findings suggest that peptide fragments are released early in emphysema and can be detected in the urine or serum (e.g., Mecham and Lang 1982). Identification of peptide relies on the presence of unusual amino acids in the elastin fragments, such as desmosine, an amino acid virtually unique to the elastin molecule.

It has been shown experimentally that treatment of animals with elastase results in elevation of elastin fragments or elastin in serum and urine, as detected by either chemical analyses or immunoassays. Although the relevance of these experimental findings to the development of emphysema in man has not been completely established, the value of these measurements is being actively investigated in individuals at high risk for the disease. Another analysis of blood or urine measured collagen breakdown through detection of hydroxyproline, alpha-1-antiprotease, and such antibodies as those against toluene diisocyanate, which have been detected in the plasma of workers occupationally exposed to the chemical.

Reproductive Markers

The development of biochemical and morphological markers for detecting the effects of environmental chemicals on the reproductive system has focused mainly on alterations of spermatic structure and function (see Wyrobek et al. 1983 for review). Measurements of such parameters as the physical properties (viscosity, liquefaction time) and chemical composition (testosterone, fructose, hyaluronidase) of seminal fluid, together with morphological and functional characteristics of sperm, have been used as indices of adverse effects, including those of environmental or occupational chemicals.

Sophisticated automated techniques have been developed for the characterization of structural aberrations and aneuploidy in sperm cells. Certain of these involve the fusion of human sperm cells with hamster ova, followed by appropriate karyotypic examinations. In addition, the use of synthetic oligonucleotide probes in conjunction with gene-mapping techniques may make it possible to detect alterations resulting from chemical insults at specific loci in DNA of sperm cells.

Perspectives for Future Research

During this century, public health efforts have increasingly emphasized the chronic diseases, which are characterized by multifactorial etiology, multistage development with long latencies, and lack of clear linkage to causative agents. Formulation of preventive strategies under these circumstances therefore has relied heavily on the use of presumptive tests, such as bioassay systems in animals and *in vitro* experimental models, in which deleterious properties of putative causative agents can be empirically characterized. Results produced in such test systems are then extrapolated to man in constructing estimates of risk resulting from environmental exposures. By virtue of the uncertainties inherent in cross-species extrapolation, the degree of certainty in risk estimation by this process is severely limited.

In order to reduce the potential health effects of environmental chemicals, the research community has therefore turned increasingly to the development of techniques for accurately measuring risk factors for disease, or precursors of disease, or early evidence of exposure to disease-causing agents. The foregoing discussion summarizes the current status of these methodologies. Elucidation of molecular and cellular bases for many chronic diseases, currently being accomplished at an impressive pace, will provide the basis for further development of markers of improved sensitivity and specificity.

The sensitivity of epidemiological studies designed to evaluate the health significance of environmental chemicals is also compromised by the lack of quantitative exposure data for individuals in exposed populations. Further development of markers of exposure, susceptibility, and effect could improve the effectiveness of conventional epidemiological investigations. In order to be maximally useful, however, the predictive power of markers must be empirically validated by appropriately designed longitudinal studies, utilizing multiple biochemical and cellular markers in human populations experiencing defined exposures. Parallel studies in animals experimentally exposed will minimize the uncertainties of interspecies extrapolation and will help to evaluate the predictive value of exposure markers for subsequent development of disease. When fully validated, these markers will greatly improve the power of epidemiological investigations to characterize environmental hazards and will aid in the development of effective measures for their control.

References

Appleton, B. S., M. P. Goetchius, and T. C. Campbell. 1982. Linear dose-response curve for the hepatic macromolecular binding of aflatoxin B_1 in rats at very low exposures. *Cancer Research* 42:3659-62.

Baselt, R. C. 1980. *Biological Monitoring Methods for Industrial Chemicals.* Davis, Calif.: Biomedical Publications.

Beck, B. D., B. Berson, H. A. Feldman, and J. D. Brain. 1983. Lactic dehydrogenase isoenzymes in hamster lung lavage fluid after lung injury. *Toxicology and Applied Pharmacology* 71:59-71.

Beland, F. A., D. T. Beranek, K. L. Dooley, R. H. Heflich, and F. F. Kadlubar. 1983. Arylamine-DNA adducts *in vitro* and *in vivo:* Their role in bacterial mutagenesis and urinary bladder carcinogenesis. *Environmental Health Perspectives* 49:125-34.

Berlin, A., M. Draper, K. Hemminki, and H. Vainio, eds. 1984. *Monitoring Human Exposure to Carcinogenic and Mutagenic Agents.* IARC publication 59. Lyon, France: International Agency for Research on Cancer.

Berlin, A., A. H. Wolff, and Y. Hasegawa. 1979. *The Use of Biological Specimens for the Assessment of Human Exposure to Environmental Pollutants.* London: Martinus Nijhoff.

Bloom, A. D. 1981. *Guidelines for Studies of Human Populations Exposed to Mutagenic and Reproductive Hazards.* New York: March of Dimes Birth Defects Foundation.

Brain, J. D. 1984. Physiology and pathophysiology of pulmonary macrophages. In *The Reticuloendothelial System,* ed. S. M. Reichard and J. P. Filkins. Vol. 7B. New York: Plenum.

Bridges, B. A., B. E. Butterworth, and I. B. Weinstein, eds. 1982. *Indicators of Genotoxic Exposure.* Banbury Report 13. Cold Spring Harbor, N.Y.: Cold Spring Harbor Laboratory.

Bryant, M. S., P. L. Skipper, S. R. Tannenbaum, and M. Maclure. In press. Hemoglobin adducts of 4-aminobiphenyl in smokers and nonsmokers. *Cancer Research.*

Busby, W. F., and G. N. Wogan. 1984. Aflatoxins. In *Chemical Carcinogens,* ed. C. E. Searle. 2d ed. Washington, D.C.: American Chemical Society.

Calleman, C. J. 1982. *In vivo* dosimetry by means of alkylated haemoglobin: A tool in the design of tests for genotoxic effects. In *Indicators of Genotoxic Exposure.* Banbury Report 13. Cold Spring Harbor, N.Y.: Cold Spring Harbor Laboratory.

Camus, A. M., A. Aitio, N. Sabadie, J. Wahrendorf, and H. Bartsch. 1984. Metabolism and urinary excretion of mutagenic metabolites of benzo(a)pyrene in C57 and DBA mouse strains. *Carcinogenesis* 5:35-39.

Davis, G. S., M. S. Giancola, M. C. Costanza, and R. B. Low. 1982. Analyses of sequential bronchoalveolar lavage samples from healthy human volunteers. *Am. Rev. Resp. Dis.* 126:611-16.

Ehrenberg, L., and S. Osterman-Golkar. 1980. Alkylation of macromolecules for detecting mutagenic agents. *Teratogenesis, Carcinogenesis and Mutagenesis* 1:105-27.

Essigmann, J. M., R. G. Croy, R. A. Bennett, and G. N. Wogan. 1982. Metabolic activation of aflatoxin B_1: Patterns of DNA adduct formation, removal, and excretion in relation to carcinogenesis. *Drug Metabolism Reviews* 13:569-90.

Evans, H. J. 1983. Cytogenetic methods for detecting effects of chemical mutagens. *Annals of New York Academy of Sciences* 407:131–41.

Evans, H. J., K. E. Buckton, G. E. Hamilton, and A. Carothers. 1979. Radiation induced chromosome aberrations in nuclear dockyard workers. *Nature* 277:531–34.

Gibson, J. F., D. Gompertz, and R. B. Hedworth-Whitty. 1984. Mutagenicity of urine from nurses handling cytotoxic drugs. *Lancet* 1:100–101.

Green, L. C., P. L. Skipper, R. J. Turesky, M. S. Bryant, and S. R. Tannenbaum. 1984. *In vivo* dosimetry of 4-aminobiphenyl via a cysteine adduct in hemoglobin. *Cancer Research* 44:4254–59.

Groopman, J. D., L. J. Trudel, P. R. Donahue, A. Marshak-Rothstein, and G. N. Wogan. 1984. High affinity monoclonal antibodies for aflatoxins and their application to solid-phase immunoassays. *Proceedings of the National Academy of Science* 81:7728–31.

Groopman, J. D., P. R. Donahue, J. Zhu, J. Chen, and G. N. Wogan. 1985. Aflatoxin metabolism in humans: Detection of metabolites and nucleic acid adducts in urine by affinity chromatography. *Proceedings of the National Academy of Science* 82:6492–96.

Hayes, W. J. 1975. *Toxicology of Pesticides.* Baltimore: Williams and Wilkins.

International Agency for Research on Cancer. 1982. *Evaluation of the Carcinogenic Risk of Chemicals to Humans.* Monographs. Lyon, France: IARC.

Kadlubar, F. F., J. A. Miller, and E. C. Miller. 1977. Hepatic microsomal N-glucuronidation and nucleic acid binding of N-hydroxy arylamines in relation to urinary bladder carcinogenesis. *Cancer Research* 37:805–14.

Latt, S. A. 1981. Sister chromatid exchange formation. *Annual Reviews* 15:11–55.

Lauwerys, R. R. 1983. *Industrial Chemical Exposure: Guidelines for Biological Monitoring.* Davis, Calif.: Biomedical Publications.

Linch, A. L. 1974. *Biological Monitoring for Industrial Chemical Exposure Control.* Boca Raton, Fla.: CRC Press.

Lutz, W. K. 1979. *In vivo* covalent binding of organic chemicals to DNA as a quantitative indicator in the process of chemical carcinogenesis. *Mutat. Res.* 65:289–356.

Mecham, R. P., and G. Lange. 1982. Antigenicity of elastin: Characterization of major antigenic determinants of purified, insoluble elastin. *Biochem.* 21:669–73.

Montesano, R., M. F. Rajewsky, A. E. Pegg, and E. Miller. 1982. Development and possible use of immunological techniques to detect individual exposure to carcinogens. *Cancer Research* 42:5236–39.

Neumann, H.-G. 1981. Significance of metabolic activation and binding to nucleic acids of aminostilbene derivatives *in vivo*. *National Cancer Institute Monograph* 58:165–171.

Neumann, H.-G. 1984. Analysis of hemoglobin as a dose monitor for alkylating and arylating agents: Review. *Archives of Toxicology* 56:1–6.

Omenn, G. S., and H. V. Gelboin, eds. 1984. *Genetic Variability in Responses to Chemical Exposure.* Banbury Report 16. Cold Spring Harbor, N.Y.: Cold Spring Harbor Laboratory.

Osterman-Golkar, S., L. Ehrenberg, D. Segerback, and I. Hallstrom. 1976. Evaluation of genetic risks of alkylating agents. Part 2. Haemoglobin as a dose monitor. *Mutation Research* 34:1–10.

Patrianakos, C., and D. Hoffmann. 1979. On the analysis of aromatic amines in cigarette smoke. Chemical studies on tobacco smoke, 65. *Journal of Analytical Toxicology* 3:150–54.

Pereira, M. A., and L. W. Chang. 1981. Binding of chemical carcinogens and mutagens to rat hemoglobin. *Chemico-Biological Interactions* 33:301-5.

Poirier, M. C. 1981. Antibodies to carcinogen-DNA adducts. *Journal of the National Cancer Institute* 67:515-19.

Randerath, K., E. Randerath, H. P. Agrawal, R. C. Gupta, M. E. Schurdak, and M. V. Reddy. 1985. Post-labeling methods for carcinogen-DNA adduct analysis. *Environmental Health Perspectives* 62:57-66.

Sabbioni, G., P. L. Skipper, and S. R. Tannenbaum. 1986. Characterization of the binding of aflatoxin B₁ to serum albumin. Abstract. Paper presented at the American Association for Cancer Research meeting, Los Angeles, California, May 7-10.

Singer, B., and D. Grunberger. 1983. *Molecular Biology of Mutagens and Carcinogens*. New York: Plenum.

Skipper, P. L., M. W. Obiedzinski, S. R. Tannenbaum, D. W. Miller, R. K. Mitchum, and F. F. Kadlubar. 1985. Identification of the major serum albumin adduct formed by 4-aminobiphenyl *in vivo*. *Cancer Research* 45:5122-27.

Sorsa, M., and H. Norppa, eds. 1986. *Monitoring of Occupational Genotoxicants*. New York: Alan R. Liss.

Törnqvist, M., S. Osterman-Golkar, A. Kautiainen, S. Jensen, P. B. Farmer, and L. Ehrenberg. 1986. Tissue doses of ethylene oxide in cigarette smokers determined from adduct levels in hemoglobin. *Carcinogenesis* 7:1519-21.

Vainio, H., M. Sorsa, and K. Hemminki. 1983. Biological monitoring in surveillance of exposure to genotoxicants. *American Journal of Industrial Medicine* 4:87-103.

Wogan, G. N., and N. J. Gorelick. 1985. Chemical and biochemical dosimetry of exposure to genotoxic chemicals. *Environmental Health Perspectives* 62:5-18.

Wyrobek, A. J., L. A. Gordon, J. G. Burkhart, M. W. Francis, R. W. Kapp, G. Letz, H. V. Malling, J. C. Topham, and M. D. Whorton. 1983. An evaluation of human sperm as indicators of chemically induced alterations of spermatogenic function. *Mutation Research* 115:73-148.

8. Biomedical Aspects of Environmental Toxicology

MICHAEL GALLO, MICHAEL GOCHFELD, AND
BERNARD D. GOLDSTEIN

*This second chapter on the human health effects of ingestion of toxic chemicals
examines diseases and disease processes. Gallo, Gochfeld, and Goldstein
introduce the basic ideas of toxicology and then examine each of the major
organ systems to describe the processes by which ingested chemicals produce
disease. Condensing an extraordinary amount of material, they describe
mechanisms of toxicity for each major organ as well as the defense mechanisms
against the disease.*

The Fundamentals of Toxicology

Toxicology is the study of the adverse effects of xenobiotics. The field
has evolved from experimental pathology, pharmacology, and biochemistry to encompass research that ranges from defining the nature of the
body's responses to xenobiotics to understanding the molecular mechanisms underlying toxic events. An important part of the toxicology of any
foreign chemical (xenobiotic) is concerned with understanding its distribution, metabolism, and excretion (ADME).

The science of toxicology underlies much of our understanding of occupationally and environmentally related diseases and plays a major role
in the development of new drugs, pesticides, food additives, and cosmetics. Toxicity studies are conducted for industrial chemicals and solvents,
and the field of industrial toxicology has expanded markedly in the past
decade due to the passage of the Toxic Substances Control Act.

The paradigms of toxicology are straightforward: (1) Each individual
chemical or physical agent has a toxicity syndrome associated with exposure to that agent. (2) The response to the agent follows a general dose-
response relationship (response increasing with dose). And (3) the re-

sponse in laboratory animals predicts the response in humans. The assumptions underlying the interpretation of the dose-response relationship are that a receptor or receptors have been occupied and that the occupation of these receptors results in a toxic response (Tallarida and Jacob 1979). The greater the percentage of receptors occupied, the greater the response, until a maximum level of response is achieved.

On the cellular level, toxic chemicals (1) interfere with cell respiration and energy-generating processes; (2) alter the structure and function of membranes; (3) disrupt cellular communication and adhesion; and (4) alter cell division, proliferation, and growth.

Several factors affect the toxicity of a compound or the response of an individual to a toxic agent. The physicochemical variables are the compound's physical and chemical state. The physiological variables (ADME) are the absorption, distribution, metabolism, and excretion of the compound by the individual. Test system variables include the sex and strain, age and weight, and nutritional status of the individual.

Physicochemical Variables

The attributes affecting the behavior of the chemical agent are relatively straightforward. The physical state of the compound determines its absorption and distribution. Solvents in the vapor state are rapidly absorbed through the lung and are dispersed throughout the body. In the liquid state they are absorbed only slowly through the lung, skin, and gastrointestinal tract. Asbestos and other solid particles are sequestered in lysosomes of the gut and lung cells; some are inactivated, while others, for yet unknown reasons—perhaps related to physicochemical variables—are associated with toxic reactions that may progress to cancer. The chemical state of a compound markedly affects its absorptivity and reactivity. The greater the polarity of the compound, the lower the lipid solubility and the lower the uptake. Nonpolar compounds generally move across membranes by simple diffusion, that is, as a function of concentration. Polar compounds, depending on charge distribution, move across membranes via energy-dependent carriers (active transport) or facilitated diffusion, and only rarely by simple diffusion (Klaassen 1986).

Physiological Variables

Several physiological factors can modify the toxicity of xenobiotics. Absorption of compounds is a function of its chemical structure, surface-to-surface interaction, solubility and polarity, acidity or basicity constant (pKa, pKb), and concentration. As stated above, the general case is that the concentration of the nonionized (or nonpolar) compound determines the rate and amount of uptake across a biological membrane system. For the most part, the range of absorptivity from greater to lesser is the lung > gut > skin (Klaassen 1986).

Distribution from these surfaces varies greatly as a function of blood supply, lymphatics, and metabolism. Compounds absorbed through the lung are rapidly distributed throughout the body because of the capillary-alveoli interface. It is for this reason that anesthetics and other inhalants are immediately active in the central nervous system and only secondarily active in the liver and kidney.

Compounds taken orally or through the skin are much more slowly distributed because they may be metabolized by the absorbing organ system, then transported to the liver via the venous return system. The passage through the liver, which is the organ with the highest concentration of xenobiotic metabolizing enzyme systems (cytochromes P-450, mixed function oxidases), results in metabolism of the compound to a more polar compound and the secretion from the liver cell as a conjugated compound. This metabolism, generally called phase 1 and phase 2 (i.e., metabolism by cytochromes P-450 followed by conjugation by transferases, respectively), leads to water-soluble compounds, which are more readily removed by the kidney and excreted in the urine. Some chemicals that are not readily metabolized by liver cells or have molecular weights greater than approximately 400 are secreted into the bile and excreted in the feces.

Metabolism does not necessarily result in the formation of a less toxic compound. In many cases the action of the cytochromes P-450 can lead to a reactive intermediate or an active oxygen species, which is either cytotoxic (kills cells), or mutagenic, or which forms covalent linkages with cellular macromolecules. These interactions occur with compounds such as vinyl chloride, ethylene oxide, acetominophen, benzo(a)pyrene, N-hexane, and the anthracycline antibiotics (Sipes and Gandolfi 1986).

The metabolism of xenobiotics is closely coupled to the general well-being of the liver. Alcohol toxicity and carbon tetrachloride intoxication cause fat accumulation, decrease cytochrome P-450 activity, and deplete the liver of glutathione, a sulfhydryl-containing compound that plays a role in detoxifying chemicals. Uncouplers of the mitochondrial bioenergetics system, such as hexachlorophene and dinitrophenol, can alter metabolism by causing toxicity and water uptake into cells. A final example of the coupling of metabolism to cellular well-being is the decreased activity of cytochromes P-450 in laboratory animals after having been fed lipotrophic diets. These diets lead to fatty livers and decreased metabolic activity.

Active oxygen species such as superoxide, hydroxyl radical, and singlet oxygen, which in some cases can be generated in the liver by disrupting metabolic processes, can cause tissue damage and possibly initiate the carcinogenesis process (Kensler and Trush 1984).

The excretory processes rid the body of not only xenobiotics or their products but normal metabolites, too. Excretory routes are urine, feces, expired air, sweat, saliva, and milk. Excretion of low-molecular-weight, water-soluble chemicals is generally through the urine. High-molecular-weight chemicals are found in the bile and are excreted via the feces. Some of these high-molecular-weight chemicals, especially those that are more lipid soluble, such as the PCBs, are excreted, or more correctly secreted, in milk. Volatile compounds such as gases, or gases dissolved in drinking water (i.e., vinyl chloride, dichloroethylene, and so on) can be excreted via the expired air. Sweating is not generally considered an excretory route. However, it is a major mechanism for control of body temperature and of ammonium and sodium ions. Sweat also serves as an excretory fluid for some sulphur-containing compounds and compounds that are generally water soluble.

Disruption of physiologic processes can markedly alter the toxicity of xenobiotics, particularly environmental chemicals, making them less or more toxic, depending on the changes in the physiology of the host. One of the most important areas of modern toxicology and risk assessment is the study of interactions of xenobiotics in animals and man. For the most part, these interactions involve the study of the effects of one or more agents on one part of the ADME system and of how these effects alter the response of another part of the system. Perhaps the greatest challenges in toxicology today are the attempt to understand interactions of several xenobiotics and the interpretation of these interactions for risk assessment.

▌Test System Variables

Understanding test system variables also leads to more accurate interpretation of the dose-response relationships and interspecies extrapolation. The variables of sex, strain, and species of animal have been explored by many investigators. If toxicology is to be a predictive science, one must understand the value of animal experimentation and the strengths and limitations of extrapolating animal results to humans. Differences and similarities between species are generally a function of the level at which a chemical interacts with the host DNA, membranes, circulating system, and so on. Vinyl chloride, for instance, is a mutagen in most test systems and causes a particular type of liver cancer in laboratory animals and man. The metabolism, distribution, and excretion of vinyl chloride appears to be similar, if not qualitatively identical, in mammals. Therefore it can be concluded that, if the data had been available, the response seen in animals could have been predicted in man.

If a chemical is handled differently by a particular species, strain, or sex of animal, the ability to predict human toxicity is problematic. An excellent example of this dilemma is 2,3,7,8-tetrachlorodibenzo-p-dioxin (TCDD), the most toxic of the dioxins. TCDD has been found to have at least a 5 thousandfold difference in toxicity across mammalian species. The toxicity varies greatly in different strains of mice, and there is at least a threefold difference in toxicity between males and females of the same species (Poland and Knutson 1982). There are several chemicals that are sex specific because of the interaction with the endocrine system. The pesticide dibromochloropropane is a testicular toxin, with no analogous effect in females, whereas TCDD has a marked effect on the female reproductive system (Gallo et al. 1986).

Age and weight also affect an animal's reaction to xenobiotics. Very young or very old animals are generally more susceptible to toxins. In the young, it is because the defense systems have not matured; in the old it is because the systems have deteriorated. These generalities apply to humans as well (Klaassen 1986).

Nutritional status, which may alter the weight of an animal independent of age, is an important variable in the response to toxic agents. The feeding of antioxidants may reduce certain responses to toxic agents in the liver. Depletion of essential elements or dietary vitamins renders an animal more susceptible to toxicity. Nutritional status must therefore be considered in evaluating the results of animal studies.

Exposure route and rate are important when interpreting the results of animal studies. Ideally, in animal experiments these should be the same as those of the human population. If the toxicity study is being conducted to determine risk from an industrial exposure, dermal and inhalation routes are most appropriate. For a drug or food additive, the oral route should be studied.

Xenobiotic Exposure

Exposure to toxic chemicals may result in both short-term and long-term responses. In the short term, the body deals with acute insults with its enormous repair and recuperative processes. However, chronic toxicity may result over the long term. One reason is an accumulation of damage from repetitive acute insults. Sometimes an acute insult is beyond the reparative processes of the host, because (1) it leads to severe tissue damage; or (2) it plants the seeds of an eventual chronic debilitating state; or (3) the appropriate repair process for protecting against acute damage is itself the basis of the disease. An example of the second is somatic mutation underlying cancer. An example of the third is the response to inhalation of noxious agents of increased production of respiratory tract mucous, which, although beneficial in the acute stage, leads to chronic bronchitis if it is persistent. Similarly, the formation of scar tissue can, if repetitive, lead to significant organ disfunction, as in chronic liver cirrhosis.

Special mention should be made of mutations induced by xenobiotics, as these are the basis of the process leading to cancer and inherited disorders. Approximately 85 percent of all cancer is due to environmental (nongenetic) factors. Most are due to life-style factors that are unrelated to exposure to an industrial chemical. The process by which chemicals produce cancer begins with a direct alteration of the DNA, the chromosomal material carrying the information of a host cell, resulting in somatic mutation. Theoretically, cancer-specific alterations of DNA can be produced by one molecule of the chemical. This theory has led to the development of "one-hit" models of cancer risk, in which exposure to any level of a pollutant carries some finite risk of developing cancer.

Such models are in contrast to noncancer end points that are not dependent on mutations and for which there is a threshold—that is, a level below which no effect is anticipated. It is likely that many cancer-causing agents do in fact have thresholds. However, prudent public policy considerations generally have led regulators to treat cancer-causing agents as if they have no threshold unless proven otherwise. In recent years it has become apparent that cancer is a multistage process and that progression through subsequent stages can be promoted by chemical compounds that do not appear to react directly with DNA. The appropriate mathematical model to assess the risk of such compounds is a matter of debate.

Each organ of the body is potentially exposed to xenobiotics or their metabolites. Each plays a potential role in the natural history (ADME) of a chemical exposure: some store and sequester the substance, other metabolize or conjugate it, yet others excrete it. In addition to its role in the tissue distribution and dynamics of chemicals in the body, each organ is the potential target of adverse effects. Examples of these adverse effects are discussed in the remainder of this chapter.

The Skin

The skin provides a first defense against chemicals in the environment. It is made up of two principal tissue layers, dermis and epidermis. The two layers function interdependently, but structurally they are markedly distinct.

The dermis, which is the undersurface of the skin, contains primarily connective tissue, fat cells, specialized glands, and the neural-vascular network. Its major components are (1) the fibrous tissues (collagen, elastin, and reticulin); (2) the neural tissues (autonomic, sensory, and connective);

(3) the appendages (sweat glands, sebaceous glands, and hair follicles); and (4) the vasculature and the cellular components (fibroblasts, macrophages, mast cells, and lymphocytes).

The epidermis contains a series of stratified layers, from the surface to the dermis. These layers are (1) the stratum corneum (cornified keratins, a special class of skin proteins); (2) the stratum granulosum (transition layer of keratinized cells); (3) the stratum spinosum (differentiated keratin); and (4) the basal layer (germinal cells). Other cell types found in the epidermis are the melanocytes, which synthesize pigments; the Langerhans cells, which are the major members of the skin's immune system; and the Merkel cells, which are sensory (nerve-conduction) cells. The epidermis is morphologically separated from the dermis by a basement membrane, which serves as a supporting structure for the entire epidermis.

The skin is selectively permeable to xenobiotics, varying in permeability according to the site on the body. Absorptivity is greatest on the abdomen, scrotum, and neck, and poorest on the palms of the hands and soles of the feet. This difference is a function of the thickness of the epidermis, primarily the stratum corneal layer.

Skin cancer is of major interest in environmental health. The primary etiologic agent for skin tumors (both basal cell and squamous cell carcinomas) is ultraviolet light from the sun, but several other agents such as X ray, oral arsenic, and poor nutrition can lead to skin tumors. The skin responds very rapidly to infrared and ultraviolet radiation (sunlight) with a phenomenon called sunburn. Sunburn is not just a reddening of the skin with localized pain and pressure sensitivity. It also involves melanogenesis (freckling and tanning), suppression of the immune system, and mutagenic events in the DNA of the basal layer. The reaction to sunlight can be exacerbated by photoactive agents such as 8-methoxypsoralen, some porphyrins, and several drugs. An increase in porphyrins (porphyria) can result from exposure to xenobiotics such as polychlorinated biphenyls (PCBs), lead, and TCDD. Some drugs that induce liver enlargement can also increase porphyrins.

The skin is the site of most occupational and household exposures and is the major site for primary irritation and localized allergic reactions. Primary irritation from detergents, appliance cleansers, and bathroom cleansers is a common occurrence. Localized allergic reactions can occur after sensitization with metals (nickel), drugs (neomycin), plants (poisoning), and several other agents (Marzulli and Maibach 1980; Shupack 1977). The skin, like all organs, has a limited way of responding to chemical insults—reddening, swelling, thickening, and thinning.

Skin irritation from chemicals is one of the most common occupational injuries that are not life threatening. Formaldehyde, which is a component of several industrial products and is used as a bactericide in dyes, textiles, deodorants, and cosmetics, is both a primary irritant and an allergen. The difference between the two responses is timing. A primary irritant causes immediate reddening, swelling, or itching, which subside in a short time and generally do not return if lower concentrations of the irritant are placed on the skin. An allergen, on the other hand, sensitizes the skin and induces reactions that appear to be irritant in nature but that grow in violence with subsequent exposures, even of lower doses. Formaldehyde, or formaldehyde-generating products such as fingernail polish, mascara, and household disinfectants, have caused serious allergic reactions. These reactions have occurred at concentrations of formaldehyde that did not cause primary irritation (Rudner et al. 1973).

Exposure to some chlorinated hydrocarbons leads to acnelike lesions called chloracne. This disease is seen in workers involved in synthesis of chemicals of which TCDD is a by-product. Other chemicals, such as PCBs and chlorinated dibenzofurans can also cause this lesion (Taylor 1979; Poland and Knutson 1982).

Xenobiotics may alter the skin in such a way as to disrupt these normal responses. Hydrocarbon solvents such as benzene, hexane, and acetone alter the lipids in the epidermis, which then allows several compounds not normally transported through the skin to penetrate to the dermis, from where it is carried throughout the body. Oxidizing agents, such as hypochlorite, and concentrated bases, such as sodium hydroxide, can disrupt the proteins of the epidermis (Emmett 1986).

The blood supply to the skin (in the dermis) is one of the richest in the body. Therefore, if a chemical can penetrate the epidermis and get to the rich vascular bed of the dermis, it will be rapidly transported throughout the body. This phenomenon is easily demonstrated in humans by the rapid excretion of solvents in expired air and in urine after the solvent has been placed on the skin. The toxicological significance of this observation is that cutaneous exposure can and does lead to systemic response. The development of scopalamine patches for motion sickness or nitroglycerin ointment for increased vasodilation makes pharmacotherapeutic use of this phenomenon. Hence risk assessment, particularly for the occupational setting, should carefully consider the role of the skin not only in local, but in systemic, toxicity.

Blood and Blood-Forming Organs

Blood consists of cells carried in a fluid known as plasma. The functions of the blood system are varied and are of importance to each organ. These include the transport of nutrients and metabolic products and the maintenance of normal fluid pressure. The production and function of blood cells and the clotting of the blood are intrinsic to hematology, the study of blood.

▌ Bone Marrow

Under normal circumstances in humans, the bone marrow is the sole source of all blood cells except lymphocytes. Marrow contains a complex mixture of cell types, which are either the direct precursors of circulating blood cells or which act, in a still uncertain manner, to nurture these precursors. At least three of the common blood cell types—the red blood cell, the platelet, and granulocytic white blood cell—are ultimately derived from a single precursor cell, known as a pluripotential stem cell. This precursor cell can differentiate within the bone marrow into any one of the earliest identifiable forms of the more mature cells. The entire process is under the control of a feedback mechanism, whereby a deficiency in a cell type leads to increased production of that cell; for example, anemia leads to increased red blood cell production. The earliest identifiable precursors go through an orderly maturation process within the bone marrow, during which their functions mature.

Bone marrow toxic substances that affect the earliest stem cells, such as benzene or X ray, tend to decrease the production of all three cell types and lead to pancytopenia. Sufficient bone marrow damage markedly decreases total bone marrow cellularity, resulting in aplastic anemia. This can be a fatal illness, particularly if an offending toxic substance is not identified and removed. Death is usually due to hemorrhage, because of lack of platelets, or to infection, due to lack of granulocytic white blood cells. Bone marrow toxic substances, including autoantibodies, can also affect the development of just one cell type, leading to anemia, leukopenia, or thrombocytopenia.

Cancer of bone marrow precursor cells can take a number of forms. Acute myelogenous leukemia is an uncontrolled proliferation of the earliest identifiable granulocytic cell precursor. Granulocytic cell types of greater maturity are found in chronic myelogenous leukemia. There is a similar neoplastic production of mature red blood cells known as polycythemia vera, as well as other far less common neoplasms of red cells and platelets. These disorders are to some extent clinically related, presumably reflecting the common nature of the stem cell. Certain of these cancers have been associated with exposure to radiation, benzene, and other aplastic agents, and to alkylating agents used in cancer chemotherapy (e.g., a patient successfully treated for Hodgkin's disease with chemotherapy has a higher than usual risk of subsequently developing acute myelogenous leukemia).

Acute myelogenous leukemia due to benzene exposure has been of particular interest from the standpoint of environmental health. Benzene is a ubiquitous environmental contaminant, being present in gasoline (1 to 5 percent of total product) and in a wide variety of chemical products and processes. In order to effectively regulate this human leukemogen, we need to know more about the mechanism by which its metabolism leads to bone marrow damage and the relationship of its aplastic to its leukemic actions (Goldstein 1983).

Another neoplasm primarily affecting bone and bone marrow is multiple myeloma. This is a neoplasm of the plasma cell, an antibody-forming cell related to the lymphocyte. An increased incidence of multiple myeloma has been reported in individuals working in chemical and other industries, but causal relationships have not been established.

In addition to acute and chronic myelogenous leukemias, there are also acute and chronic lymphatic leukemias. The lymphatic leukemias differ greatly from each other and from the myelogenous leukemias. Acute lymphatic leukemia is the commonest form of childhood leukemia. Chronic lymphatic leukemia is a disease of older age groups and often is of minimal clinical consequence. There are also a variety of other lymphatic tumors, known as lymphomas, which may sometimes be observed in the bone marrow. As we become more knowledgeable about lymphocytes and related cells, it has become easier to differentiate the various types of lymphoma. Certain types of lympho-proliferative disorders have been associated with exposure to benzene and other solvents or with particular occupations, but the causal relationships are not proven.

▌ Red Blood Cells

The primary purpose of red blood cells is to carry oxygen. Over 90 percent of the cell protein is in the form of hemoglobin, which has the property of binding with oxygen in the lung and releasing the oxygen in the tissues. This oxygen-carrying capacity can be interfered with by a number of toxic agents. Among these is carbon monoxide, which combines with the oxygen-combining site of hemoglobin, thereby preventing oxygen from being carried. The affinity of hemoglobin for carbon monoxide is approximately 200-fold greater than oxygen. Therefore, breathing 0.1 percent carbon monoxide (a thousand parts per million) in a 20 percent oxygen atmosphere would lead to 50 percent of the hemoglobin being bound to the carbon monoxide (carboxyhemoglobin: COHb) and 50 percent to the oxygen. This is a fatal level, inasmuch as carbon monoxide also interferes with the release of the remaining oxygen from hemoglobin at the tissue level. Fortunately, it requires eight to sixteen hours, depending upon respiratory rate, to achieve a steady state—otherwise smoking one cigarette would be fatal. Children, in part due to their relatively high respiratory rate, are particularly susceptible to high levels of carbon monoxide. At lower levels, individuals with preexisting cardiovascular disease seem particularly at risk (see below). There is a background level of about 0.5 percent COHb due to the formation of carbon monoxide during the metabolism of normal body constituents.

The normal function of the oxygen-combining site of hemoglobin also depends on the presence of iron in reduced ferrous form. Oxidation to the ferric state produces methemoglobin, a brownish hemoglobin that cannot carry oxygen. There are a number of chemicals, including aniline dyes and nitrites, that can produce significant, even life-threatening, levels of methemoglobin. Methemoglobin is continuously found in normal red cells in small amounts (0.5 percent) due to the steady-state oxidation of iron in hemoglobin. Its presence is counteracted by an enzyme in the red cell (methemoglobin reductase), which functions to keep it at normal level. Individuals with inherited low levels of this enzyme are particularly susceptible to methemoglobin-causing chemicals. Infants also appear to be deficient in the ability to fully reduce methemoglobin and thus have a greater sensitivity (Smith 1980).

Xenobiotics may also destroy red cells before the end of their normal 120-day survival period in the circulation. Anemia can thus be caused by the failure of the bone marrow to produce sufficient red cells or by the early destruction of red cells within the circulation, the latter being known as hemolysis. There are two general types of hemolysis: intravascular and extravascular. Intravascular hemolysis occurs when there is sufficient damage to the red blood cell membrane to allow direct release of hemoglobin into the circulating blood. Release of sufficient hemoglobin into the blood to overwhelm normal body-clearance mechanisms may produce acute kidney failure. A chemical notorious for producing this problem is arsine gas, which appears to make the red cell swell rapidly and then burst. Arsine is used commercially and may also be produced inadvertently when an arsenic-containing compound undergoes reduction (e.g., addition of acid).

Extravascular hemolysis is a more common phenomenon. The reticuloendothelial system, and particularly the spleen, has the function of destroying partially damaged red blood cells. Toxic substances that alter the red blood cell to an extent less than that causing immediate loss of hemoglobin may produce anemia through extravascular hemolysis. A high dose of a hemolytic agent may lead to intravascular hemolysis, a low dose to extravascular hemolysis.

There are a number of inherited disorders that lead to hemolysis. These include genetic alterations leading to changes in the amino acids of hemoglobin and red blood cell enzymes, particularly those enzymes responsible for energy metabolism and for protection of the red cell against oxidant stress. Much has been learned about genetics by studying hemoglobin disorders in which there is inadequate synthesis or an altered protein. Many hemoglobin alterations are silent, in that there is no or negligible clinical significance to these particular replacements of one amino acid with another. On the other hand, certain amino acid substitutions have never been observed, presumably because they so severely impair the oxygen-carrying capacity of hemoglobin that fetal development is precluded.

In the case of sickle cell disease, the replacement of glutamic acid with valine on the beta chain of hemoglobin results in an abnormal hemoglobin, which has the property of unwanted precipitation in the circulation. As is generally true with inherited disorders of this type, sickle cell trait confers a survival advantage despite the generally poor outcome of the disease. The survival advantage is protection against infection with malaria. Another inherited change that produces protection against malaria is glucose-6-phosphate dehydrogenase (G6PD) deficiency. This is inherited as a sex-linked recessive and is relatively common, being present in one in seven black males and one in fifty black females in the United States. Individuals with this variant of G6PD deficiency are at greater risk of hemolyzing with oxidant drugs. While there has been some speculation in the literature that inhaled oxidant gases might also produce hemolysis in G6PD deficiency, this in essence can be excluded as a reasonable possibility (Amoruso et al. 1986).

▌ White Blood Cells

The largest number of circulating white blood cells are the type known as polymorphonuclear (PMN) leukocytes, which function to phagocytize and destroy invading microbes. Along with basophils and eosinophils, which are active in certain allergic-type responses, the PMNs make up a class of white blood cells known as granulocytes. Somewhat related are monocytes, which, like PMNs, function as phagocytic cells—capable of destroying invading microbes but also involved in long-term immune responses. Numerically the second largest white cell type in the blood are the lymphocytes. Once thought to be a relatively homogenous cell type, it is now clear that there are many different subsets of lymphocytes, all of which participate in the immune response (see below).

▌ Platelets and Blood-Clotting Proteins

The clotting of blood is a complex phenomenon under fine control. It is a necessary response to bleeding but potentially harmful should clotting begin under normal conditions. A major cellular component of a clot is the platelet, a circulating blood cell. Various plasma proteins also play major roles in the sequence of events, leading to a fibrin meshwork being laid down to support the clot and close the wound. Numerous drugs, including aspirin, are known to alter blood coagulation. There is little evidence that blood coagulation is affected to any great extent by known environmental agents.

The Immune System

The immune system classically has been considered the primary body defense against invading organisms. It is a finely balanced network of different cell types in many body organs. The cell types include phagocytic white blood cells and lymphocytes, which are found in the blood, bone marrow, spleen, lymphoid system, and portals of entry such as the gut and lung. The first job of the immune system is to recognize the difference between host and foreign agents and to rid the body of the latter.

Rapid advances have been made in recent years in understanding the dynamics of the immune system. The underlying cellular basis for long-recognized variations in immunological response to different agents is now being unravelled. These advances have led to a rapid increase in knowledge of immunotoxicology. Agents foreign to the body, such as bacteria, evoke a complex response. Phagocytic cells such as granulocytes and macrophages actively reach out and destroy the invaders through a complex series of reactions, including the release of cytotoxic enzymes and oxidizing free radicals. Different types of lymphocytes participate in the process. B lymphocytes produce antibodies against antigenic foreign material. T lymphocytes, of which there are a variety of subtypes with different functions, modulate the entire process through the secretion of compounds that mediate the activity of various portions of the immune system.

Dysfunction of the immune system can cause a variety of problems. Hypersensitivity is the state of enhanced sensitivity to specific molecules and is often known as allergy, a common problem in both the workplace and among the general population. Four types of hypersensitive responses to chemicals have been described: (1) bronchial asthma from inhaled allergens; (2) production of cytotoxic antibodies; (3) formation of antigen-antibody complexes; and (4) contact dermatitis, a form of cell-mediated delayed hypersensitivity (Coombs and Gell 1975; Luster and Dean 1982).

Suppression of the immune system can be caused by a variety of chemicals, including therapeutic drugs that may be chosen for this property. The use of immunosuppressive therapy in recipients of organ transplants has had the side effect of an increased incidence of infections, often by microbes usually harmless to a normal host, and there has been a higher risk of cancer in long-time survivors of kidney transplantation. Xenobiotics have also been shown to interfere with the function of phagocytic cells responsible for the killing of bacteria.

Autoimmune disorders are those in which a component of the immune system reacts against the host. A variety of drugs and chemicals have been shown to produce autoimmune disease, such as systemic lupus erythematosis and autoimmune hemolytic anemia. The possible role of environmental chemicals in these and related conditions, such as rheumatoid arthritis, warrants serious consideration.

Our ability to finely measure this complex system of cells and chemical mediators has led to a marked increase in the number of studies evaluating the possible role of chemical agents in changing one or more parameters of immune function. Unfortunately, studies on many of these parameters have been inadequate in defining normal limits or in validating the relevance of deviations from control values. The foremost current challenge is to interpret associations between pollutant exposure and altered parameters of cellular or humoral immunity.

The Respiratory System

The respiratory system functions to provide the body with oxygen and to remove carbon dioxide. Inhaled air moves through the upper respiratory tract—nose, mouth, pharnyx, and larynx—through the trachea and into the bronchial system. Each bronchial division leads to two smaller bronchi and eventually into air sacs known as alveoli. Each alveolus has a thin layer of cells, under which is a blood capillary. Gas exchange consists of inhaled oxygen diffusing from the air within the alveolus through the alveolar and capillary membranes into the red blood cell, while carbon dioxide from the blood moves across the membranes, into the air sac, and is then expired. This delicately balanced process is dependent on a number of factors, including good respiratory muscle mechanics, patent airways, proper anatomical relationships within the alveolus, and appropriate distribution of capillary blood flow.

Air pollution is not a new phenomenon. Study of primitive tribes in New Guinea has shown a very high incidence of emphysema, presumably related to indoor use of crude cooking fuels in the absence of chimneys. A number of respiratory tract mechanisms protect against such air particles. At one end, the nose is an excellent filter, the nasal turbinates imparting a swirl to the entering air, leading to a high rate of particle deposition on the moist nasal mucosa. The bronchial tree also secretes mucus. And it contains cilia, which beat upward, moving particles deposited in the bronchial tree (including bacteria) up to the mouth, to be swallowed. The alveolar macrophage is a major line of defense in the lower respiratory tract. It engulfs bacteria (which are relatively large) and other particles. It kills bacteria in part through a process similar to that occurring in circulating white blood cells. But all of these protective processes can be interfered with by air contaminants.

The excellent vascularity of the lung makes it a major portal of entry into the body for certain toxic compounds, which are able to pass un-reacted through the lung and into the body, where they circulate until reaching target organs. Those airborne contaminants that have adverse effects in the lung either tend to be relatively reactive, with the lung being the first target of opportunity, or tend to be particulate in nature and un-able to readily penetrate beyond the lung surface.

The diameter of the airways in the respiratory tract is under fine con-trol and varies during the respiratory cycle. Mild construction of the air-ways is a reflex response to a number of situations, including apprehen-sion, cold air, and noxious environmental stimuli. Airway constriction is also the basis for symptoms occurring in asthma attacks and chronic bron-chitis. Accordingly, public health approaches to the regulation of air-borne contaminants often have the goal of preventing additional bronchial constriction in susceptible populations.

Other aspects of lung dynamics pertinent to toxicology include the lung's capability of metabolizing many foreign compounds and the rela-tionship of respiratory rate to toxic effects. A fundamental concept of toxi-cology is that toxicity is dependent upon dose to the target site. Toxicity can thus be affected by metabolism or by the extent and rate of respiration, the latter depending upon a variety of factors including disease and exer-cise. The greater activity and hence greater respiratory rate of children ac-counts in part for their enhanced susceptibility to air pollutants.

Much information about respiratory toxic substances has come from the recognition of effects in workers exposed to relatively high pollutant levels. A wide range of effects has been noted, including (1) cancer due to compounds such as asbestos and arsenic; (2) fibrosis of the lung from as-bestos and other mineral agents; (3) nonspecific irritant effects due to a variety of reactive chemicals; and (4) allergic sensitization from com-pounds such as toluene diisocyanate. Considered below are some com-pounds under regulation by EPA and present in the general environ-ment—usually at levels much below those in the workplace.

▌ Primary Air Pollutants

The Clean Air Act of the United States identifies a number of primary air quality pollutants for which ambient standards have been set. These are ozone, nitrogen dioxide, sulfur dioxide, total suspended particles, car-bon monoxide, and lead.

Ozone

Ozone is one of the most potent oxidizing agents known. It is highly irritating to the lung, producing pulmonary edema, a condition in which fluid enters the alveolar spaces. The lethal dose for this effect in animals is in the range of 4 to 8 parts per million (ppm) for four hours. The highest recorded concentrations in the general outdoor environment have approached 1 ppm for one hour in Southern California. The U.S. air quality standard for ozone is 0.12 ppm for one hour, not to be exceeded more than once yearly. Relatively low-level effects of ozone include biochemical changes observed in animal lungs; acute bronchoconstrictive effects in human volunteers experimentally exposed for a few hours, usually while exercising; and a suggestion of effects observed in epidemiological studies of Southern California residents, with children particularly at risk. An additional aspect of ozone toxicology is its ability, similar to that of nitrogen dioxide, to potentiate lethal bacterial pneumonia in laboratory mice. This occurs at levels of ozone as low as 0.08 ppm and appears to be due to an interference in the ability of alveolar macrophages to kill inhaled bacteria. A particular point of concern is the potential, based on its oxidant effects, that long-term, low-level exposure to ozone may produce chronic effects.

Nitrogen Dioxide

Nitrogen dioxide is also an oxidant, although much weaker than ozone. In addition, it is an acid anhydride. The U.S. nitrogen dioxide standard is 0.05 ppm as an annual average. More recent regulatory efforts have focused on the development of shorter-term nitrogen dioxide standards, in part because this compound has an acute bronchoconstrictive effect on humans while they are exercising. Nitrogen dioxide, like ozone, is able to potentiate bacterial infections in mice, apparently through interfering with the ability of alveolar macrophages to kill inhaled bacteria. There is some evidence in epidemiological studies that nitrogen dioxide exposure may also potentiate respiratory tract infections in humans (U.S. Environmental Protection Agency 1982). Recent studies of this controversial subject have focused on the potential for such effects occurring indoors in the presence of gas stoves, kerosene heaters, and other appliances that may release substantial amounts of nitrogen dioxide. For instance, during cooking on a gas stove levels of nitrogen dioxide may approach 1 ppm, and the kitchens of many homes have around-the-clock nitrogen dioxide levels that exceed the U.S. outdoor standard (National Research Council 1981).

Sulfur Dioxide and Particles

Sulfur dioxide and particles are part of a gas-aerosol complex resulting from the combustion of fossil fuels in stationary sources, such as power plants, industries, and homes. These pollutants were primarily responsible for the air pollutant disasters in the past, including the great London smog episode, which took perhaps 3 thousand lives a little over three decades ago. Sulfur dioxide is very water soluble and is scrubbed out in the upper airways. For many years this was believed to limit its toxicity, and the observed epidemiological association between sulfur dioxide and adverse pulmonary effects was considered to be an association in which sulfur dioxide was serving as a surrogate for other more harmful components of the gas-aerosol complex. Recently, however, it has become apparent that sulfur dioxide itself, at concentrations approaching those in the vicinity of sources such as power plants, can produce acute airway constriction in humans while they are exercising.

Other components of the gas-aerosol complex, including a variety of respirable particles also produce respiratory bronchial constriction. Many of these are sulfates derived from the atmospheric oxidation of sulfur dioxide. Respirable sulfates have a wide range in potency to produce airway constriction, depending upon the associated cation and such factors as size, solubility, and pH—the more acid particles, such as sulfuric acid, being the most potent (Amdur 1974). Respirable particulate nitrates derived from the oxidation of gaseous oxides of nitrogen also contribute to the potency of the gas-aerosol complex in producing bronchial constriction.

Lead

The realization that airborne lead makes a substantial contribution to total body burden of lead in the general population has produced regulatory action that has substantially decreased lead levels in gasoline in recent years. The major source of lead in lead poisoning is by ingestion rather than through inhalation.

▌ Toxic Air Pollutants

Under the Clean Air Act, all airborne compounds not regulated as primary air pollutants are subject to control through a separate regulatory mechanism. These compounds have collectively become known as toxic air pollutants or hazardous air pollutants and represent a broad collection of chemical agents. As the compounds tend to be present at levels well below those for which there are workplace standards, attention has been focused on presumed cancer-causing compounds, such as benzene, and on compounds that tend to accumulate in the body, such as mercury.

Risk assessment, a formal methodology to quantify risk due to relatively low levels of pollutants, has provided a valuable tool to make decisions about regulating toxic air pollutants. In the case of benzene, the projection of lives saved by various control strategies was of importance in making decisions about which benzene source to control (Anderson et al. 1983; Goldstein 1986).

The Cardiovascular System

The cardiovascular system includes the heart and blood vessels. Relatively little research has been done to explore the potential role of environmental toxic substances in this system. Chemical compounds such as ergot alkaloids and perhaps lead can affect the blood pressure, presumably by altering vascular resistance. Long-term exposure to carbon disulfide has been associated with heart disease (Beauchamp et al. 1983). Individuals with preexisting heart disease are among those particularly at risk to stationary source, fossil fuel air pollutants, such as sulfates (as indicated by increased mortality and morbidity of this population during severe smog episodes). Impaired circulation within the heart muscle (arteriosclerotic heart disease) may produce the anginal symptom of chest pain with exercise, exposure, or with any stress-induced increased oxygen demand. Individuals with this disorder tend to be susceptible to even low levels of carbon monoxide, which decreases the blood's oxygen-carrying capacity. In essence, the decrease in oxygen in the blood in conjunction with the rigid, narrowed coronary arteries lead to a lesser degree of exercise tolerance.

It has been proposed that the underlying change in the wall of the artery that leads to arteriosclerosis is a benign tumor and, based on preliminary evidence, that the process may be initiated by the circulation of environmentally derived mutagens. Cardiovascular disease remains the leading cause of death in the United States. Much more needs to be known about the potential role of environmental chemicals.

The Liver

The liver plays a fundamental role in a variety of physiologic and metabolic processes. It functions in the metabolism of carbohydrates, lipids, and proteins, in the synthesis and degradation of hormones, in the regulation of the blood volume, and in the metabolism of xenobiotics. Because it is supplied by both the hepatic arterial circulation and the portal vein draining the intestines, the liver is the first organ to be reached by the myriad compounds absorbed through the intestines. Xenobiotics entering the body by other routes (skin, lungs) are also transported to the liver through the blood. The liver is the major organ where foreign compounds undergo metabolism, but it also has the potential of activating many toxic substances by metabolizing inactive substances into toxic metabolites

(Plaa 1986). Major works on hepatotoxicity include Farber and Fisher (1979) and Zimmerman (1978).

Consideration of the role of the liver in environmental toxicology must focus on two aspects: (1) the role of the liver in increasing or decreasing the toxic potential of xenobiotics; and (2) the liver as a target organ, which means it is vulnerable to the toxic effects of chemicals.

Understanding the microarchitecture of the liver is important to understanding its function and susceptibility to toxic substances. The liver is divided into lobules. Under a microscope these lobules appear as hexagons, the corners of which are marked by a group of three vessels, the large portal vein, a smaller hepatic artery, and a branch of the bile duct. The vein and artery carry nutrient-rich blood and freshly oxygenated blood, respectively, into the lobule. Bile produced in the liver cells is gathered, conducted away from the lobule into the bile ducts, and is ultimately conducted to the gall bladder. Blood is simultaneously delivered to several adjacent lobules, flows through the lobules, and eventually drains into the central vein, which leads into the hepatic vein and ultimately to the vena cava.

It has long been recognized that different parts of the lobule differ in susceptibility to various toxic substances. Some chemicals produce their major damage in the cells immediately around the central vein (centrolobular necrosis), whereas others damage cells closer to the portal triad (periportal necrosis). Until recently, the common belief was that characteristics of blood flow and metabolic change were the passive determinants of where injury occurs within the lobule. Recent research has demonstrated that within the lobule there are differences in the metabolic activity of different cells (Rappaport 1979; Schiff 1982).

Enzyme systems in the hepatocytes act on a wide variety of substrates. Exposure to certain substances stimulates the production of additional amounts of enzyme, hence the term *inducible enzymes.* The inducibility of hepatocellular enzymes varies among individuals, depending not only on genetic factors but on environmental factors as well.

The metabolic activity of the liver is often considered under two phases. In phase 1, the mixed-function oxidase (MFO) enzyme system calls upon the cytochrome P-450 system. Together these oxidize many xenobiotics, forming among other compounds some toxic or bioactive free radicals. Phase 2 reactions involve the conjugating of various small molecules to carrier molecules (usually proteins or carbohydrates) in the blood, which facilitate their excretion.

Although surgical excision of three-fourths of the liver mass may have little impact on health or on clinical assessments of liver function, a single exposure to a virus or a hepatotoxin may result in such massive cellular damage that many aspects of liver function are affected. One can directly visualize the clinical impact of many of these adverse effects. For example, damage that interferes with the MFO (phase 1) system may result in failure to properly metabolize hormones such as estrogens. In the male this leads directly to a characteristic feminization syndrome, including gynecomastia (breast enlargement), loss of body hair, and change of voice.

Damage to the phase 2 system is readily seen as jaundice. The liver cells are responsible for attaching or conjugating molecules of bilirubin to molecules of a carbohydrate. This renders the insoluble bilirubin sufficiently soluble to be excreted via the kidney, thereby preventing a buildup of excessive amounts of bilirubin in the blood and tissues (which results in jaundice). Since bilirubin is a major breakdown product of hemoglobin, and since the body is constantly turning over hemoglobin, the excretion of bilirubin is a full-time job, and failure of the conjugation mechanism is soon manifest as jaundice.

A third example can be seen when the liver's ability to synthesize the protein albumin is inhibited. This protein is a major component of the blood plasma and provides the osmotic pressure necessary to maintain blood volume. When albumin synthesis is reduced, the concentration of albumin in the blood declines, and water tends to move out of the bloodstream into the tissues. This creates a reduced blood volume as well as an apparent accumulation of edema fluid in the tissues.

There are several important reasons why the liver is a vulnerable target organ: (1) foreign compounds concentrate in the liver; (2) many xenobiotics are excreted in the bile, and thus find their way through the liver; and (3) the liver is the major organ for metabolism of xenobiotics. This vulnerability is enhanced in individuals who possess certain risk factors, such as poor nutrition, and varies among individuals because of heredity, age, sex, and endocrine factors, and various disease states.

Types of Hepatotoxicity

The major pathologic categories of xenobiotically induced liver disease include (1) cancers of the liver; (2) cytotoxicity and toxic hepatitis; (3) fatty liver; (4) cirrhosis of the liver; and (5) biliary proliferation leading to cholestasis (Popper and Schaffner 1959).

Cancers of the Liver

The epidemiologic investigation of liver cancer has been hampered by the fact that many other cancers metastasize to the liver, causing death. Hence many death-certificate liver cancers did not actually arise in the liver. In Africa, primary liver cancer is a common disease associated with environmental agents such as aflatoxin B_1, viruses, and parasitic diseases. In other areas, primary liver cancer is uncommon. Wogan (1976) reviewed the causes of liver cancer, summarized below.

Cirrhosis of the liver is an important precondition for cancer, although it is not clear to what extent. The relationship of toxic substances such as alcohol and aflatoxin B_1 and infections such as hepatitis B_1 to both liver cirrhosis and liver cancer require clarification. Aflatoxin B_1 is clearly a hepatocarcinogen in animals, and its implication in human cancers is based largely on epidemiological studies linking high frequencies of hepatocellular carcinoma to areas where the aflatoxin content of the diet is high. The role of hepatitis B_1 in the occurrence of cancer is also inferred from epidemiological data. For most other animal liver carcinogens, there is little direct evidence linking them to cancer in human populations, although prudence guides us to view such substances with extreme suspicion.

Several other hepatocarcinogens are known that do not lead to cirrhosis and that affect different target cell populations. One of the classic detective stories in occupational medicine was the discovery that exposure to vinyl chloride monomer causes angiosarcoma, an otherwise extremely rare liver cancer. The existence of three cases of this rare disease in one factory population called attention to this relationship, which was subsequently confirmed by examination of other populations exposed to vinyl chloride. In fact, this is one of the "sentinel" cancers: a cancer so rare in the unexposed population that it immediately points to a significant toxic exposure.

This discovery, verified in laboratory studies, led to a lowering of the allowable exposure limit (threshold limit value) for the vinyl chloride monomer to one part per million. The fact that no recent cases have been discovered, despite substantially improved surveillance, is dramatic evidence that lowering the allowable level has had an effect in preventing angiosarcoma. The fact that the disappearance of the disease occurred less than a decade after imposition of the new standard is important evidence that vinyl chloride is a tumor promoter.

Inorganic arsenic and thorium as well as vinyl chloride monomer can induce angiosarcoma but, interestingly, none of these three substances is clearly associated with hepatocellular carcinoma. Thus there is a discrete target cell population within the liver. Since the same vascular tissue exists in other organs, why have the few angiosarcomas been reported only in liver? Is it simply that they are readily detectable or quickly fatal there? Or is it the role of the liver to activate some substance that localizes the angiosarcoma to that organ?

Cytotoxicity and Toxic Hepatitis

In addition to cancer, there are several major manifestations of liver toxicity. The death of hepatocytes resulting from exposure to toxic chemicals is a dramatic event. Liver necrosis is often fatal, whether it stems from viruses or from chemicals. And toxic hepatitis is relatively frequent, although fulminant and fatal poisonings occur infrequently.

Fatty Liver

A variety of substances that interfere with metabolism lead to the condition known as steatosis, or fatty liver. This condition can result from chemical interference with the synthesis, transport, or release of fat. Beginning with the appearance of small fat droplets in the cell, the accumulation increases until the nucleus is squeezed to the periphery and the entire body of the cell appears under the microscope as a clear, nonstaining fat droplet. Such cells are called signet rings. Further progression involves the rupture of liver cells and the coalescence of fat into macroscopic globules (Zimmerman 1978).

Cirrhosis of the Liver

Cirrhosis involves the replacement of the normal architecture of the liver with bands of fibrous scar tissue. Such bands often constrict areas of liver cells, leading to pressure necrosis and eventually hepatic insufficiency. Cirrhosis actually involves several pathogenic processes with the common feature of extensive infiltration of fibrous tissue. It may follow any process that damages liver cells (Schiff 1982). It in turn compresses cells and interferes with their function. Cirrhosis may be fatal in and of itself or may predispose to cancer.

Biliary Proliferation and Cholestasis

A number of substances, particularly some drugs, induce a hypersensitive response of the bile canaliculi, leading to a proliferation of these small ducts within the liver lobule. The ducts are often not open, and the movement of bile from the liver cells to the gall bladder is slowed (cholestasis). The newly synthesized bile continues to accumulate in the liver cells and extracellular fluid, and the pressure from this accumulating fluid compresses the cells, leading in the most serious cases to pressure necrosis. The bile accumulation is accompanied by jaundice and is often reversible upon cessation of exposure to the causative agent.

This proliferation can arise in response to certain chemicals, notably chlorpromazine. It is idiosyncratic in its occurrence, affecting relatively few people who take the medication, and appears to involve a sensitization (see also Plaa and Priestly 1976).

▌ Categories and Examples of Hepatotoxins

There are so many toxic substances that can damage the liver that it is useful to divide these into categories. One classification is predictability, adapted from Zimmerman's (1978) textbook on liver disease:

Characteristics of Predictable Toxic Substances	Characteristics of Unpredictable Toxic Substances
Clear dose-response relationship	No dose-response relationship
Toxic to most humans	Toxic to only a few, susceptible, humans
Good animal models exist	Good animal models do not exist
Steatosis (fatty liver) results	Cholestasis results
Easily replicable effects	No easily replicable effects

The primary distinction between the two categories is that some substances are predictably hepatotoxic, inducing a dose-related effect in most exposed individuals, while other substances are benign to most individuals but induce disease in a few highly susceptible individuals. (The terminology for these categories is unfortunately confused. The terms *direct* and *indirect* sometimes appear in this context, but they also indicate toxic substances that act directly on the liver versus those that act through a metabolite. Plaa 1986 used the terms *Type I* and *Type II,* but as Zimmerman showed, the two categories are not discrete.)

Extensive lists of hepatotoxins are given in textbooks. The several examples selected for discussion here illustrate toxic substances that require activation (carbon tetrachloride), that are carcinogenic (aflatoxin B_1), that are predictable (all except for halothane), and that are unpredictable (halothane).

Carbon Tetrachloride

Among the numerous chemicals with documented liver toxicity, carbon tetrachloride, until recently a common household solvent and industrial chemical, is perhaps the best known (Recknagel 1983). Exposure to carbon tetrachloride in poorly ventilated facilities was once commonplace. An interesting feature of this toxicity is the clear evidence that the vulnerability of the liver was enhanced by prior exposure to alcohol.

This substance provides good evidence of the importance of metabolic activation, because a metabolite, rather than the parent compound, is responsible for the damage. If animals are pretreated with an unrelated substance that induces MFO enzymes, they suffer greater necrosis, because a more toxic metabolite is produced. Conversely, if the production of MFO enzymes is inhibited, there is a protective effect. The mechanism by which carbon tetrachloride damages cells is believed to involve metabolism of this compound to a free radical, which causes lipid peroxidation in the cell membrane (Alpers et al. 1968).

Aflatoxin B_1

Although this compound is not of major concern in North America as either an occupational or an environmental toxic substance, there are two reasons for considering aflatoxin B_1: (1) it is among the most toxic natural compounds known; and (2) it is widespread in certain parts of the world and may contribute significantly to liver disease and liver cancer.

Aflatoxin B_1 is a mycotoxin produced by cultures of certain species of *Aspergillus* mold. Traces of aflatoxin B_1 and other fungal toxins are found in many stored foods where molds grow: peanuts, ground nuts, soy beans, and many grains. Acute toxic hepatitis, liver cancer, and cirrhosis are the major conditions attributed to this compound. Major outbreaks of aflatoxin B_1 poisoning are difficult to document, but it is known that an outbreak of acute aflatoxin B_1 toxicity in India in 1974, attributed to contaminated corn, claimed about 400 lives.

Alcohol

Alcohol is still the most common substance of abuse. Approximately 3 percent of the U.S. population can be classified as excessive users of alcohol. Liver disease may develop after only a few months of hard drinking. About a third of heavy drinkers get alcoholic hepatitis, and a tenth get cirrhosis. The threshold dose for significant toxicity is approximately eighty grams (about three ounces) a day over a one-year period (Zimmerman 1978). Liver cell necrosis and the toxic effect is potentiated by poor nutrition.

Halothane

Historically, the hepatotoxicity of anesthetics was recognized since the earliest days of anesthesia, with postsurgical deaths from severe jaundice associated with chloroform poisoning. Recognition of this relationship was complicated by the fact that postsurgical jaundice could also arise from excessive internal hemorrhage, hemolysis, stress, or perhaps infection. A number of chlorinated hydrocarbon anesthetics, such as trichloroethylene, divinyl ether, and tribromomethanol were too hepatotoxic for extensive application.

After World War II, a number of compounds were introduced for anesthesia, including enflurane, methoxyflurane, and halothane, the last rapidly ascending to the position of a safe and reliable compound. Following its introduction in the mid-1950s, there appeared sporadic reports of fatal cases of jaundice. These accumulated slowly, only 7 by 1961, but over 400 by 1966, and about 1 thousand by 1971. There are three important reasons for the slow increase of cases: (1) Halothane is simply not very toxic, and susceptibility is a rarity. (2) Toxicity usually occurs in individuals who have had previous exposure to halothane; hence it was inevitably a number of years before individuals had their second surgical experience. (3) Anesthesiologists and surgeons were so confident of the safety of halothane that postsurgical jaundice was likely to be attributed to some other cause.

Nonetheless, by the early 1970s the conclusion that, in some individuals, repeated exposure to halothane might be fatal became inescapable. Out of thirteen published studies, twelve reported that at least 60 percent of such patients had had opportunity for sensitization to halothane through one previous exposure.

The Kidney

The kidney plays a primary role in several major physiologic functions. As one of the body's main excretory organs, it is the route for removing those waste products that can be made water soluble. Along with the lung, it is responsible for maintaining the acid-base balance of the body within relatively narrow limits. Along with the liver, it is responsible for the homeostatic regulation of the extracellular fluid volume, blood volume, and electrolyte balance. Certain hormones are secreted by the kidney, and others are excreted by it—hence it plays a role in the endocrine regulation of the body, and particularly the regulation of blood pressure.

Unlike the liver, which appears relatively homogeneous to the naked eye, the kidney has readily apparent differentiation. The three major zones are the outer layer or cortex, an inner zone or medulla, and the central pelvis, which receives the urine formed in the kidney and funnels it down the ureter to the bladder.

The functional unit of the kidney is the nephron. It consists of a vascular component, a filtration unit (the glomerulus), and a collection and adjustment unit (the tubules). Freshly oxygenated blood from the renal artery transports to the nephron the myriad products, necessary and also unwanted, upon which the nephron acts. As the artery enters the glomerulus it divides into a fine capillary tuft, which provides a very extensive membrane area through which the watery component of the blood and most small molecules are "filtered." Many substances are "pushed" into the glomerular space by a combination of hydrostatic and osmotic pressure, larger proteins and other molecules remaining in the blood. The capillaries of the tuft now rejoin as an efferent arteriole, which, leaving the glomerulus, plunges downward along the tubular system, where it forms additional capillaries that lie in intimate contact with the tubules (Tisher 1976).

The glomerular filtrate now consists of much of the liquid portion of the blood plus many organic and inorganic molecules. These begin their passage down the descending loop of the tubule, passing out of the cortex, where the glomeruli are found, into the medulla, which comprises most of the tubular elements of the nephron. As the dilute urine passes down the nephron, it runs parallel to the concentrated blood in the efferent arteriolar system. Here the high osmotic pressure of the blood assures that most of the filtered water will pass out of the tubule back into the bloodstream. With it will go many molecules important to life—glucose, sodium, potassium, and so on. At the same time, some molecules too large to be filtered, may be actively secreted by the tubular cells into the urine.

The interchange of materials between the bloodstream and the tubule is a complex interaction of passive and active transport systems, the latter being energy dependent. The final product, urine, exits from the tubular component of each nephron into a collecting duct, which drains it first into the renal pelvis and ultimately into the bladder. This final urine is a highly concentrated product that contains many naturally occurring waste products, a few necessary molecules, and whatever xenobiotics or metabolites have been rendered water soluble. Many drugs, for example, not themselves water soluble, form soluble metabolites that are excreted in the urine. In order for the reabsorption of water to occur, the tubular epithelium must be permeable to water. This is under control of the antidiuretic hormone. Individuals deficient in this pituitary hormone are virtually unable to reabsorb water and, instead of the normal one liter per day of urine, may excrete more than twenty liters.

In summary, then, the nephron contains (1) a vascular component that delivers waste products, returns the reabsorbed or secreted products to the circulation, and provides the necessary oxygen and energy sources for the maintenance of the kidney tissues; (2) a glomerulus, where the bloodstream is filtered and where the urine flow begins; and (3) the tubular complex, where the constitution of the urine is carefully adjusted.

Adjacent to the glomerular cells are a small collection of endocrine cells, the juxtaglomerular apparatus. These cells manufacture the enzyme renin (not to be confused with rennin involved in the digestion of milk). This is the major humoral mechanism influencing blood pressure and electrolyte balance. Renin converts the substrate angiotensinogen into angiotensin I, which is in turn cleaved to produce angiotensin II. This chemical is a potent vasoconstrictor, which in its own right can lead to increased blood pressure. In addition, this stimulates the release of aldosterone from the adrenal gland, and this hormone then acts on the kidney tubule to promote the reabsorption of sodium, which in turn increases the reabsorption of water and also increases blood pressure.

❚ The Kidney as Target Tissue

Several factors render the kidney unusually susceptible to the toxic effects of compounds that reach it (Hook and Hewett 1986):

1. Since it receives 25 percent of the cardiac output each minute, a large amount of any xenobiotic in the bloodstream will quickly reach the kidney, assuring the renal cells a high level of exposure.
2. The kidney has a high rate of aerobic (oxidative) metabolism, which is easily interfered with by a variety of compounds. Since maintenance of renal viability and function is dependent on this metabolism, any inhibition compromises the kidney cells.
3. The kidney cells require abundant energy, particularly for transport of substances across the tubular epithelium.
4. During urine formation, there is a high degree of concentration, such that any toxic substances that are filtered (but not reabsorbed) will reach high concentrations in the tubules.
5. Many toxic compounds are specifically excreted through the kidney.
6. There is a vast membrane area within the kidney, particularly in the glomerulus; this tissue is highly susceptible to processes or substances—particularly certain allergenic compounds—that damage membranes.

Although one may speak of the kidney as a single target, each component of the nephron is a discrete target tissue and each is susceptible to a certain spectrum of nephrotoxins that act with various mechanisms. These mechanisms of nephrotoxicity (Hook and Hewitt 1986) are listed below:

1. The constriction of blood vessels decreases renal blood flow, thereby decreasing glomerular filtration and urine flow. This leads to a buildup of natural and nonnatural toxic waste products in the body. If severe, the reduced blood flow can lead to ischemia and necrosis.
2. The extensive membrane system of the glomerulus is vulnerable to immunotoxic effects, which alter the membrane properties, allowing macromolecules and even red blood cells to pass out of the bloodstream into the urine.
3. Some substances act directly on the kidney tubule, or even on a specific segment of the tubule, affecting specific aspects of secretion and resorption.

Nephrotoxins

Metals, antibiotics, and glycols are toxic to the nephron. The nephrotoxic metals include mercury, cadmium, and lead, each of which has its different propensities and risks.

Mercury has a high affinity for the sulfhydryl groups of proteins and therefore binds avidly to albumin and to the red cell membrane. It accumulates rapidly in the renal cortex, but it is the nephron tubule that suffers, for at appropriate levels of mercury the tubular epithelial cells die and the tubules appear to fall apart (Ganote et al. 1974). If the individual survives, the tubules regenerate, and normal nephron function may resume. The effects of acute and chronic mercury exposure differ somewhat. Interference with tubular function results in failure to reabsorb as much water as usual. Thus mercurials have a significant diuretic function and were long used as the primary diuretic in clinical medicine.

Much of the cadmium in the body is bound to a low-molecular-weight, sulfhydryl-rich protein known as metallothionein. This binding reduces the toxicity of the free cadmium, but excessive buildup results in the release of significant amounts of cadmium by mass action. Unlike mercury, which is rapidly excreted, cadmium is lost from the body only slowly.

Lead acts specifically on the epithelial cells of the proximal component of the tubule. Microscopically, one sees characteristic inclusion bodies within the nuclei, while functionally the transport of molecules such as amino acids is reduced. Mitochondria are damaged, and cells undergo autolysis.

In high doses, the aminoglycoside antibiotics Gentamycin and Kanamycin—which are also ototoxic—bind to renal tissue, accumulate in the tubular cells, and damage the proximal tubule. Tetracyclins also damage the proximal tubule. On rare occasions, penicillins have been implicated in an allergic inflammatory renal disease. Amphoteracin B can damage both proximal and distal tubular cells.

Glycols, which are alcohol compounds, are also associated with severe tubular damage, often accompanied by the formation of oxalate crystals in the tubules. The damage occurs, however, even if crystal formation is blocked.

One unifying pattern in nephrotoxicity is that the glomerular filtration rate (initiation of urine formation) declines. Additional damage may include leakage of fluid out of tubules due to epithelial damage, obstruction of urine flow by cellular debris in the tubule, endothelial swelling, reduced glomerular permeability, and vasoconstriction of the afferent arterioles. Such damage may result in the cessation of urine formation or acute renal failure, with a resultant buildup of toxic constituents in the body.

The Nervous System

The nervous system is unique in its cellular makeup and function. The system is made up of specialized cells, which have both physical and electrical (conduction) functions. The nervous system is divided into two anatomical categories and several functional categories. The anatomical categories are the central and peripheral nervous systems (CNS and PNS, respectively). The functional categories can be distinguished as voluntary versus involuntary and sensory versus motor.

The entire nervous system can be thought of as a very complex electric power grid. The CNS includes the brain, brainstem, and spinal cord. The PNS comprises the nervous tissue emanating from the spinal cord to the organs and tissues of the body. In keeping with the analogy of the electrical grid, there are relay stations in the system, called ganglia. These function to transfer and distribute information (nerve impulses) over specific areas of the grid without affecting other tissues in the same locale. Some nerves, particularly long nerves in the PNS, have an insulation layer (the Schwann cells and myelin sheath), which prevents nerve impulses from "short circuiting" and enhances the rapid conduction of impulses. If this insulation is damaged, the nerve and the tissue it innervates will have reduced function.

Most nerves are bundles of a functional unit called the neuron, which is made up of a cell body with nucleus, an axon or long shaft for transport and distance, and a terminal end of connecting fibers, called dendrites. The dendrites interact with dendrites of other neurons by electrical and chemical communication across defined spaces (synapses).

Nervous tissue, particularly in the brain, requires high levels of oxygen to function properly. Anoxia (lack of oxygen) is a highly toxic state to the nervous system, and any xenobiotic that compromises oxygen flow to the brain can seriously damage the tissue. Chemicals such as cyanide and carbon monoxide are extremely potent, because they induce a marked lack of oxygen particularly in the brain.

Substances that result in neurotoxicity demonstrate amazing site and fiber specificity. The sense organs, the cochlea in the inner ear, and the retina in the eye are examples of highly differentiated nervous tissues that are markedly injured by agents that have little or no effect on other nervous tissue. The cochlea is permanently damaged by loud noises, for example, such as rifle shots, the noise in a steel-manufacturing plant, or a jackhammer at work on a city street. And the retina can be permanently damaged by ultraviolet wavelengths in sunlight. The cochlear nerves are also exquisitively sensitive to certain types of antibiotics, such as Kanamycin and Gentamycin, and the retina is damaged by the antimalarial drug chloroquine (Hobbs et al. 1959; Hawkins 1976).

Other classic neurotoxins include lead, the toxic effects of which have been known for many centuries. It is hypothesized that the downfall of Rome resulted in part from the deleterious effects of lead from aquaduct pipes. Low-level exposure of infants to lead, either by inhalation or ingestion, results in permanent learning disabilities.

The Mad Hatter in Lewis Carroll's *Alice in Wonderland* was thought to represent the manifestations of poisoning by mercury, which was used to make felt in the hat industry early in industrial revolution. Mercury has also been determined to be the cause of Minamata disease in Japan. This tragic disease occurred following mercury pollution of water and fish from an uncontrolled effluent. Mercury compounds have been used to prevent fungal infestation of stored seed, but the use of such seed for food has resulted in severe poisoning in the United States and the Middle East (World Health Organization 1976).

Several drugs and industrial chemicals also have a variety of adverse effects on the nervous system. Some organophosphate pesticides have induced permanent peripheral and central neuropathies after being consumed by cattle and humans. These neuropathies occur in the long nerves of the hind limbs and appear to progress toward the spinal cord (hence the misnomer "dying-back syndrome"). Recent evidence has shown that damage first occurs near the central compartment but is not manifest there. The classic chemical to cause this type of disease is triorthocresyl phosphate (TOCP). Early outbreaks of TOCP poisoning in the United States during Prohibition was termed the "ginger-jake" syndrome and resulted from the consumption of TOCP in ginger beer (Spencer and Schaumberg 1980).

Alcohol has specific effects on the nervous system, which result in permanent damage. These effects can be exacerbated by malnutrition, and the alcohol-malnutrition neurotoxic syndrome is often seen in chronic alcoholic patients. Several widely used neuroleptic drugs have caused a Parkinsonlike syndrome. Recent evidence has shown that this effect can also be induced by some "street" drugs that chemically resemble Demerol. All these drugs block the uptake or release of some normal brain chemicals, a blockage that leads to the Parkinsonlike disease (Heikkila et al. 1984; Langston et al. 1983).

Mention must be made of poisoning by organophosphate insecticides (malathion, parathion), since these are widely used in agriculture. These compounds generally have little permanent effect on the structural integrity of the nervous system but profoundly interfere with the chemical neurotransmitter function of the nervous system, leading to weakness, paralysis, and sometimes death (Hayes 1982).

Many other xenobiotics are neurotoxic, but it is the purpose of this short section to present the reader only with the diversity of the problem.

In addition, neuroscience must unravel the mysteries of neural function before we can understand the neurotoxic manifestations of xenobiotics.

The Reproductive System

Reproductive toxicology is concerned with the effect of toxic substances on reproduction and on the reproductive system. Adverse birth outcomes can result from effects of xenobiotics on the mother, on the developing embryo and fetus, on the father, and on the neonate. The effects on the mother may affect the gametes (eggs and sperm), may arise via the placenta, or may affect accessory organs. In the male, the major adverse reproductive effects occur after insult to the gonads or the secondary sex organs.

Adverse birth outcomes not related to gonadal toxicity generally result from maternal exposure. These adverse outcomes manifest as low birthweights, delayed calcification of bone, spontaneous abortion, and fetal death. Agents or conditions that first alter the health of the mother and consequently affect the fetus are poor nutrition, drugs, alcohol, stress, and dehydration. Agents that directly damage the fetus at doses that do not affect the mother are classified as teratogens. An example is smoking. Few laboratory studies have tested the hypothesis that a combination of toxic compounds exacerbate the effects of a teratogen, but if other toxic effects can be used as models, then exposure to complex mixtures may well contribute to teratogenesis.

Many compounds that are classic teratogens in one species have little or no detectable effects in other species. One of the best examples is the drug Thalidomide. This compound is a marked human teratogen, the administration of which resulted in thousands of seriously malformed babies. However, in laboratory animals, Thalidomide is only slightly toxic to the fetus and in many species does not cause any reproductive effects until maternally toxic doses are administered. Carbaryl, the active ingredient in the insecticide Sevin, is teratogenic in dogs and fetotoxic in rabbits but does not have these effects in monkeys and rats. Aspirin is a potent teratogen in rats but not in mice, monkeys, and dogs. Some epidemiology studies have implicated aspirin as a possible cause of low birth weights, but none of these studies indicate that aspirin is teratogenic in humans.

Gonadal toxicity may or may not result in adverse birth outcomes. If a compound destroys sperm or spermatogenesis, it will inhibit conception but will not result in an adverse birth outcome unless it causes sele chromosomal aberrations resulting in lethal or nondisjunctional diseases, such as trisony-21. Another well-established antispermatogenic compound is the insecticide dibromochloropropane. This chemical, also an alkylating agent, can reach the basal cells of the testes and block the formation of sperm. Several chemicals with estrogenic activity also adversely affect the spermatogenic process, but these compounds generally work through a central mechanism at the level of the hypothalamus or the anterior pituitary. Diethylstilbestrol and estradiol are two examples of the latter case.

The toxicology of the female gonadal system is emerging as one of the most interesting fields in modern toxicology. It was thought for many years that the ovary was well protected from xenobiotics and that adverse effects would be secondary to the toxicity of some other organ. With the advent of oral contraceptives, this line of thinking has changed drastically.

It has been shown in recent years that, besides chemicals with toxic effects on the pituitary-gonadal axis, there are chemicals that are not hormonal but are toxic to the developing ova. Oocyte maturation is an ongoing process, which results in the expulsion of fertilizable ova into the Fallopian tube. During this process, chemicals, including drugs, can be toxic to the ova or the ovarian stroma. Some of the prime examples of ovarian toxicity are seen after chemotherapy with such agents as radiation, cyclophosphamide, and busulfan. Treatment of young women with these agents has resulted in some cases of permanent sterility. There are also reports in the literature that some polycyclic aromatic hydrocarbons directly affect the oocytes. Some of these compounds, such as benzo(a)pyrene and dimethylbenz(a)anthracene, are products of combustion.

Embryos that are severely damaged or that fail to develop are usually aborted early in development by a rather effective quality control system. Certain defects, however, are not incompatible with gestation, and such birth defects are vivid reminders of the vulnerability of reproduction.

The medical and scientific significance of these observations is that the reproductive system and its product, the embryo and fetus, are not spared from the toxicity of xenobiotics but rather may be selected targets for some classes of agents. Toxicologists and developmental biologists must work more closely to understand the mechanisms of action of reproductive toxic substances.

Conclusion

Our knowledge of the biomedical aspects of environmental toxicology is rapidly increasing. There are two major reasons for this. One is the almost headlong pace of advances in basic biological sciences, which provides the underpinning for understanding the mechanisms by which chemical and physical compounds produce their adverse effects. The second is the recognition that such information is an absolute requirement for appropriate regulation of environmental chemicals. It has become more than apparent that the enormous expenditures required for the management of environmental risk warrant mounting a major research effort to understand the basic biomedical effects of xenobiotics (Upton and Goldstein 1984).

References

Alpers, D. H., M. Solin, and K. J. Isselbacher. 1968. The role of lipid peroxidation in the pathogenesis of carbon tetrachloride-induced liver injury. *Molecular Pharmacology* 4:566–73.

Amdur, M. O. 1974. Cummings Memorial Lecture: The long road from Donora. *American Industrial Hygiene Association Journal* 35:589–97.

Amoruso, M. A., J. Ryer, D. Eastson, G. Witz, and B. D. Goldstein. 1986. Estimation of risk of glucose-6-phosphate dehydrogenase deficient red cells to ozone and nitrogen dioxide. *Journal of Occupational Medicine* 28:473–79.

Anderson, E. L., and the Carcinogen Assessment Group of the U.S. Environmental Protection Agency. 1983. Quantitative approaches in use to assess cancer risk. *Risk Analysis* 3:277.

Beauchamp, R. O., Jr., J. S. Bus, J. A. Popp, and C. J. Boreiko. 1983. A critical review of the literature on carbon disulfide toxicity. *CRC Critical Review of Toxicology* 11:159–278.

Coombs, R. R. A., and P. G. H. Gell. 1975. Classification of allergic reactions responsible for clinical hypersensitivity and disease. In *Clinical Aspects of Immunology,* ed. P. G. H. Gell, R. R. A. Coombs, and P. J. Lachman. Philadelphia: Lippincott.

Emmett, E. A. 1986. Toxic responses of the skin. In *Toxicology,* ed. C. D. Klaassen, M. O. Amdur, and J. Doull. New York: Macmillan.

Farber, E., and M. M. Fisher. 1979. *Toxic Injury of the Liver.* New York: Marcel Dekker.

Gallo, M. A., E. J. Hesse, G. J. Macdonald, and T. H. Umbreit. 1986. Interactive effects of estradiol and 2,3,7,8-tetrachlorodibenzo-p-dioxin on hepatic cytochrome P-450 and mouse uterus. *Toxicology Letters* 32:123–32.

Ganote, C. E., K. A. Reimer, and R. B. Jennings. 1974. Acute mercuric chloride nephrotoxicity: An electron microscopic and metabolic study. *Laboratory Investigation* 31:633–47.

Goldstein, B. D. 1983. Clinical hematotoxicity of benzene. *Carcinogenicity and Toxicity of Benzene.* Vol. 4. Princeton: Princeton Scientific Publishers.

———. 1985. Risk assessment and risk management of benzene by the Environmental Protection Agency: Risk quantitation and regulatory policy. Banbury Report. Cold Spring Harbor, N.Y.: Cold Spring Harbor Laboratory.

———. 1986. Critical review of toxic air pollutants—Revised. *Journal of Air Pollution Control Association* 36:367.

Hawkins, J. E. 1976. Drug ototoxicity. In *Handbook of Sensory Physiology,* ed. W. D. Keidel and W. D. Neff. Vol. 5/3. Heidelberg: Springer.

Hayes, W. J. 1982. *Pesticides Studied in Man.* Baltimore: Williams and Wilkins.

Heikkila, R. E., L. Manzino, F. S. Cabbat, and R. C. Duvoisin. 1984. *Nature* 311:467–69.

Hobbs, H. E., A. Sorsky, and A. Friedman. 1959. Retinopathy following chloroquine therapy. *Lancet* 2:478–80.

Hook, J. B., and W. R. Hewitt. 1986. Toxic responses of the kidney. In *Toxicology*, ed. C. D. Klaassen, M. O. Amdur, and J. Doull. New York: Macmillan.

Kensler, T. W., and M. A. Trush. 1984. Role of oxygen radicals in tumor promotion. *Environmental Mutagenisis* 6:593–616.

Klaassen, C. D. 1986. Distribution, excretion, and absorption of toxicants. In *Toxicology*, ed. C. D. Klaassen, M. O. Amdur, and J. Doull. New York: Macmillan.

Langston, J. W., P. Ballard, J. W. Tetrud, and I. Irwin. 1983. *Science* 219:979–80.

Luster, M. I., and J. H. Dean. 1982. Immunological hypersensitivity resulting from environmental or occupational exposure to chemicals: A state of the art workshop summary. *Fundamental Applied Toxicology* 2:327–30.

Marzulli, F. N., and H. I. Maibach. 1980. Contact allergy: Predictive testing of fragrance ingredients in humans by draize and maximization methods. *Journal of Environmental Pathology and Toxicology* 3:235–45.

National Research Council. 1981. Board on Toxicology and Environmental Health, Committee on Indoor Pollutants. *Indoor Pollutants*. Washington, D.C.: National Academy Press.

Plaa, G. L. 1986. Toxic responses of the liver. In *Toxicology*, ed. C. D. Klaassen, M. O. Amdur, and J. Doull. New York: Macmillan.

Plaa, G. L., and B. G. Priestly. 1976. Intrahepatic cholestasis induced by drugs and chemicals. *Pharmacology Reviews* 28:207–73.

Poland, A., and J. C. Knutson. 1982. 2,3,7,8-tetrachlorodibenzo-p-dioxin and related halogenated aromatic hydrocarbons: Examination of the mechanism of toxicity. *American Review of Pharmacology and Toxicology* 22:517–54.

Popper, H., and F. Schaffner. 1959. Drug-induced hepatic injury. *Annals of Internal Medicine* 51:1230–52.

Rappaport, A. M. 1979. Physioanatomical basis of toxic liver injury. In *Toxic Injury of the Liver*, ed. E. Farber and M. M. Fisher. New York: Marcel Dekker.

Recknagel, R. O. 1983. A new direction in the study of carbon tetrachloride hepatotoxicity. *Life Sciences* 33:401–8.

Rudner, E. J., et al. 1973. Epidemiology of contract dermatitis in North America. *Archives of Dermatology* 108:537–40.

Schiff, L. 1982. *Diseases of the Liver*. Philadelphia: Lippincott.

Shupack, J. L. 1977. The skin as a target organ for systemic agents. In *Cutaneous Toxicity*, ed. V. A. Drill and P. Lazar. New York: Academic Press.

Sipes, I. G., and A. J. Gandolfi. 1986. Biotransformation of toxicants. In *Toxicology*, ed. C. D. Klaassen, M. O. Amdur, and J. Doull. New York: Macmillan.

Smith, R. P. 1980. Toxic responses of the blood. In *Casarette and Doull's Toxicology*, ed. J. Doull, C. D. Klaassen, and M. O. Amdur. New York: Macmillan.

Spencer, P. S., and H. H. Schaumberg. 1980. Classification of neurotoxic disease. In *Experimental and Clinical Neurotoxicology*, ed. P. S. Spencer and H. H. Schaumberg. Baltimore: Williams and Wilkins.

Tallarida, R. J., and L. S. Jacob. 1979. *The Dose Response Relation in Pharmacology*. New York: Springer-Verlag.

Taylor, J. S. 1979. Environmental chloracne: Update and overview. *Annals of New York Academy of Sciences* 320:295–307.

Tisher, C. C. 1976. Anatomy of the kidney. In *The Kidney*, ed. B. B. Brenner and F. C. Rector. Philadelphia: W. B. Saunders.

Upton, A. C., and B. D. Goldstein, eds. 1984. *Human Health and the Environment: Some Research Needs.* Report of the Third Task Force for Research Planning in Environmental Health Sciences, U.S. Department of Health and Human Services. Washington, D.C.: Government Printing Office.

U.S. Environmental Protection Agency. 1982. *Air Quality Criteria for Oxides of Nitrogen.* EPA-600/8-82-026. Washington, D.C.: EPA.

Wogan, G. N. 1976. The induction of liver cell cancer by chemicals. In *Liver Cell Cancer,* ed. H. A. Cameron, D. A. Linsell, and G. P. Warwick. Amsterdam: Elsevier.

World Health Organization. 1976. *Environmental Health Criteria: Mercury.* Geneva: WHO.

Zimmerman, H. J. 1978. *Hepatotoxicity.* New York: Appleton-Century-Crofts.

9. Cleanup of Contaminated Sites

NORTON NELSON, SCOTT BAKER, STEVEN P. LEVINE,
LILY YOUNG, JOSEPH O'CONNOR, RONALD D. HILL,
ADEL SAROFIM, AND DAVID GORDON WILSON

Chapter 9 turns to the problem of the cleanup of toxic waste dumps. The chapter begins with the question of whether cleanup is warranted and then addresses the problems and difficulties of cleanup. Nelson and coauthors address a wide range of topics: protection of workers at the toxic waste site; biological degradation of the chemicals; various disposal methods; and recycling. Each discussion is based on an extensive body of technological knowledge.

This chapter is restricted in the sense that it is primarily concerned with the cleanup of disposal sites where waste materials have been deliberately or accidentally placed and where the need may arise to remove, rebury, or dispose of them by other more durable techniques. Sometimes, of course, the sites of contamination may be inadvertent, through spills or illegal dumping. With some exceptions, this chapter is not concerned with cleanup of contaminants polluting the water or air except as that pollution may occur through inadequate disposal. It does approach, in general terms, the metabolic processes in aquatic organisms that lead to the degradation of contaminating chemicals.

Since the passage of the superfund act (U.S. Environmental Protection Agency 1982), national concern over the magnitude of the problem and the reliability of the disposal techniques has steadily mounted. Lack of public confidence in the durability and safety of the disposal practices has led Congress to add significant funds for health-related research.

The section by Scott Baker calls attention to the massive dimensions of the problem both in the quantity of waste and in the number of waste

---

This section was prepared by Norton Nelson.

sites—and hence the necessity to establish priorities. Whether a cleanup of a contaminated site is required depends upon estimates of health risks. The level of contamination often demands risk assessment techniques at the frontier of those available. Thus one of the major research needs is the refinement, in both specificity and sensitivity, of these techniques. Although the emphasis here is on health risk as a basis of determining the need for cleanup, obviously there are factors, such as threats to the natural environment.

Should it be determined that a cleanup is required, then it is clearly imperative to accomplish it in such a way that injury to the cleanup crew is avoided. This is dealt with in the section by Steven Levine, which considers worker safety, reliability of garments and respirators, and transport procedures. Improvement in these tools and procedures is required to ensure safety for the workers without needless complexity.

The next problem is disposal of the contaminated waste. The objective here should always be reduction in the toxicity and in the amount of materials requiring disposal. To this end, a variety of procedures are being used or are being considered. One approach is microbial biodegradation— that is, the use of living systems to reduce the toxicity of contaminants. The section by Lily Young considers these processes. The deliberate use of microorganisms for reducing the toxicity or waste is under active study in many areas, including altering organisms through biotechnology to improve the efficiency of these procedures.

Joseph O'Connor, in the following section, considers the metabolic processes by which aquatic vertebrates and invertebrates alter toxic contaminants. Aquatic contamination may be incidental rather than direct, for example, in runoff of pesticides from agricultural land. In other cases it is deliberate, through the discharge of industrial waste directly into aquatic systems.

The section by Ronald Hill considers both older procedures and newer modifications aimed at improvement. Many of these procedures must be regarded as of uncertain reliability even under the best circumstances. However, they may be the only economically feasible options at this time. These approaches involve landfills of much more sophistication than those used in the past: natural and artificial caverns, deep-well injection, and solidification techniques, including encapsulation and chemical inactivation.

The last section, by Adel Sarofim and David Wilson, deals with the most attractive technology for reduction in toxicity, namely, recycling of a toxic product back into the primary system or into alternate processes that may make practical use of the waste material while at the same time reducing the amount and toxicity of material requiring disposal. This section also deals with incineration, perhaps one of the oldest technologies for reduction of waste materials. It has become increasingly apparent that the demands placed on successful incineration are greater than was earlier supposed. This section reviews the considerations required to ensure maximal destruction of toxic materials without, in the process, generating new toxicants.

Clearly, the objective among these options is the eventual elimination of materials requiring disposal, namely, such complete reuse that only nonhazardous materials remain; it is to be hoped that, in some cases, such options may have economic utility. We are, however, still a long way from such a satisfactory goal.

Health Appraisal and the Need to Clean Up

More than six-billion tons of waste are produced in the United States each year, including agricultural, commercial, industrial, and domestic waste (figure 9.1). While problems of pollution from all sources and in all environmental compartments are significant, it is those problems associated with hazardous waste, largely land based, that have most recently captured society's attention because of emerging understanding of their

Figure 9.1. Hazardous waste generated in the United States each year.

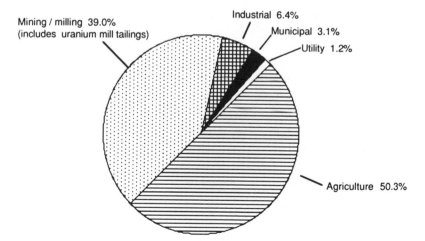

Mining / milling 39.0%
(includes uranium mill tailings)

Industrial 6.4%

Municipal 3.1%

Utility 1.2%

Agriculture 50.3%

Note: Excluded high-level radioactive waste. (*Source:* U.S. Environmental Protection Agency 1984a.)

This section was prepared by Scott Baker.

size, cost to remediate, and potential threat to public health and the environment. Years of disposal practices, both irresponsible and those carried out by the standards of the time, have left a burdensome legacy needing costly and complex cleanup.

We need to clean up existing hazardous wastes and control the disposal of newly generated wastes because of their potential health threat. Accordingly, the common goal of governmental organizations like the Environmental Protection Agency (EPA), the Agency for Toxic Substances and Disease Registry (ATSDR), and the National Institute for Environmental Health Sciences (NIEHS) is protection of public health and the environment from the potential dangers posed by hazardous waste. These organizations attempt to determine the relationship between exposure and health for existing hazardous waste sites so that the federal agencies responsible for cleaning up wastes can assess the work and the priority to be given to each site.

▌Appraising a Waste Site

The need to clean up a given hazardous waste site is based on several factors: the degree of contamination (extent, medium, the number of chemicals at the site, and the geographical area of coverage); the likelihood of spread; the likelihood or degree of human exposure; the intrinsic toxicity of chemicals at the site; and the overall health threat to potentially exposed populations (figure 9.2). While the focus of this section is on the health threat posed by hazardous waste, a composite of precedent conditions as illustrated in figure 9.2 determines the degree of this threat and the priority for cleanup.

Assessing the need to clean up a site requires collecting, cataloguing, and appraising data. Because much of this requires intervention by government on behalf of the public welfare, laws, regulations, and procedures have been established to systematize and record all events that occur between the reporting of a possible hazardous waste site and the decision to

Figure 9.2. Factors determining the need to clean up.

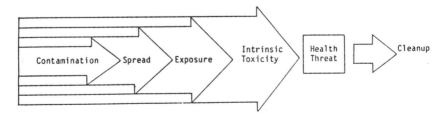

clean it up. The enabling legislative authority for government to clean up hazardous waste sites is embodied in the superfund program, established by Congress in the Comprehensive Environmental Response, Compensation, and Liability Act (CERCLA) (U.S. EPA 1982). The government's guide in its exploration of potentially hazardous sites is the National Contingency Plan. The plan delineates which authorities are responsible for abandoned or uncontrolled waste sites and defines criteria and methods for removal of wastes or for remedial response. The plan limits long-term, superfund-financed cleanup actions to sites included on the National Priorities List. This list designates the worst of the nation's known sites contaminated with hazardous substances.

The overall assessment starts with a report to a local, state, or federal authority of possible contamination, triggering a succession of activities, which may lead to a decision to clean up the reported site (figure 9.3). The discovery list maintained by EPA contains some 26-thousand reported sites. These sites are subjected to a preliminary assessment to ascertain the size of the site, contaminating parties, types and quantities of waste, local hydrological and meteorological conditions, and environmental impact. At the ensuing site inspection, evidence of contamination, such as effects on vegetation, is gathered, along with soil and water samples for laboratory analysis. Inspectors determine the possibility of contamination of the surrounding environment.

With this information in hand, sites are ranked for hazard according to type, quantity, and toxicity of waste, the number of people potentially exposed, the likely pathways for exposure, the vulnerability of underlying aquifers, and other relevant factors. If the hazard ranking is high enough to place the site on the National Priorities List, a carefully designed field

Figure 9.3. Steps in cleaning up a hazardous waste site.

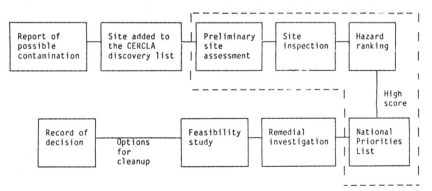

Note: Hatched area denotes activities related to health appraisal.

study—a remedial investigation—is conducted to provide precise data on the types and quantities of waste through extensive sampling and analyses of waste, soil type, water drainage patterns, and environmental or health threats. Cleanup approaches are then identified in a feasibility study, comparing their relative effectiveness and cost. The appropriate cleanup method is then selected and carried out.

The Hazard Ranking System (HRS) determines the eligibility for site placement on the National Priorities List. However, each state is allowed to designate one state priority site, regardless of its ranking. The HRS was designed to help fulfill the superfund requirement that at least four-hundred high-priority sites be identified. This scoring system allows priorities to be made among several thousand widely varying hazardous waste sites. As of June 1986, the National Priorities List contained 888 sites.

The ranking system does not determine if cleanup is possible or worthwhile or the amount of cleanup needed. Rather, it measures the relative severity of the problems at the site and the likelihood and potential magnitude of exposure to hazardous substances for humans and sensitive environments. Preliminary assessments and site inspections provide information for the system, which then produces three scores that measure the possibility of (1) hazardous substances spreading from the site through ground water, surface water, or air, and reaching populated areas; (2) people coming in direct contact with hazardous substances; and (3) fire or explosion caused by hazardous substances. The second and third scores are used to identify sites that need removal actions. Only the first score is used to place sites on the National Priorities List and is generally called the HRS score.

The Hazard Ranking System was not designed to distinguish between the risks presented by two sites with similar scores, but it is a meaningful indicator of large differences in risk. The scores are weighted to increase those given to sites that threaten densely populated areas, that have a greater likelihood of exposure to the affected population, or that contain large volumes of waste. Sites are placed on the National Priorities List only if they receive a ranking score of 28.5 or more (on a scale of zero to 100), except when designated by a state as a priority site regardless of the score (U.S. Congress 1985).

▌ Appraising Human Health Risks

One of the most important steps in evaluating a hazardous waste site problem is determining the effect the site has on human health. Detailed health considerations in the cleanup investigation occur principally during the remedial investigation; the evidence is cursorily evaluated in the preliminary site assessment and the site inspection. Although it is apparent that hazardous waste sites can endanger human health, there are medical and scientific uncertainties concerning the relationship between exposure to toxic substances and adverse health effects. Establishing links between this exposure and specific adverse health consequences involves the assessment of rapidly changing technical and medical data.

To help resolve this issue, the superfund act directed the Department of Health and Human Services to carry out various health-related studies on the relationship between toxic substances and illness and to develop national registries of persons exposed to toxic substances and who have serious diseases and illnesses. The studies include laboratory projects and chemical testing to determine relationships between exposure to toxic substances and illness. The exposure registries are being established by ATSDR at hazardous waste sites where there is a strong indication of substantial human exposure, with the hope of establishing a sound scientific basis for investigating the possible correlation between exposure and health effects among persons living near the sites.

Within the framework presented in figure 9.3, EPA and ATSDR have different but somewhat overlapping roles in the health assessments collectively factored into the decision-making process. ATSDR uses a hazard assessment approach, while EPA relies on a more broadly based approach, which includes a health risk assessment obtained by multiplying the degree of hazard by the size of the population exposed. From a management perspective, the two health assessments can reinforce each other in the event of cleanup, minimizing both potential and immediate health impacts. The approaches use monitoring, modeling, exposure, hazard, and dose-response data to obtain health assessments.

The ATSDR approach provides a means for making cleanup decisions based on the potential public health impact. As a result, its site-specific analysis and short-term and immediate orientation places a premium on the present population. (ATSDR's data collection and registries will provide a scientific knowledge base for future long-term studies.) EPA extends the public health assessment to an expression of risk, which, along with environmental concerns, cleanup costs, and institutional controls, determines the extent of cleanup needed, the technically feasible choices, and the best approach to restoring the site. As such, EPA's focus is on long-term protection of populations residing in the area of a site now or in the future. These two approaches combined give a conservative estimate of public health risk, affording both immediate protection for the existing population and long-term protection through stipulations intended to assure that no further cleanup will be necessary.

The health hazard appraisal conducted by ATSDR can include as many as four activities—a general health advisory, a pilot study, a more detailed health study, and a registry; these are conducted heirarchically, depending on the degree of concern about a given site and the need for detailed analyses.

The health advisory contains three elements: (1) an expression of the inherent hazard of each compound present at the site, including its explosivity, flammability, radioactivity (alpha, gamma, including radon daughters), irritancy, and toxicity (carcinogenicity, mutagenicity, or teratogenicity); (2) a determination of the potential for human exposure through ingestion, inhalation, and dermal contact from air, water, and soil at the site and through bioconcentration in the food chain; and (3) a characterization of the population potentially at risk, with consideration of such factors as age, dietary habits, and child-bearing status.

The pilot study includes preliminary estimates of human uptake of chemicals of concern in individuals most likely to have received the highest exposure, definition of a boundary around the population potentially at risk, and a community survey for behavioral effects and the presence of specific symptoms or diseases. The assumptions about exposure pathways may be altered when closer scrutiny reveals that there is biotransformation of the waste to metabolites. If concern is high, a confirmatory procedure may be conducted to look for evidence of uptake (residues, biomarkers, or clinical signs) in a group presumed to have had high exposure.

An ensuing detailed study includes a more comprehensive laboratory determination of exposure and uptake, case-control or cohort epidemiologic studies, and organ-specific tests for such health endpoints as chromosomal abnormalities, neurobehavioral effects, dysfunction of the immune system, pulmonary effects, and kidney function.

A registry for long-term observation, to determine whether a relationship exists between exposure to a contaminated site and health, can then be established. The registry can aid in follow-up screening for cancers or such reproductive outcomes as low birth weights, spontaneous abortions, infant mortality, birth defects, and developmental disabilities. Such a registry should indicate if a cleanup action is effective in reducing health impacts. It can also serve as a preventive tool by foretelling serious disease (cancer cells in the urine may forecast bladder cancer). The health advisory and pilot study contribute to EPA's hazard-ranking score. Should the chemical make the National Priorities List, a more detailed health study conducted by ATSDR may be necessary for the remedial investigation.

Since enactment of CERCLA in 1980, two schools of thought have emerged on the most appropriate approach to assessing the need for cleaning up hazardous waste. One emphasizes site-specific health and exposure considerations. The second emphasizes engineering parameters such as environmental monitoring, chemical migration patterns, and soil chemistry. Each approach may lead to different conclusions about the need for cleanup. In cases where, despite high health hazard, engineering evaluations estimate the potential for exposure (and therefore risk) as low, more meaningful indications of risk can be obtained by considering pathways of waste movement from source to surrounding populations. The end result is a greater interplay between the environmental engineers, who are concerned with the impacts of the waste site on the environment as it affects people indirectly, and the health experts, who are concerned with the waste site as it affects people directly.

The level of cleanup sought has a direct bearing on the extent to which cleanup will protect public health, and conversely the thresholds used in health appraisals have a direct bearing on the level of cleanup sought. In the absence of superfund cleanup standards, standards for other environmental laws are applied to waste sites. While these cover many chemicals, they do not address all substances and conditions found at hazardous waste sites. There is currently no consensus on appropriate site cleanup, owing largely to the fact that little information exists on how hazardous waste sites affect human health.

Research is needed to develop sentinel toxicity surveillance systems for rapid identification of potential human health risks at waste sites. Additional toxicity studies are needed to assess the hazard potential of priority chemicals at waste sites, as well as the health effects of chemical mixtures. To provide timely and less costly results, early-detection methodologies need to be developed for human health effects, along with more sensitive tests for monitoring humans in epidemiology studies.

The Health and Safety at Hazardous Waste Sites

The single most basic problem in industrial hygiene at hazardous waste sites is the unknown composition of the materials being handled (Levine and Martin 1985). This is almost always true for drum and tank materials at superfund sites and is frequently true at licensed disposal sites. The consequences of this lack of knowledge, for both the on-site worker and the surrounding community, are that the following cannot be readily chosen: (1) personal protective equipment (PPE) for worker protection; (2) air-monitoring methods for worker breathing zones, work areas/unit processes, and the site fenceline and downwind communities; (3) medical surveillance strategies for site workers and the potentially exposed communities.

These questions and related, equally important, questions are dealt with in a number of publications (Levine and Martin 1985; U.S. Department of Health and Human Services 1984, 1985; and Schwope et al. 1981).

This section was prepared by Steven P. Levine.

The interagency guidance manual (U.S. DHHS 1985) provides an overview for each of the subject areas discussed in the other reference materials. The information in this document represents the most recent consensus of scientific opinions.

This section first discusses the question of the perception of hazard at hazardous waste sites and at the "traditional" workplace. Second, reasons are given for the lack of knowledge of the contents of drums and tanks. Then, the questions of PPE, air monitoring, and medical surveillance are discussed and related to information given in the interagency guidance manual and other reference documents.

▌ Perceived Hazard

Equally important to the technical questions of personnel and community protection at hazardous waste sites is the question of perspective and perceived danger. There is no fundamental reason why a hazardous waste site cannot be viewed as a collection of unit processes (Cralley and Cralley 1983; Shreve and Brink 1977). Certainly, if the traditional industrial hygiene triad of recognition, evaluation, and control can be applied to such diverse workplaces as metal foundries, phosphorus furnaces, and pesticide intermediate plants (U.S. Department of Health, Education, and Welfare 1976; Olishifski and McElroy 1977), the same principles can be applied to hazardous waste sites. Traditional workplaces have generally been more hazardous than hazardous waste sites. Indeed, the recent Bhopal incident resulted in far more serious consequences than has any incident at a hazardous waste site (*Chemical Engineering News* 1985; Union Carbide 1985; *New York Times* 1985).

However, "several factors distinguish the hazardous waste site environment from other occupational situations involving hazardous substances. One important factor is the uncontrolled condition of the site. . . . Another factor is the large variety and number of substances that may be present at the site. . . . The combination of . . . these conditions results in a working environment that is characterized by numerous and varied hazards which:

—May pose an immediate danger to life and health.
—May not be immediately obvious or identifiable.
—May vary according to the location on site and the task being performed.
—May change as site activities progress (U.S. DHHS 1985).

▌ Materials Analysis

One of the basic problems in industrial hygiene at hazardous waste sites is that the materials being handled are of unknown composition

(Levine and Martin 1985). The question is, why is this the case when analysis methods for environmental samples are well established. In order to answer this question, an understanding of the processes involved in hazardous waste cleanup should be reviewed. Briefly, one of the principal unit processes at a hazardous waste site is that of drum bulking (U.S. DHHS 1985), at which drums and tanks that are excavated or otherwise found on a site are brought to a central staging area. The drums are opened and sampled and then moved to a second staging area until the results of the laboratory analysis are received. At that point, all wastes are recontainerized in compatible chemical groups, since mixtures of uncompatible hazardous wastes have the potential for fire, explosion, violent reaction, and the release of toxic dusts, mists, fumes, and gases. Disposal of these bulked wastes is far more cost effective than disposal of individual drums. Incompatible wastes, however, must be segregated rather than bulked.

Chemical compatibility testing is not as extensive as gas chromatography–mass spectrometry (GC-MS) or inductively coupled plasma emission spectrometry (ICP). Rather, chemical compatibility testing follows a flow chart scheme, which ultimately classifies the material into categories such as acid, base, organic, chlorinated organic, oxidizer, sulfide-cyanide, and so on. The objectives of compatibility testing are (1) to allow the bulking of wastes without generating an explosion or releasing hazardous gases and (2) to divulge enough about the characteristics of the waste to complete the shipping manifest.

Compatibility testing accomplishes these objectives, but its use from an industrial-environmental standpoint is limited. For example, a drum categorized after compatibility testing as nonhalogenated organic may contain the slightly toxic chemical toluene, the moderately toxic chemical benzaldehyde, the highly toxic chemical parathion, or a mixture of all three.

Ideally, the two objectives of compatibility testing should be met in about a day and at a minimal cost. An on-site mobile laboratory that can analyze 100 to 200 samples a day with GC-MS or ICP would take far longer than a day to analyze a ten-thousand-drum site, with an average of two phases per drum. And the cost, between $100 and $1,000 per sample, would result in an analytical cost for the site in the range of millions of dollars. Both such cost and such turnaround time are unacceptable. In addition, these complete analysis methods may fall short in actual performance. GC-MS, the most frequently used method, does not detect labile, polar, or high-molecular weight (polymeric) materials. A paint sludge, for example, may be misidentified even after extensive analysis.

Thus compatibility testing procedures should be carefully chosen and followed (see Levine and Martin 1985; U.S. DHHS 1984; Puskar et al. 1986; U.S. Environmental Protection Agency 1984c, 1985a).

| Personal Protective Equipment, Air Monitoring, and Medical Surveillance

The interagency guidance manual (U.S. DHHS 1985) summarizes the subject of personal protective equipment:

> Use of PPE is required by OSHA regulations in 29 CFR 1910 and reinforced by U.S. EPA regulations in 40 CFR 300 which include requirements for all private contractors working on Superfund sites to conform to applicable OSHA provisions and any other . . . requirements deemed necessary by the . . . agency overseeing the activities.
>
> No single combination of protective equipment . . . is capable of protecting against all hazards. Thus, PPE should be used in conjunction with other protective methods. The use of PPE can itself create significant worker hazards, such as heat stress, physical and psychological stress, and impaired vision, mobility, and communication. In general, the greater the level of PPE, the greater are the associated risks. . . . Over-protection as well as under-protection can be hazardous and should be avoided. . . .
>
> A written PPE program should be established for work at hazardous waste sites. . . . A comprehensive PPE program should include hazard identification; medical monitoring; environmental surveillance; selection, use, maintenance, and decontamination of PPE; and training.

Selection of PPE can best be accomplished by reference to the selection guides from the National Institute for Occupational Safety and Health (NIOSH) and American Conference of Governmental Industrial Hygienists (see U.S. DHHS 1984 and Schwope et al. 1981; for summaries and extensions of these guides, see Levine and Martin 1985 and U.S. DHHS 1985).

Schwope et al. (1981) developed the permeation testing protocol used by the American Society for Testing and Materials and NIOSH for PPE garments and gloves. All PPE materials must undergo appropriate testing to the expected challenge chemicals. The problem at a hazardous waste site, of course, is that the challenge chemical is not known (even though informed guesses can be made). Furthermore, the success of decontamination procedures cannot be quantitatively determined (although U.S. DHHS 1985 recommends optimal decontamination procedures). These facts almost force the use of disposable garments, which, at present, must be made of Saranex-Tyvek. Schwope thoroughly characterized this garment material in a manner not yet available for any other disposable fabric.

Turpin developed the Environmental Protection Agency's standard operating procedures for the designation of safe work practices, air monitoring, and PPE at hazardous waste sites (U.S. EPA 1984c). All the procedures are based on levels of protection, with level A being the highest level and level D being used when minimal protection is required. These protocols were refined and extended in the interagency guidance manual (U.S. DHHS 1985). A significant change was the modification of the requirement that airborne total hydrocarbon values be used as criteria for choice of PPE. A summary of this revised protocol is given in table 9.1.

This protocol became the standard used at all hazardous waste sites simply by default. Turpin developed it in "real time," when it was sorely needed. Had he waited for the normal rulemaking process, we might still have no protocol.

The assumption in his protocol is that a full-face respirator (for acid

Table 9.1. Protocols for the four levels of protection for personal protective equipment

Level and Hazard Criteria	Personal Protective Equipment

Level A
  Possibility of more than 19.5% O_2
  Possibility of immediate danger to life and health
  Harmful or unidentified vapor, gas, or splash
  High-hazard chemical
  High splash potential
  Confined space
	Fully encapsulated garment; self-contained breathing apparatus (pressure demand)

Level B
  Possibility of more than 19.5% O_2
  Possibility of immediate danger to life and health
  Harmful or unidentified vapor, gas, or splash
	Impermeable garment; self-contained breathing apparatus (pressure demand)

Level C Possibility of more than 19.5% O_2	Impermeable garment; full-face respirator for particulates, acid gas, and organic vapor
Level D Less than 19.5% O_2	Hard hat, safety shoes, and so on

Source: U.S. Department of Health and Human Services 1985.

gas, organic vapor, and particulates) and a five-minute self-contained air
escape pack is inadequate for use by workers at a hazardous waste site,
since there is almost never a guarantee that conditions of immediate danger to life and health will not occur. Since real-time air-monitoring methods are at present inadequate for speciation and quantitation, air-monitoring data must be developed by nonreal time methods (Levine et al. 1985a,
1985b; Levine and Martin 1985), which do not provide the information
necessary to protect the workers on a daily basis. This forces the use of a
self-contained breathing apparatus, which cuts down on productivity and,
in combination with the protective garment, results in a high probability of
the workers suffering from heat stress (Levine and Martin 1985; U.S.
DHHS 1984, 1985).

Furthermore, the lack of real-time air-monitoring data forces the use
of highly conservative guidelines for community evacuation in case of an
airborne release. Unfortunately, the decision to evacuate a community
from the downwind area of a hazardous waste site may be made on the
basis of community activist sentiment rather than on any sound air-monitoring data. Since one of the main stumbling blocks to adopting an alternative to the standard operating procedure is the total lack of knowledge of
the contents of the drums and tanks, a remedy might be to significantly
increase the analytical capability at each site. At present, the only significant capability on site is a mobile laboratory for compatibility testing. It
may well be that it is cost effective to field a second mobile laboratory,
equipped with a gas chromatograph, a mass spectrometer, and a Fourier
transform infrared spectroscope (FTIR). The presence of two mobile laboratories, one for compatibility testing and one for more extensive analysis,
might yield the critical mass of skilled analytical manpower on a site to
allow for near real-time air monitoring. For example, GCs equipped with
gas sampling loops, calibrated for a variety of compounds and compound
classes, and equipped with flame ionization detector, electron capture detector, nitrogen-phosphorus detector, or flame photometric detector,
could be placed at appropriate unit processes within a site. Lines for transmission of computer information (RS232) could be run to the mobile laboratory for monitoring, data collection, or alarm. Similarly, a high-resolution FTIR (Herget and Levine 1986) or a tandem mass spectrometer–mass
spectrometer system (MS-MS) could be used for this purpose. Certainly,
small alarm devices, such as the Drager/Ecolyzer series 100 compound-
specific monitor or the GCA Mini-RAM dust monitor, could be properly
calibrated and placed on workers for continuous use.

Lack of knowledge of the contaminants in the air and of the materials
in drums and tanks also affects the design of a medical surveillance program for on-site workers and members of the surrounding and downwind

community. The interagency task group (U.S. DHHS 1985) came to the following conclusions:

> A medical program is essential to assess and monitor workers health and fitness both prior to employment and in the course of work; to provide emergency and other treatment as needed; and to keep accurate records for future reference. In addition, OSHA recommends a medical evaluation for employees required to wear a respirator. . . . Information from a site medical program may also be used to conduct future epidemiological studies; to adjudicate claims; to provide evidence in litigation; and to report workers' medical conditions. . . .
>
> A medical program should be developed for each site based on the specific needs, location, and potential exposures of employees. . . . The program should be designed by an experienced occupational health physician . . . in conjunction with the Site Safety Officer. . . .
>
> A . . . medical program should provide the following components:
> —Surveillance
> —Treatment
> —Recordkeeping
> —Program review.

Designing a medical surveillance program for the site workers and for the community is a difficult task (Levine and Martin 1985; U.S. DHHS 1985; Melius and Halperin 1982). In traditional industrial hygiene practice, medical screening is based on the known toxic effects of specific chemicals, on the assumption that the type and duration of exposure to those substances are known. Even then, many surveillance programs are based on unvalidated screening protocols.

For both on-site workers and the community, the identity, duration and route of exposure are unknown. Therefore, there is little rational basis for defining a surveillance protocol. Despite these factors, Melius and Halperin (1982) suggested the following steps for on-site workers, which are outlined only briefly here:

1. The focus of preemployment screening should be on determining if the worker is physically fit for the assigned work. Since the worker will be wearing extensive PPE and subject to heat stress, the principal focus should be on the pulmonary and cardiovascular system. In addition, it may be desirable to perform baseline medical screening and biological monitoring tests, although there are no clear guidelines for prescribing specific tests. Monitoring tests are described, along with the option of archiving blood samples for analysis after on-site work is

completed in case the worker is later suspected of having been exposed to certain chemicals (see also U.S. DHHS 1985).

2. The frequency and content of periodic and postemployment screening of hazardous waste workers will depend on the nature of their work.

One of Melius and Halperin's conclusions is that "any testing employed be specific for the possible medical effects of the worker's exposure. The application of a large batch of medical tests in an attempt to cover all of the possible medical effects of the multitude of potential exposures facing the worker is not very useful."

▌ Conclusions

1. The industrial hygiene problems encountered at hazardous waste sites can be solved by using the traditional triad of recognition, evaluation, and control for the unit processes in use at such sites. Evaluation is the single most difficult step, since the identity of the materials in drums and tanks at these sites is unknown.
2. The methods of analysis now used for waste chemicals at hazardous waste sites are compatibility testing and GC-MS testing, which are inadequate for the task. New methods may help to remedy this problem.
3. Methods of analysis used for on-site and fenceline air monitoring are also inadequate, since there are no available methods that can be used for both speciation and quantitation in real time. Experimental methods such as MS-MS and high-resolution FTIR may soon be available at these sites.
4. The consequences of the lack of adequate analysis and monitoring methods are (1) PPE are overly protective, leading to the potential for heat stress, decreased productivity, and related problems; (2) medical surveillance cannot be adequately defined because of a lack of knowledge of the types of chemicals and of the duration and route of exposure of workers and the community. Nevertheless, limited guidelines can be provided for a surveillance program.

Microbial Biodegradation

One of the major differences between macroorganisms and microorganisms in the metabolism of toxic chemicals is that microorganisms have the capability to mediate the complete mineralization of many toxic or-

This section was prepared by Lily Young.

ganic chemicals to carbon dioxide and water. This is largely because, notwithstanding their toxicity, many of the toxic compounds can serve as the carbon source for growth and energy for microorganisms, which is not the case with other organisms. This capability has long been exploited for the treatment of municipal and industrial wastes in facilities designed to optimize the microbially mediated processes of biodegradation.

The same degradative capacity used for treatment of wastes is present in the environment. However, conditions are subject to environmental variability and are frequently not ideal with regard to such factors as pH, temperature, oxidation-reduction potential, adsorption, solubility, immobilization, essential nutrients, and competition. Nonetheless, it is well accepted that much of the restorative capacity of the environment following chemical contamination is dependent on microbial activity.

Once a chemical is released into the environment, it can be removed by several means. For example, evaporation favors low-boiling-point compounds, diluting such contaminants and transferring much of them into a different environmental compartment. Dissolution favors soluble compounds, which are generally of low molecular weight (mw), since solubility is inversely proportional to mw and serves to dilute them. Chemical-physical degradation can decompose some compounds, for example, those that are particularly sensitive to light and air. For the most part, however, microbiologically mediated degradation is the major means of removal of contaminant organic chemicals from the environment.

Metabolism by higher organisms, as discussed elsewhere in this section, is largely mediated by liver enzymes and serves a very different function. Namely, metabolites are formed from toxic chemicals largely to make them more soluble or more reactive and, hence, more mobile. Metabolism, then, is a detoxification strategy to eliminate toxic chemicals from the body. In fact, the metabolism of many hydrocarbons by fungi and algae are mediated by biochemical mechanisms more closely related to those of mammalian systems than to those of bacteria, which are able to carry out a complete mineralization.

▌ Microbiologically Mediated Degradation Strategies

Polynuclear Aromatic Hydrocarbons

The biochemistry of aerobic metabolism of a wide variety of toxic aromatic compounds has been well documented (Cerniglia 1984; Gibson and Subramanian 1984; Gibson 1976; Colwell and Sayler 1978; Fewson 1981). Recognizing that there can be specific differences in metabolism, depending on the species and on the compound, some of the salient features of aromatic hydrocarbon metabolism can be illustrated with two examples, benzene and phenanthrene.

As illustrated in figure 9.4, oxygen is required as a reactant in the metabolic pathway for benzene catabolism, in addition to it being used as an electron acceptor for respiration. The intermediate, a cisdihydrodiol, is uniquely different from the transdihydrodiols formed from benzene by both mammalian and fungal systems. In fact, formation of the transdihydrodiol intermediate is preceded by that of benzene epoxide, a highly reactive structure, which can undergo several transformations, including formation of a glutathione conjugate and covalent binding to nucleic acids and proteins. This latter set of reactions is thought to be associated with genotoxicity (see Cerniglia 1984). In addition, mammalian and fungal systems do not mediate aromatic ring fission. By dehydrogenation of the cisdihydrodiol, on the other hand, bacteria mediate the formation of catechol, which then serves as the precursor for ring fission, also requiring oxygen as a reactant. After ring fission, further metabolism then yields

Figure 9.4. Alternative pathways utilized by mammals and bacteria for oxidation of benzene.

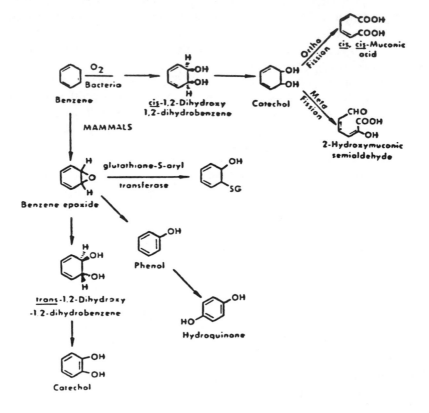

metabolites such as acetate, succinate, or pyruvate, which are readily incorporated into known metabolic pathways leading to carbon dioxide or other cellular compounds.

Phenanthrene metabolism by bacteria proceeds along a parallel though more protracted pathway. Oxygen again is a reactant in the formation of a cisdihydrodiol, which is followed by the sequential fission of one ring at a time of the polynuclear aromatic hydrocarbon (PAH) structure. Pathway differences are apparent, depending on the bacterial species. Intermediates released during fission of each of the rings are then further metabolized by constitutive metabolic pathways, as with benzene.

The higher molecular weight PAHs are less readily metabolized by bacteria. This is thought to be, at least in part, a function of insolubility, such that the compounds are not readily available to the bacteria, and a function of size, which inhibits transport across the cell membrane. For example, although several cisdihydrodiol intermediates have been documented, the metabolism of benzo(a)pyrene by bacteria is not well understood (Cerniglia 1984).

Chlorinated Aromatic Compounds

It is generally agreed that the chlorinated aromatic ring is more resistant to microbial biodegradation than the nonchlorinated structure. For compounds such as polychlorinated biphenyls, the greater the degree of chlorine substitution, the less biodegradable the compound (Gibson and Subramanian 1984; Reineke 1984). In general, chlorine substitution impairs the activity of the usual ring metabolism enzymes by, for example, impeding the electrophilic attack of the dioxygenases and interfering with oxygen binding (Knackmuss 1981). Nonetheless, chlorinated aromatic compounds are subject to both aerobic and anaerobic metabolism by bacteria, and for many compounds complete mineralization occurs.

Two approaches have emerged with regard to biodegradation of this group of chemical contaminants by bacteria. In some cases, specific enzyme systems have developed in response to the chlorinated compounds, while in other cases, they may be fortuitously attacked by enzymes involved in the metabolism of related nonhalogenated structures.

Under aerobic conditions, studies with pure and mixed cultures have shown several strategies for metabolism, some more complete than others. For example, many halogenated aromatic compounds are partially oxidized to a corresponding halogenated catechol. The latter is not further metabolized (figure 9.5), most likely because it is a potent inhibitor of catechol dioxygenase (Gibson and Subramanian 1984).

If ring fission does take place, in most cases the halogen remains attached and is released in a later step in the pathway. After dechlorination takes place, complete metabolism of the ring fission metabolites can pro-

Figure 9.5. Reactions involved in the oxidation of halogenated benzenes by *Pseudomonas putida*.

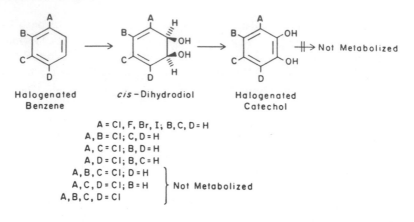

Halogenated Benzene   *cis*-Dihydrodiol   Halogenated Catechol

A = Cl, F, Br, I; B, C, D = H
A, B = Cl; C, D = H
A, C = Cl; B, D = H
A, D = Cl; B, C = H
A, B, C = Cl; D = H
A, C, D = Cl; B = H   } Not Metabolized
A, B, C, D = Cl

ceed through known metabolic pathways. In some instances, dechlorination of the aromatic structure under aerobic conditions occurs before ring fission, after which ring fission then can proceed in the usual manner (Reineke 1984). Hence there are mechanisms for the partial and complete oxidation of chlorinated and other halogenated aromatic structures by microorganisms.

Polychlorinated biphenyls (PCBs) are widely recognized toxic contaminants, which appear to be highly persistent in the environment. Laboratory studies with microbial populations, however, indicate that substantial degradation can take place. Commercial PCBs are a mixture of congeners with one to five chloro substituents on each of the rings. Degradation is highly structure dependent.

In general, degradation decreases with increased chlorination; PCBs with unequal distribution of chloro substituents are more readily metabolized with the attack directed at the least substituted ring (see figure 9.6); the 2,4-dichloro substitutions are readily subject to meta ring fission; the orthosubstituted congeners tend to be highly resistant to degradation; and major differences between different bacterial species are apparent (Safe 1984a; Chatterjee and Chakrabarty 1981). These laboratory studies appear to confirm the observation that the more highly chlorinated PCBs accumulate in the environment (Safe 1984b). Several bacterial strains have recently been isolated that can metabolize the highly chlorinated congeners, and they may prove to be useful in the treatment of contaminated areas (Unterman et al. 1985; Bopp et al. 1986). Others have isolated strains highly active on Arochlor 1260 and have used them successfully in activated sludge treatment of up to 400 ppm PCB (Kopecky 1984).

Figure 9.6. Metabolic sequences for the degradation of polychlorinated biphenyls by *Alcaligenes* sp. Y42 and *Acinetobacter* sp. P6.

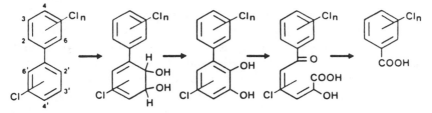

Note: n=1-4. (*Source:* Young 1984.)

The chlorinated dibenzo-p-dioxins—present at Love Canal, N.Y., Times Beach, Mo., and Seveso, Italy—are particularly persistent and highly toxic. TCDD, the tetrachloro-substituted dioxin, is extremely toxic and microbiological studies thus far indicate that little, if any, biodegradation takes place (Philippi et al. 1981). This is an example of a synthetic chemical for which there is no biologically produced related compound and for which there are apparently no enzyme systems capable of metabolizing it.

Anaerobic Environments

If rapid degradation does not occur in the aerobic regions of the environment, contaminant chemicals can then enter the anaerobic zones. Anaerobic conditions commonly exist in soils and sediments. In addition, anaerobic degradation processes are important for the design of sewage digesters and municipal landfills. Of current concern is the increasing contamination of groundwater sources by chemicals from known and unknown disposal sites. Deep aquifers are generally oxygen depleted, while many aquifers have regions of little or no oxygen (Bitton and Gerba 1984). With half the U.S. population (and three-fourths of the U.S. public water supplies) dependent on groundwater, its chemical contamination is likely to be a serious public health problem for the next generation.

In the absence of oxygen, degradation of contaminants such as chlorinated and unchlorinated aromatic compounds cannot be mediated by the oxygenase mechanisms so thoroughly documented under aerobic conditions. In fact, only relatively recently has it been accepted that many aromatic chemicals can undergo anaerobic metabolism (see Young 1984). Interestingly, for several compounds, degradation is more readily achieved under anaerobic than under aerobic conditions. Anaerobic conditions are also quite varied. In the absence of molecular oxygen, nitrate, sulfate, or carbonate can serve as alternative electron acceptors in oxidation-reduction reactions, yielding nitrogen gas or ammonia, hydrogen sulfide, and methane, respectively. A variety of species of microorganisms have the capability of using one of these alternative electron acceptors.

Laboratory studies have shown that the anaerobic pathways of metabolism have several key steps, which are unique. As summarized in a general scheme in figure 9.7, first, substituents removal and simplification takes place, followed by ring reduction and saturation of the double bonds. Unlike the reaction pattern that is found with aerobic degradation schemes, ring fission does not occur with the aromatic structure but, rather, after reduction of the aromatic ring to the cyclohexane structure (Young 1984; Evans 1977). Clearly, the degradation pathways are quite different; however, little information is available on the biochemical mechanisms responsible for the reactions. In part, this may be because much of the initial work relied on mixed cultures, making it difficult to carry out enzyme studies. In addition, it is inherently difficult to work with oxygen labile enzymes.

Many chlorinated aromatic compounds, known to be more resistant to biodegradation under aerobic conditions, were fortuitously found to be readily dechlorinated under anaerobic conditions. As illustrated in table 9.2, the number of chloro substituents does not appear to be important. Substitutions in the para or ortho positions, however, appear to be more resistant. Nonetheless, under these methanogenic conditions, once the chloro substituents are removed, further metabolism—including ring fission and complete metabolism to carbon dioxide and methane—takes place (Suflita et al. 1982; Young 1984). The chlorinated alkene, perchloroethylene—widely used in the dry cleaning industry—is anaerobically de-

Figure 9.7. Anaerobic-catabolic pathways of aromatic acids and phenols.

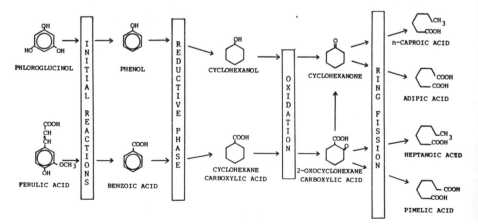

Table 9.2. Fate of chlorobenzoates under anaerobic conditions with lake sediment and sewage sludge inocula

Compound	Fate or Products Formed
2-Chlorobenzoate	No metabolism
3-Chlorobenzoate	→ Benzoate, CO_2, CH_4
4-Chlorobenzoate	No metabolism
2,4-Dichlorobenzoate	No metabolism
2,5-Dichlorobenzoate	→ 2-Chlorobenzoate
2,6-Dichlorobenzoate	No metabolism
3,4-Dichlorobenzoate	→ 4-Chlorobenzoate
3,5-Dichlorobenzoate	→ 3-Chlorobenzoate → benzoate → CO_2, CH_4
2,3,6-Trichlorobenzoate	→ 2,6-Dichlorobenzoate

Source: Young 1984.

chlorinated, whereas it is quite resistant under aerobic conditions (Vogel and McCarty 1985).

Pesticides known to be persistent, such as DDT, lindane, aldrin, and endrin, have been reported to undergo dechlorination under anaerobic conditions (see Young 1984). In fact, evidence indicates that subjecting persistent chemicals such as methoxychlor and chlorophenols to an anaerobic-aerobic cycle appears to enhance their biodegradation. For methoxychlor, initial incubation under anaerobic conditions yielded dechlorination. Subsequent aerobic incubation resulted in a fifteen- to seventy-fold increase in decomposition; whereas aerobic incubation alone yielded no change (Fogel et al. 1982). Chlorophenolic wastes from pulp and paper processing subjected to an anaerobic fluidized bed connected in series to an aerobic trickling filter showed 95 percent removal of the highly toxic chlorophenols, whereas, again, each process alone was unable to effect any removal of the chlorophenols (Hakulinen and Salkinoja-Salonen 1982).

▌Treatment and Cleanup

Clearly, it would be better and even easier perhaps to prevent toxic chemicals from getting into the environment, with the use of proper and innovative treatment processes, than it is to remove them once they are there. Biological waste treatment processes have been widely used for many years in the treatment of municipal sewage. Industries have successfully applied the major microbiological and engineering principles of domestic waste treatment to the treatment of particular organic chemical wastes. Interest appears high and research in this area is active (Hertzbrun et al. 1985; Deshpande et al. 1985). Aerobic and anaerobic processes are being examined for both relatively well-defined wastes such as penta-chlorphenol (Guthrie et al. 1984; Hichman and Novak 1984) and unde-fined wastes such as landfill leachates (Kosson and Ahlert 1984; Venka-taramani and Ahlert 1984).

The microbiological treatment of toxic or hazardous chemicals is of current interest because it is one of the few processes that can transform such chemicals into nontoxic components. In addition, biological pro-cesses are generally among the least costly methods. Most chemical and physical processes either transfer the chemical from one component to an-other (e.g., from soluble to solid) or are more costly and energy intensive. There is commercial interest in using microbiological means of contami-nant treatment; for example, it has been reported that PCB was success-fully removed from 68 thousand liters of contaminated oil with a microbio-logical preparation (Chemical Engineering 1984b). Another example is the successful on-site treatment of a 23-thousand-gallon spill of formaldehyde (Johnson and Thomas 1984).

The efficacy of biological treatment once a contaminant gets dissemi-nated into the environment has yet to be systematically and carefully evalu-ated. There are commercial companies that treat chemically contaminated areas; treatment appears to be most effective when the contamination is localized and confined (*Chemical Engineering* 1984a). The need for *in situ* and on-site treatment of groundwaters and soils is apparent, is gaining attention, and is stimulating research (McMurtry and Elton 1985; Kosson and Ahlert 1984; Keenan et al. 1984; Michelson et al. 1984; Kopecky 1984).

Experimental treatments of contaminated soil, using strains of bacte-ria capable of metabolizing the chemicals in question, have been success-ful; after microbiological treatment, plants that were highly sensitive to the contaminant could grow in the soil (Karns et al. 1984). These bacteria were not genetically altered by molecular procedures but, rather, acquired the genetic ability to metabolize the chemicals by natural selection controlled in the laboratory: the necessary genes were thus "naturally" acquired, rather than artificially engineered in the laboratory. Thus it is not clear if the use of these strains in the environment would require the same strict regulatory oversight criteria as would the dissemination of genetically engi-neered bacteria.

The use of genetically engineered organisms for human and environ-mental benefit holds much promise and potential. However, without the context of experience, it is far from certain whether the benefits outweigh the risks. Certainly, for contaminant treatment and environmental reme-diation purposes, the development of molecularly engineered organisms has a role. It is likely that contamination by a single major component would be more treatable with an engineered strain developed for that contaminant than with undefined mixtures of strains. It is also likely that genetically altered organisms for contaminant treatment would be applied in a closed and confined process long before they would be used in the open environment. The caution urged by ecologists with regard to the use of molecularly developed genotypes is well taken, for there are many examples of deleterious and unforeseen consequences caused by the parallel, though not equivalent, situation of introducing nonindigenous species into an environment (see Alexander, 1984). However, the future gains with molecular biology hold great promise and must be explored. Clearly, there is a need to recognize and acknowledge that this process must be undertaken with great care and caution.

Last, the resiliency of the environment in the face of the chemical, physical, and biological onslaughts from human civilization should give us much encouragement. By learning more about how the natural environment responds to these stresses (and we are far from knowing enough), we can expect to identify some of the best strategies for cleaning up our environment.

Biodegradation and Biotransformation

Virtually all foreign chemicals (xenobiotics, including toxicants, mutagens, carcinogens, drugs, and other substances) are subject to degradation and transformation by organisms in the environment. There are, however, qualitative and quantitative differences between bacteria (prokaryotes) and higher organisms (eukaryotes) in the manner in which degradation and transformation of persistent toxicants takes place. In the strict sense of the term, degradation is metabolism to mineral components; it takes place only within bacterial and fungal groups (Alexander 1973; Brink 1981; Borouin et al. 1985; Ghosal et al. 1985). The metabolism of persistent compounds in higher organisms is generally restricted to transformation, the production of polar intermediate products suitable for excretion (Malins 1977; Thakker et al. 1981; Conney 1982).

▌ Persistent Environmental Toxicants

Persistent environmental toxicants are defined as compounds having a half time for disappearance from the environment, due to natural processes, of more than one year (Doull et al. 1980; O'Connor and Kneip 1986). The persistent contaminants of greatest concern in environmental

---

This section was prepared by Joseph O'Connor.

health are chlorinated hydrocarbons (pesticides, PCBs, dioxins) and higher molecular weight polycyclic aromatic hydrocarbons (PAHs), including such compounds as benzo(a)pyrene, methylbenzanthracenes, and other carcinogenic and potentially carcinogenic compounds. The ultimate fate of such persistent compounds is transport through soils, water, and atmosphere to their environmental sinks—the sediments and water column of surface water bodies (Risebrough et al. 1968; Wasserman et al. 1975, 1979).

A major route for human exposure to toxicants such as PCBs, organochlorine insecticides, and dioxins is through the ingestion of contaminated fish and shellfish (Nelson 1972; Nisbet and Sarofim 1972; Schwartz et al. 1983; Belton et al. 1985a, 1985b). Detailed descriptions of the exposure, assimilation, retention, and elimination of persistent compounds by fishes and shellfish have been published (Pizza and O'Connor 1983; Mackay and Hughes 1984; Thomann and Connolly 1984; Connolly and Winfield 1984; Varanasi et al. 1984). Reference to these publications will provide the reader with the means to estimate the body burden in aquatic organisms of persistent environmental toxicants under a variety of exposure conditions and time periods. Figure 9.8 provides a schematic representation of the major pathways followed by persistent contaminants from their sources, through the environment, to humans. Collected data on the physical and chemical fate of these compounds and compound classes in natural environments may be found in Callahan et al. (1979). Research on these topics is regularly published in periodicals such as *Chemosphere* and *Environmental Science and Technology*.

The contaminants discussed in this section include the chlorinated pesticides of the DDT family (DDT, DDE, DDD, DDA, and methoxychlor), chlorinated cyclodienes (aldrin, dieldrin, chlordane, and so on), the polychlorinated biphenyls (PCBs), chlorinated dibenzodioxin dioxins

Figure 9.8. Pathways followed by persistent contaminants.

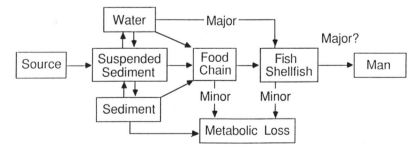

(*Source:* O'Connor and Kneip 1986.)

(PCDDs), and selected polycyclic aromatic hydrocarbons (PAHs). The primary organisms considered are fishes, although data from other taxa are included.

Persistent organic compounds may be categorized as moderately to highly nonpolar, lipophilic, and sparingly soluble in water. Their accumulation by aquatic organisms occurs by equilibrium partitioning between the aquatic medium and the tissues of the organisms in question (Hamelink et al. 1971; Clayton et al. 1977; Spacie and Hamelink 1982; Mackay 1982; Mackay and Hughes 1984). Although heated debate continues on the relative importance of uptake from food compared to uptake from water, the three long-term consequences of frequent exposure of aquatic organisms to lipophilic, persistent contaminants from either source are generally the same. (1) Body burdens (tissue concentrations) increase rapidly, with a preference for accumulation in lipid-rich tissues and fat depots (Norstrom et al. 1976; Pizza and O'Connor 1983; Thomann and Connolly 1984). (2) Pathways for elimination following tissue disposition are from the tissues to blood and thence to liver, bile, and alimentary tract, for final excretion to the environment (Varanasi and Gmur 1980; Malins et al. 1985; O'Connor and Pizza in press). (3) Elimination half times are generally quite long (Oliver and Niimi 1985) except for the rapidly transformed PAH compounds. For the PAHs, parent compound mass may decline rapidly, but metabolites, some of which are highly toxic, may accumulate to high levels (Gmur and Varanasi 1982; Malins et al. 1985; Moese and O'Connor 1985).

❙ Generalized Concepts of Biotransformation

Once accumulated, persistent toxicants are subject to metabolism by a variety of enzymes following a biphasic scheme:

$$\text{Compound} \xrightarrow{\text{Phase 1}} \text{Metabolite} \xrightarrow{\text{Phase 2}} \text{Conjugate.}$$
(Deactivation; sometimes activation) (Endogenous substrate; deactivation)

Phase 1 reactions (hydration, hydroxylation, epoxidation, and epoxide hydration) occur in the liver, kidney, and digestive tract. They are mediated in large part by a suite of enzymes known as the microsomal oxidases. For contaminants such as the PCBs, DDE, and probably the dioxins, phase I metabolism proceeds at such slow rates in fishes and invertebrates that the effect on tissue disposition and overall body burden is trivial (Guiney and Peterson 1980; Lech and Bend 1980; Pizza and O'Connor 1983; Thomann and Connolly 1984; Melancon and Lech 1983). In such cases, contaminant body burdens are determined by the frequency and magnitude of the dose and by the inherent rate constant for elimination of the parent compound (Pizza and O'Connor 1983; O'Connor and Pizza 1986, in press). In the case of PAHs, however, phase 1 reactions in fish may proceed rapidly, yielding measurable quantities of metabolites within minutes after assimilation (Krahn et al. 1984; Stein et al. 1984; Varanasi et al. 1985; Moese and O'Connor 1985).

Phase 2 reactions are generally conjugation reactions, with glucuronides being the dominant conjugates formed. Glucuronide conjugation is mediated by a range of transferase enzymes; glutathione and glycosylation conjugations also occur in aquatic organisms (Malins et al. 1979; Lech and Bend 1980; Varanasi et al. 1985). Some metabolic products of phase 1 reactions may be eliminated from fishes without conjugation (Melancon and Lech 1976; Malins et al. 1979; Stein et al. 1984; Moese 1986).

The microsomal monooxygenases responsible for the transformation of persistent toxicants in aquatic organisms are referred to as the cytochrome P-450-dependent, mixed-function oxidases (Stegeman et al. 1979). The cytochromes P-450 are assumed to have lipophilic and toxic xenobiotics of natural origin as their normal substrates (Nakatsugawa and Morelli 1976; Conney 1982). Their principal components were determined for mammalian systems in the 1950s (Mason 1957; Hayaishi 1962) and generalized for the fishes through the efforts of Stegeman and co-workers (Stegeman 1981, 1983; Stegeman et al. 1979, 1985, 1986). These oxidative xenometabolic enzyme systems facilitate the deactivation and elimination of not only naturally occurring substrates but also insecticides, industrial pollutants, drugs, and other chemicals of human manufacture.

Various environmental chemicals are known to induce the cytochrome P-450 monooxygenase systems in fishes as well as in mammals (Bend and James 1978). In mammals, five different cytochromes P-450 have been identified that may increase in response to specific classes of chemicals (Ryan et al. 1979, 1980, 1982). Of these, the cytochrome P-450b system is induced in rat liver microsomes by exposure to phenobarbital and other organic compounds with basically globular structure (Conney 1982). Cytochrome P-450c monooxygenases are induced in rat liver microsomes exposed to compounds that have a coplanar, or flat, structure; this includes PAHs such as methylcholanthrene, benzo(a)pyrene, and chlorinated aromatic compounds such as 2,3,7,8-tetrachlorodibenzo-p-dioxin (TCDD; see Conney 1982; Safe 1983, 1984a). Poland and colleagues (Poland et al. 1979; Poland and Glover 1977) listed according to their structural characteristics a number of chlorinated organic compounds likely to act as inducers of monooxygenase systems. These included not only the PAHs and certain of the dioxins but also several coplanar PCBs.

Safe (1983, 1984a) noted that the most potent inducer of cytochrome P-450c (P-448) in mammals is TCDD. Other inducers of P-450c may be predicted based upon their structural similarity to TCDD. Thus the PCB congener 3,3′,4,4′-tetrachlorobiphenyl, an approximate isostereomer of TCDD, is a potent inducer, as are certain of the PAHs (figure 9.9; Safe 1984). Melancon and Lech (1983) showed that 3,3′,4,4′-tetrachloro-biphenyl is a potent P-450 inducer in rainbow trout and carp. Stein et al. (1984) showed that the cytochrome P-450 system induced by PCBs in English sole increased the transformation of BaP by aryl hydrocarbon hydroxylase and was the same P-450 system induced by BaP administered alone, or in combination with PCBs.

Klotz and colleagues (Klotz et al. 1983; Klotz and Stegeman 1984; Stegeman et al. 1985, 1986) purified five cytochromes P-450 from a marine fish (scup, *Stenotomus chrysops*). The cytochrome P-450e isolated and purified by Klotz and Stegeman (1984) was inducible by exposure of the fish to methylcholanthrene and is similar to the P-450 system induced in trout (Williams and Buhler 1983). Fishes and other aquatic organisms appar-

Figure 9.9. Halogenated aromatic compounds that are approximate isostereomers of 2,3,7,8-TCDD.

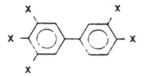

3,3′,4,4′,5 – Pentahalobiphenyl

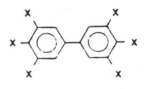

3,3′,4,4′,5,5′ – Hexahalobiphenyl

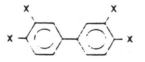

3,3′,4,4′ – Tetrahalobiphenyl

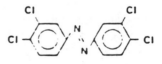

3,3′,4,4′ – Tetrachloroazobenzene

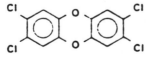

2,3,7,8 – Tetrachlorodibenzo-p-dioxin

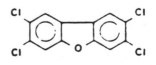

2,3,7,8 – Tetrachlorodibenzofuran

(*Source:* Safe 1984.)

ently do not possess a cytochrome P-450 monooxygenase system inducible by phenobarbital-type inducers.

Once induced, the major activity of the cytochrome P-450e monooxygenase system in fishes and crustaceans appears to be the hydroxylation of aryl hydrocarbons (aryl hydrocarbon hydroxylase, or AAH; see Malins 1977; Bend and Foureman 1984; Lech and Bend 1980; Melancon and Lech 1983). Within the diversity of 20 thousand to 30 thousand species of fish, however, there exist substantial differences in both inducibility of P-450 monooxygenase systems and their efficacy in transformation reactions. Bend and Foureman reported that only a few of several fish species studied were induced to synthesize high levels of P-450 after environmental exposure to PAH compounds. Stegeman et al. (1986) reported the induction of cytochrome P-450e in a deep ocean fish and concluded that this was evidence for the penetration of biologically active PCB congeners to the abyssal ocean. The cytochrome system induced by PCBs in deep ocean fish was the same P-450e system identified in other species as metabolizing aryl hydrocarbons to biologically active forms (Stein et al. 1984).

Metabolism and Biotransformation of Toxic Chemicals by Aquatic Species

Different classes of persistent organic toxicants are metabolized and transformed in different ways in aquatic organisms. A summary table (table 9.3) provides a generalized overview of biotransformation reactions, enzymatic pathways, transformation products, and probable fates for some persistent compounds.

Most of the persistent contaminants examined in this section are subject to metabolic transformation by mixed-function oxidases located in or on cellular microsomes. DDT is an exception, however, in that the most common DDT isomer, p,p'-DDT, is transformed to p,p'-DDE by a nonmicrosomal enzyme, DDT-dehydrochlorinase. The isomer p,p'-DDE is the most common DDT metabolite found in the environment and in biota. Other members of the DDT family, however, may be subject to microsomal oxidation and elimination as metabolites of increased solubility (methoxychlor, table 9.3).

Certain of the cyclodiene pesticides may be transformed to products more toxic than the parent compounds (aldrin to dieldrin, heptachlor to heptachlor epoxide; see table 9.3 and figure 9.10). Other cyclodienes are hydrated, hydroxylated, and dechlorinated by microsomal oxidases, leading to the formation of soluble compounds suitable for excretion. Dieldrin and heptachlor epoxide may be transformed by epoxide hydrases to intermediates, referred to as arene oxides, which have the potential to interact with DNA and RNA (table 9.3).

Table 9.3. Pathways and fate of persistent organic compounds in aquatic organisms

Compound and Enzymatic Pathways	Products and Fate
p,p'-DDT	
Nonmicrosomal; DDT dehydrochlorinase	p,p'-DDE
Microsomal oxidation	Kelthane
p,p'-DDE	
Little or no biotransformation	Essentially stable in fat depots
Methoxychlor	
Microsomal oxidation; O-dealkylation	Hydroxy products of increased solubility
Nonmicrosomal; dechlorination and dehydrochlorination	Glucuronide conjugates
Aldrin	
Microsomal epoxidation	Transformation to dieldrin
Heptachlor	
Microsomal epoxidation	Transformation to heptachlor epoxide
Endrin, Chlordane, Kepone, Mirex	
Microsomal oxidation: hydrases, hydroxylases, dechlorinases	Products of increased polarity and solubility: carboxylic acids, glucuronides, glutathoine conjugates
Dieldrin, heptachlor epoxide	
Microsomal oxidation: epoxide hydrases, hydrases	Arene oxides subject to rearrangement and possible DNA adduct formation
PCBs	
Microsomal oxidation: AHH, hydroxylation	Hydroxy and dihydroxy products; possible formation of arene oxide intermediates; glucuronide conjugates; phenols
Dioxins	
Microsomal oxidation: AHH, hydroxylation	Arene oxide intermediates; possible DNA adduct formation; glucuronide conjugation
PAHs	
Microsomal oxidation: AHH	Hydroxylation; possible arene oxide formation; glutathione conjugates; sulfate conjugates; formation of diols, dihydrodiols, and diolepoxides; possible DNA adduct formation

Sources: Walker 1975; Khan 1977; Khan et al. 1977; Nakatsugawa and Morelli 1976; Kapoor et al. 1970; Van Veld 1980; Matthews 1983; Hutzinger et al. 1972; Lech and Peterson 1983; Stein et al. 1984; Melancon and Lech 1983; Safe 1983, 1984a; Poiger and Buser 1983; Neal 1985; Sawahata et al. 1982; R. Lee et al. 1972; Krahn et al. 1984; Varanasi and Gmur 1981; Malins et al. 1985; Varanasi et al. 1985.

Figure 9.10. Metabolism of dieldrin and endrin.

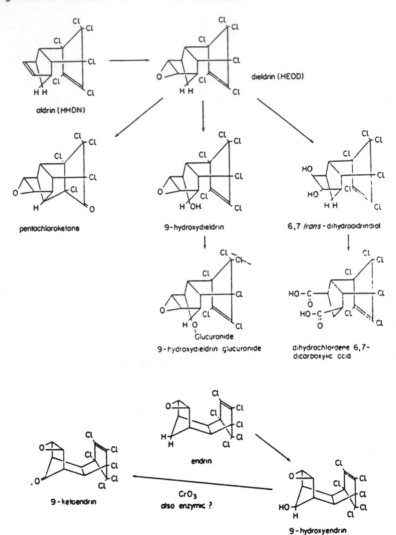

Note: All of these transformations are known to occur in male rats *in vivo*, with the following reservation: 9-hydroxydieldrin glucuronide has been reported as a metabolite *in vitro* with rat liver preparations; there is also evidence that it is excreted in the bile by rats, but this is not conclusive. Although 9-ketoendrin is excreted *in vivo* by rats, its formation from 9-hydroxyendrin has not been proved. (*Source:* Moriarty 1976.)

The metabolic transformation of PCBs, dioxins, and PAHs follows similar pathways in most aquatic organisms. Compounds with great planarity may induce cytochrome P-450e activity and may be subjected to metabolism with aryl hydrocarbon hydroxylase (table 9.3). AHH, however, may lead to the formation of arene oxide intermediates, possible DNA adduct formation, and the potential for genotoxic effects (table 9.3).

▌ Summary and Conclusions

Persistent and widely distributed toxic chemicals have several common characteristics: (1) They are generally not metabolized to their mineral components by eukaryotic organisms. (2) They are bioaccumulated by fishes and invertebrates. And (3) they are partially metabolized or biotransformed into forms suitable for excretion from the organism. For a number of chemicals, such as cyclodienes, PCBs, dioxins, and PAHs, transformation products may be more toxic than the parent compound.

Biotransformation in aquatic organisms generally follows the same pathways identified for mammals: exposure to the toxic chemical results in the induction of microsomal monooxygenase systems leading to the formation of conjugates of the transformed chemical and subsequent elimination from the body. In some cases, reactive intermediates are formed that are capable of binding with cellular macromolecules such as DNA and RNA. Under such circumstances, there exists the potential for chronic effects, including the induction of neoplastic growths. Also, reactive intermediates may be transported to the human population through the ingestion of seafood products contaminated with bioactivated molecules.

Only part of the contaminants in the environment of man can be cleaned from the environment. To a very large extent, chemicals that have been introduced to the environment over many years from diffuse or uncontrolled sources cannot be "cleaned up." Rather, they persist in the environment for long periods of time, until natural processes of biodegradation and transformation lead to their decomposition. Whereas bacterial dioxygenase systems are capable of eliminating persistent contaminants, animal monooxygenase systems transform persistent pollutants to compounds that are only slightly more soluble in water and only slightly more subject to mineralization. These biotransformation processes proceed at a relatively slow rate in aquatic systems and cannot be expected to have a major effect on the elimination of persistent toxic substances from natural surface waters.

Disposal Methods

This section deals with four disposal options for hazardous waste: landfills, geologic formations, chemical stabilization and solidification, and chemical treatment. Landfilling has been the traditional method of disposing of hazardous waste. Improper disposal into the land, however, has led to groundwater and surface water pollution. As a result of such environmental damages, Congress placed stringent criteria on landfills in the Hazardous and Solid Waste Amendments of 1984 (U.S. Congress 1984). Geologic formation disposal includes the placement of hazardous waste in injection wells, salt formations, and underground mines. Chemical stabilization and solidification includes processes that reduce the hazard potential of a waste by converting the contaminants into their least soluble, least mobile, or least toxic form. Chemical treatment comprises technologies either to prevent the release of hazardous materials into the environment or to alter their nature so they no longer pose an environmental problem.

▌ Landfills

A report by a task force of the American Institute of Chemical Engineers (1986) drew some thought-provoking conclusions about landfills:

> Use of impoundments and landfills for the management of hazardous waste is greatly affected by two somewhat conflicting facts: (1) there will always be a need to dispose of residues in the environment; and (2) all land disposal schemes are ultimately subject to some form of failure in terms of releases of contaminants to the environment. The first statement is true by virtue of the fact that some toxic constituents cannot be destroyed, do not have sufficient utility in commerce for recycle, and their production cannot be eliminated by process modification. . . . The second statement has been hotly debated, but cannot be denied if a sufficiently long-term view is taken. . . . Hazardous waste management in the future should be based on two guiding principles: (1) the volume and/or intrinsic hazard of wastes requiring ultimate disposal should be minimized; and (2) ultimate disposal technology should be designed to minimize the effects of anticipated failure modes.

The 1984 amendments to the Resource Conservation and Recovery Act placed significant restrictions on those wastes that can be disposed into

---

This section was prepared by Ronald D. Hill.

landfills and on minimum technology requirements for landfill design, construction, and operation. The numerous reported cases of groundwater pollution resulting from poorly designed and operated landfills have led to a dual approach for decreasing the environmental risks associated with landfills. The first approach is to ban landfilling of hazardous wastes with uncertain long-term persistence, toxicity, mobility, and propensity to bioaccumulate, unless these undesirable characteristics are corrected. The second approach is to construct and operate landfills so that hazardous substances are not released to the environment and to monitor landfills so that corrective actions can be taken if releases do occur.

Placement of liquids into landfills is considered undesirable because of their potential to migrate; also, liquids may leach other wastes within the landfill and cause them to migrate. Because of these concerns, the disposal of bulk or noncontainerized liquid hazardous waste or free liquids contained in hazardous waste have been prohibited since 1985. In addition, EPA has promulgated regulations that minimize the disposal of containerized hazardous liquid waste. These regulations prohibit the disposal of liquids that are absorbed in materials that biodegrade or release liquids when compressed during routine landfill operations.

The EPA has developed a list of wastes prohibited from landfills, based on the criteria previously given. The first wastes considered for banning (November 1986) were those containing dioxins or solvents. The second group of wastes (the California List) will be ruled upon by July 1987. Following is the California list and the concentrations at which they would be banned:

1. Free cyanides ($\geq$ 1,000 mg/l)
2. PCB ($\geq$ 50 mg/l)
3. pH ($\leq$ 2 mg/l)
4. Arsenic ($\geq$ 500 mg/l)
5. Cadmium ($\geq$ 100 mg/l)
6. Chromium VI ($\geq$ 500 mg/l)
7. Lead ($\geq$ 500 mg/l)
8. Mercury ($\geq$ 20 mg/l)
9. Nickel ($\geq$ 134 mg/l)
10. Selenium ($\geq$ 100 mg/l)
11. Thallium ($\geq$ 130 mg/l)

By May 1987, EPA is to review and rank all other hazardous wastes and determine their status for landfill disposal. Landfill disposal even of banned wastes is possible if they are pretreated to specific levels or standards established by the EPA, or if the disposer can demonstrate to the EPA or the state regulatory agency that such disposal will not endanger human health and the environment.

The second approach to insure that landfills do not cause environmental damage is the use of "minimum technology requirements." Since May 1985, new landfills must have double liners, leachate collection systems above and beneath the liners, and groundwater monitoring systems. During the active life of a landfill the bottom liner is to prevent or minimize the release of leachates. Any moisture that enters the landfill from precipitation or the waste is collected in the leachate collection system and removed to a treatment system (Shuckrow et al. 1983). Once the landfill has been filled, a cover is placed over it to prevent moisture from entering. If the cover is operating properly, free liquids that may be in the landfill will be removed in time, and leachate production will cease. Thus the key to a successful landfill is proper design, installation, and maintenance of liner and cover systems.

Figures 9.11 and 9.12 illustrate the double-liner concepts required to meet the standards set in the Hazardous and Solid Waste Amendments. In essence, the second liner is redundant; it is there in case the first liner fails. Liners are constructed of two materials, a flexible membrane and compacted, low-permeability soil. The EPA has published several documents on the use of clay and flexible membranes as liners (Goode and Smith 1984; Roy et al. 1985; Roberts 1984; Haxo 1983; Moore 1983).

Flexible membrane materials being manufactured and marketed vary considerably in physical and chemical properties, methods of installation, costs, and resistance to wastes. The durability and service life of a liner

Figure 9.11. Landfill double-liner system using two flexible membranes and compacted, low-permeability soil.

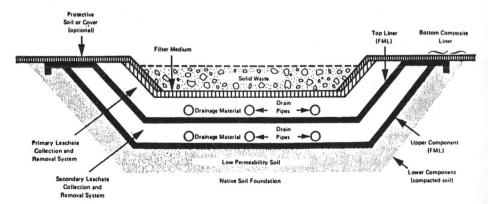

Note: Drawing is not to scale.

Figure 9.12. Landfill double-liner system using one flexible membrane and compacted, low-permeability soil.

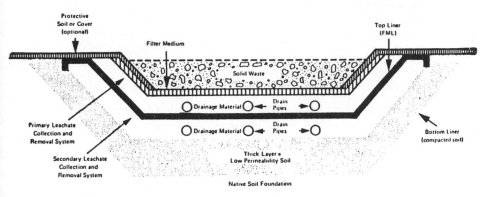

Note: Drawing is not to scale.

depend to a great extent on the specific liquids that contact it; no single material can resist chemical attack by all wastes. The compatibility of a liner with a specific waste is one of the first factors a designer must consider in planning a specific landfill site. Each of these factors must be considered in the design and material of the liner. However, proper installation is easily as important as proper selection of material and design (see U.S. EPA 1985a).

Intact flexible membrane materials are impermeable to liquids, but the membrane can be permeated through physical, biological, and chemical means, as shown below:

Physical means
1. Puncture
2. Tear
3. Creep
4. Freeze-and-thaw cracking
5. Wet-and-dry cracking
6. Differential settling
7. Thermal stress
8. Hydrostatic pressure
9. Abrasion

Biological means
10. Microbial attack

242 NORTON NELSON AND COLLEAGUES

Chemical means
11. Ultraviolet attack
12. Ozone attack
13. Hydrolysis
14. Ionic species attack
15. Extraction
16. Ionic species incompatibility
17. Solvents

Low-permeability, compacted soils have been a common liner material for years. However, all soils have some finite leakage rate. For example, soils with a permeability of 1×10^{-7} centimeters per second (a value commonly recommended for liners) have a seepage rate of seventy-nine gallons per acre per day under a one-foot head of waste. Thus in the design of a soil liner, the capacity of the surrounding environment to assimilate the leakage must be considered. The suitability of a soil as a liner material is usually based on laboratory permeability testing. There is evidence that permeabilities measured in the field are higher than those found in the laboratory, because the rigorous laboratory conditions cannot be duplicated in the field. There also is evidence that wastes, especially concentrated wastes, interact with the soil, causing an increase in permeability. Thus it is recommended that permeability tests be conducted with the specific waste leachate that will be present in the landfill (see American Society for Testing and Materials 1981, 1985; Acar and Seals 1984; Bowders et al. 1986; Brown and Anderson 1983; Haxo et al. 1984; Daniel and Trautwein 1986).

Landfill covers are similarly multilayered systems, designed to (1) exclude surface waters from contacting the landfilled waste, (2) act as a barrier to human or animal contact with the waste, and (3) prevent uncontrolled releases of vapors to the environment.

Figure 9.13 presents a schematic diagram of the elements of a multilayered cover system. All cover systems need a surface layer for vegetative support and protection of the hydraulic barrier. Filter layers serve to separate fine materials from coarse materials and to prevent fine materials from clogging the drainage layer. The biotic-barrier layer (largely conceptual at present) hinders plant roots and burrowing animals from disrupting the layers below, particularly the hydraulic barrier. The drainage layer intercepts downward-percolating water and conveys it laterally out of the system. The hydraulic barrier (flexible membrane liner) controls water percolation. The foundation (buffer) layer isolates the hydraulic barrier from the wastes and also provides mechanical support. The gas-control layer intercepts gases generated by the wastes and conducts them to the atmosphere through venting mechanisms. (See Lutton 1982; McAneny and Hathaway 1985; Schroeder et al. 1984).

Figure 9.13. Schematic of a landfill cover.

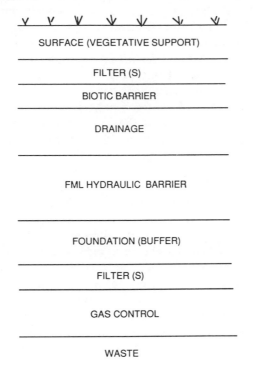

SURFACE (VEGETATIVE SUPPORT)

FILTER (S)

BIOTIC BARRIER

DRAINAGE

FML HYDRAULIC BARRIER

FOUNDATION (BUFFER)

FILTER (S)

GAS CONTROL

WASTE

Geologic Formations

Injection wells have been a popular waste disposal method for some time. In 1981, an estimated 2.8 percent of the chemical industry's hazardous wastes were disposed of in this manner (Chemical Manufacturers Association 1983). The long-term or permanent storage of hazardous waste in underground mines also has been proposed for a number of years. The EPA has conducted a number of feasibility studies on the subject, which have shown mine storage to be a viable option (Stone et al. 1985). Only one underground mine—a salt mine in West Germany—currently is being used. In recent years there have been several proposals to use salt domes, both existing cavities and new ones opened through solution mining.

Injection Wells

The technique of injecting liquid waste through wells into subsurface geologic formations is based on the concept that these geologic strata do not have any potential beneficial uses. The practice is used widely by the oil industry to dispose of brine. Since the 1950s, there has been a steady increase in the use of wells for disposal of other industrial waste. Over 250 wells containing 150 different chemical compounds are now operating.

The geologic formation is the key factor in the success injection well disposal. Desirable attributes for an underground reservoir are uniformity, large area, substantial thickness, high porosity and permeability, low pressure, a salaquifer (an aquifer containing brackish water, salt water, or brine), separation from fresh-water horizons, adequate overlying and underlying aquicludes (strata that confine water), no poorly plugged openings into the reservoir, and compatibility between the mineralogy and fluids of the reservoir and the injected waste.

Injection well disposal is not without controversy. Proponents argue that it is a safe, economical method to dispose of a variety of wastes, while opponents are concerned with groundwater pollution and future use of the aquifer. Some states have limitations on the types of wastes that can be injected—for example, chlorinated hydrocarbons. Injection wells that have created environmental problems have been located in unsuitable geologic settings or have been poorly engineered and installed for the existing geologic conditions. Good engineering and construction of an injection well are critical to its success. The first concern in planning, construction, and operation is the protection of potable waters and economically valuable minerals. The second concern is the prevention of corrosion of the tubular works and cementitious materials used in the well itself.

Mines

At this time, the EPA has no regulations concerning underground mine storage of hazardous waste. The 1984 amendments to the Resource Conservation and Recovery Act (RCRA) prohibited the disposal of bulk or noncontainerized liquid hazardous waste in salt domes, salt beds, underground mines, and caves as of November 8, 1984, until the EPA promulgates performance and permitting standards for such facilities.

For underground mine storage, the hazardous waste is packed in a solid form, transported into the mine, and placed in prepared rooms. The rooms are filled with wastes compatible with one another and then sealed off. The atmosphere in a properly selected mine is dry, so the drums have an indefinite life unless they are corroded from the inside. The drums can be retrieved from the mine at any time.

Although several firms in the United States have considered mine disposal, no mine disposal sites are currently in operation. The Herfa-Neurode facility in the Republic of West Germany has run satisfactorily since its startup in 1972. About 270 thousand tons of hazardous wastes have been placed in this mine over a period of ten years; the present annual volume is 35 thousand to 40 thousand tons. Reuse of stored waste is possible, and more than 1 thousand tons have been retrieved.

Salt, potash, and gypsum mines have been identified as having the greatest potential for waste storage. Salt deposits, especially, have many advantages, including their wide distribution throughout the United States, which means they are likely to be in close proximity to industrial areas. The technique for developing a salt mine is to drill into a salt mass, pump fresh or low-salinity water into the hole, and carry the dissolved salt to the surface as a brine solution. The hole gradually enlarges and eventually forms a useful cavern. After the cavern has been plugged with cement, the plastic nature of the salt under strata pressure provides an effective seal. Three factors are necessary for successful salt-cavern construction: (1) sufficiently thick and structurally sound salt at a proper depth and without excess interbedded insolubles; (2) an adequate supply of raw water for leaching the salt, and (3) an environmentally and economically sound means of disposing of the resulting brine. Several methods exist for injecting hazardous wastes into solution-mined salt caverns. Three are discussed here briefly.

In a brine-balanced cavern, the waste slurry is injected through the well casing with a pump, displacing the brine, which flows up the well casing to a brine-holding pond. Caverns using this concept have a very long life, because the stress on the salt walls is small; furthermore, this method permits the use of very large caverns. If the waste slurry is significantly heavier than saturated brine, the waste can be injected into the top of the cavern, displacing saturated brine up the casing string. If the specific gravity of the waste is close to or less than that of the saturated brine, the waste slurry must be weighted so that it is significantly heavier than the brine and sinks to the bottom of the cavern. The floating brine is then displaced from the top of the cavern through the well casing. Contamination of the brine by the waste is possible using this method.

In an atmospheric-pressure cavern, the brine is pumped out by means of a submersible pump and directed to disposal. Chemically compatible liquid and pumpable slurry wastes are then injected into the cavern through the well. Displaced vapors or gases are collected and are either sent through a scrubber or burned in an approved flare. A cavern exposed to such atmospheric pressure must be limited in size to maintain structural integrity. No brine contamination occurs, but a scrubber and flare are required. Hazardous wastes can be mixed with a cement or polymer slurry before injection to provide permanent solidified storage for liquid and slurry wastes and to reduce risks from earthquakes or inadvertent drilling into the cavern.

In a gas-pressure cavern, the brine is displaced by an inert gas and injected into a remote brine-disposal well. The cavern is sealed at the point of minimum pressure, then liquid and slurry wastes are injected into the cavern until the inert gas reaches maximum pressure. Gas balancing permits the use of a smaller cavern than brine balancing, and a larger cavern than the atmospheric method. Gas balancing eliminates the possibility of brine contamination and the need for a scrubber and flare.

▌ Chemical Stabilization and Solidification

Stabilization refers to those techniques that reduce the hazard potential of a waste by converting the contaminants into their least soluble, least mobile, or least toxic form. The physical nature and handling characteristics of the waste are not necessarily changed by stabilization. Solidification refers to techniques that encapsulate the waste in a monolithic solid of high structural integrity. The encapsulation may be of fine waste particles (microencapsulation) or of a large block or container of wastes (macroencapsulation). Solidification does not necessarily involve a chemical interaction between the wastes and the solidifying reagents but may involve mechanically binding the wastes into the monolith. Contaminant migration is restricted by vastly decreasing the surface area exposed to leaching or by isolating the wastes within an impervious capsule (Cullinane and Tones 1985).

Most stabilization and solidification systems available today are proprietary processes, involving adding absorbents and solidifying agents to wastes. Often the process is changed to accommodate specific types of wastes. Most processes fall within a few generic types, with proprietary additives added by different companies. The performance of a specific system may vary widely from that of its generic type, but the general characteristics of a process and its products can be discussed. Waste stabilization and solidification systems that have potentially useful application for hazardous waste include

1. Sorption
2. Processes using lime or cement plus fly-ash pozzolana (any siliceous and aluminous substance that chemically reacts with slaked lime to form a cementitious compound)
3. Thermoplastic microencapsulation
4. Macroencapsulation
5. Vitrification

Sorption

Sorption involves the adding of a dry, solid substance to liquid or semiliquid wastes to take up free liquid and to improve the handling characteristics of the wastes. The sorbent may hold the fluid as capillary liquid or may react chemically with it. Common natural sorbents include soil, fly ash, bottom ash, cement kiln dust, and lime kiln dust. Synthetic sorbents are also available, but due to their relatively higher cost, they are less commonly used as solidification agents.

Sorbents, especially natural ones, are in wide use at hazardous waste landfills. In many cases, however, the sorbed wastes remain subject to leaching, and the landfill liner and leachate collection system are relied on to prevent contaminant migration. Sorbents that act like sponges and only soak up the liquids are prohibited by the RCRA amendments of 1984.

Lime-Based and Cement-Based Techniques

These processes involve mixing wastes with hydrated lime and natural or artificial silicic material (pozzolana). Natural pozzolana include some volcanic tuffs and diatomaceous earth. Artificial pozzolana include blast furnace slag, ground brick, and some fly ashes from the burning of coal.

Lime and fly-ash-pozzolana processes involve mixing wastes with natural or artificial pozzolana and hydrated lime. A number of waste treatment processes employ portland cement as the solidifying agent, often with a pozzolanic material (such as fly ash) added to improve strength and increase durability. Other forms of silica or clay may also be added to alter performance. The type of portland cement can be selected to favor particular cementation reactions, thus avoiding interference from incompatible compounds. Cement-pozzolana techniques, with or without waste-specific additives, are among the most common offered by solidification vendors. However, because of their higher cost, they are less often used than lime-pozzolana techniques.

In both techniques, the suspended solids in the waste slurry become incorporated into the hardened concrete matrix. Most multivalent toxic metals are transformed into their low-solubility hydroxides or carbonates by the high pH of the cement mixture, and some metal ions may become integrated into the mineral crystals within the cement. Some materials, such as sulfides (except sodium sulfide), asbestos, and latex, can increase the strength and durability of cemented wastes. Other compounds can interfere with the solidification process. Still others, such as soluble salts of manganese, tin, zinc, copper, and lead, can increase setting times and greatly decrease physical strengths. Impurities such as organic matter, silts, some clays, and other insoluble materials fine enough to pass a no. 200 mesh sieve, can coat larger particles and weaken the waste-cement bond, delaying setting.

Thermoplastic Microencapsulation

Thermoplastic microencapsulation involves mixing dried wastes with a heated thermoplastic material such as bitumen (asphalt), paraffin, polyethylene, polypropylene, or sulfur-amended asphalt, and placing the mixture in a container or mold. The most commonly employed material is asphalt. Microencapsulation techniques, developed originally for radioactive waste disposal, are adaptable to highly soluble toxic substances, which are not amenable to lime-based or cement-based techniques. The greatest limitation to use of these techniques is their relatively high cost because of the need for specialized mixing equipment and highly trained operators and the need to dry the wastes before mixing with the thermoplastic. Consequently, these techniques are used mainly to achieve complete containment of special waste types.

Macroencapsulation

Macroencapsulation, often referred to as jacketing, is a technique for isolating wastes by completely surrounding them with a durable, impermeable coating. One such technique involves sealing the wastes in a drum made of or lined with polyethylene. Another technique involves drying the wastes, mixing them with polybutadiene, and compressing the mixture into a block. The block is then placed in a mold lined with powdered polyethylene and heated under pressure. The resultant product is a block with a thin polyethylene coating fused to it.

Vitrification

Another solidification technique is vitrification. Wastes are mixed with silica, heated to extremely high temperatures, and allowed to cool into a glasslike solid. A variation of this technique, using graphite electrodes driven into buried wastes, allows *in-situ* vitrification. All vitrification systems employ some type of hood to capture and treat the fumes and vapors given off during operation. Because these systems are energy intensive, and thus costly, they are generally considered only for radioactive or extremely dangerous wastes.

▌ Chemical Treatment

Chemicals have the ability to alter the nature of materials, and this accounts for the rather wide applicability that chemical treatment has in hazardous waste destruction (U.S. EPA 1983, 1986). It is possible, for example, to chemically convert the pesticide ethylene dibromide (EDB) to the salt potassium bromide (which has economic value) and the gas acetylene. Other chemical approaches modify hazardous materials so that they become nontoxic. Glycol-based chemical reagents, for example, remove a chlorine atom from 2,3,7,8-dioxin, converting it to a nontoxic adduct. Here, chemical and biological methods can complement each other, for once a single chlorine atom is removed from the dioxin molecule, the partially dechlorinated dioxin is much less toxic to microorganisms and is consequently subject to natural biological decomposition to harmless salts and gases (DeRenzo 1978). A brief review of the major chemical treatment processes follows.

Chemical Oxidation

Ions or compounds can be chemically oxidized to render them nonhazardous or to make them more amenable to removal or destruction. During the process, the chemical oxidizing agent is itself reduced.

Chemical oxidation has been used to treat hazardous organic and inorganic contaminants in aqueous solution. Its major use has been for treating cyanide in metal-plating wastes. In this process, chlorine gas, chlorine dioxide, or hypochlorite (sodium or calcium) destroy cyanide (CN^-), which is converted to nitrogen gas (N_2) and carbon dioxide gas (CO_2). Other, less-common oxidants, include potassium permanganate ($KMnO_4$), hydrogen peroxide, and ozone. Potassium permanganate has been used experimentally for destruction of trace organics (including aldehydes, mercaptans, phenols, and organic acids) in aqueous hazardous waste and drinking water. It has also recently been used to treat nonchlorinated pesticides.

Chemical oxidants are relatively nonselective and may oxidize other compounds present in the wastes before oxidizing the contaminant of concern. As a result, this process has limited application for slurries, tars, and sludges, which may contain large amounts of oxidizable components. It is most useful for dilute aqueous wastes.

Ozonation is appropriate for aqueous streams that contain less than 1 percent oxidizable compounds. Ozone can be used to break down refractory organics in wastes before they are subjected to biological or other treatment. Biorefractory compounds in aqueous wastes contaminated with toluene diisocyanate, ethylene glycol, or ethylene dichloride are oxidized to a biodegradable form by ozone. Ozonation improves the biotreatability of water containing styrene by transforming it to a compound such as benzoic acid. It can also be used to oxidize untreated organics left after biological or other treatment processes.

A combination of ultraviolet radiation and ozone has been demonstrated to economically treat certain halogenated organics, including aldrin, chlorinated phenols, dieldrin, endrin, ethylene dichloride, kepone, methylene chloride, PCB, DDT, and pentachlorophenol. Aldehydes, ketones, alcohols, aromatic hydrocarbons, ethers, carbonyl compounds, chlorinated aromatics (pesticides), nitroso compounds, and saturated hydrocarbon groupings are all oxidizable with ozone. Bis (2-ethylhexyl) phthalate, benzene, anthracene, benzo(a)pyrene, benzo(k)fluoranthene, pyrene, benzoic and perbenzoic acids, styrenes, and aqueous wastes from petrochemical processes producing toluene diisocyanate, ethylene glycol, styrene monomers, and ethylene dichloride have also been successfully treated by ozonation before biological treatment.

Chemical Reduction

Chemical reduction involves the transfer of reactive electrons from one compound to another and is used to either render compounds nontoxic or to enable compounds to undergo chemical destruction or physical removal. Metals, in particular hexavalent chromium, are reduced through the addition of a compatible reducing agent—for example, reduced sulfur compounds. Requirements for specific pH solutions and agitation must be met to ensure successful chemical reduction.

Chemical reduction is best applied to liquid wastes free of organic compounds. It is widely used in industry to control hexavalent chromium waste, and to remove or recover mercury from mercury cells used in chloralkali manufacturing. Chromium is usually reduced by sodium sulfite salts or sulfur dioxide. Iron, aluminum, and zinc have also been identified as potential chrome-reducing agents. Caustic sodium borohydride ($NaBH_4$) has been commercially employed to reduce mercury to elemental form, allowing its recovery. $NaBH_4$ is also used on a commercial scale to reduce soluble lead, including organolead salts from tetraalkyl and aqueous wastes from lead manufacturing, and to reduce and recover silver from photographic operations.

Chemical reduction is also a common technology for reducing complexed or chelated metals, such as copper and nickel, found in aqueous metal-plating wastes. The solution's pH is adjusted to break the metal-chelate bond; then the reducing agent is added to reduce the metal and precipitate it out of solution. Filtration often follows. Chemical reduction has limited application to treatment of slurries, tars, and sludge, because surface contact is difficult to achieve between the reducing agent and the hazardous constituent. Solid hazardous materials must be liquified before treatment by reduction. Because reducing agents are not selective, organic compounds present in the treated solutions decrease destruction efficiency and may liberate offensive odors.

Neutralization

While relatively straightforward in theory, neutralization continues to be one of the most common and critical processes used in the hazardous waste treatment industry. It involves combining a hazardous waste stream with either an acid or a base to adjust liquid pH to acceptable levels. Neutralization may be required before waste treatment to protect downstream equipment and to optimize treatment performance. The pH of an acid or base should not be confused with its acidity or basicity, which is the volume of base or acid required to reach a specified pH. The desired pH is usually between 6 and 9, and the reaction products include water, salts, and solids precipitated by pH-dependent solubility reactions.

Neutralization is most commonly performed in corrosion-resistant tanks, although ponds and limestone filter beds are also used. Lime, calcium hydroxide, caustic soda, soda ash, and ammonium hydroxide are common bases used for neutralization; sulfuric acid, hydrochloric acid, and nitric acid are common acids.

Chlorinolysis

In the chlorinolysis process, chlorine reacts with chlorinated hydrocarbon wastes at temperatures of 500° to 800° C and pressures of a thousand pounds or greater per square inch gauge. The reaction products include carbon tetrachloride (CCl_4), perchloroethylene, trichloroethylene, anhydrous hydrogen chloride, unreacted hydrocarbons, and unreacted chlorine. The process steps include (1) pretreatment of the wastes by filtration or distillation to remove water, solid materials, and incompatible compounds extraneous to the process; (2) reaction with chlorine; (3) distillation to separate the reaction products; and (4) absorption of the hydrochloric acid solution that is produced.

Generally, chlorinolysis is suitable for treating chlorinated wastes and residues, including but not limited to wastes from the production of pesticides, vinyl chloride, herbicides, and solvents. The thirteen pesticides amenable to chlorinolysis are aldrin, chlordane, DDD, DDT, ethylene dichloride, benzene hexachloride, heptachlor, lindane, o- and p-dichlorobenzene, pentac, perthane, and TCBB (GCA Corporation 1984). Wastes to be used as feedstock should contain only hydrogen, carbon, and chlorine. Other substances, such as sulfur, could result in corrosion; and phosphorus, nitrogen, or oxygen could result in the production of unwanted byproducts. In addition, feed streams must contain less than 5 percent aromatic compounds in order to limit the reaction temperature to the design temperature. Pretreatment is required to remove undesirable compounds. Chlorinolysis is done on a large scale, requiring an adequate continuous supply of chlorinated wastes to make the process feasible.

Wet Air Oxidation

Wet air oxidation is the aqueous phase oxidation of dissolved or suspended organic or inorganic substances at elevated temperature (177° to 315° C) and pressure (300 to 3,000 psi). Elevated pressure is used to keep the water in its liquid state, allowing organic destruction to proceed at lower temperatures than would otherwise be necessary. Water serves to moderate the oxidation rate, removing excess heat of reaction (Kiang and Metry 1982). Oxygen is incorporated as the oxidizing agent. Feed materials are pressurized and pumped to a heat exchanger, which preheats the feed and cools the effluent in the reactor vessel. Additional heat is added as needed to the preheated feedstock or the reactor vessel. Air or oxygen is injected either prior to the heat exchanges or into the reactor. Reactor effluent not sufficiently cooled in the heat exchanges may require additional cooling. The effluent then travels through a pressure control valve to reduce its pressure to a normal atmospheric level. After pressure letdown, the vapor and liquid components of the cooled effluent are separated. The vapor passes through an air pollution control system, which may include a water scrubber and an activated carbon adsorption system or an off-gas incinerator. The aqueous effluent stream, which might contain low-molecular-weight organic acids, may be discharged to a subsequent treatment process for further treatment.

Wet air oxidation oxidizes hazardous wastes to less toxic substances: reduced sulfur compounds, such as sulfides and mercaptans, to inorganic sulfates; cyanides to carbon dioxide plus ammonia or nitrogen gas; chlorinated hydrocarbons to hydrochloric and simple organic acids; and metals to metal salts (Canney and Schaefer 1983). Certain highly chlorinated aromatic organics, such as pentachlorophenol, PCBs, and DDT, are resistant to destruction by conventional wet air oxidization. However, a proprietary cocatalyst system at bench scale showed greater than 99.5 percent destruction of these compounds at 275° F.

Wet air oxidation can be used to oxidize any material, organic or inorganic, with an approximate value of ten thousand and a hundred thousand milligrams per liter (California Department of Health Services 1984). It is best suited to cyanide destruction and to pretreatment of organics containing aqueous hazardous wastes too toxic for biological treatment or too dilute for incineration (Canney and Schaefer 1983). The process is well established for treatment of municipal sludges and industrial wastes; over 180 installations are in operation or under construction. But its commercial application to hazardous waste has been limited to date.

Dechlorination

Dechlorination uses chemical reagents to remove chlorine from chlorinated molecules, to break apart chlorinated molecules, and to change the molecular structure of the molecule. Metallic sodium is the typical reagent used to strip the chlorine away from constituents to form sodium chloride. Other proprietary reagents are often used in conjunction with metallic sodium to further treat the dechlorinated constituents. The majority of dechlorination research has been aimed at the detoxification of polychlorinated biphenyls (PCBs). This research is applicable to many chlorinated organic molecules—for example, the detoxification of 2,3,7,8-tetrachlorodibenzo-p-dioxin (referred to as dioxin).

A number of companies and research institutions have investigated dechlorination processes. Four of the more common dechlorination technologies include the Acurex process, the Sunohio PCBX process, the PPM process, and the APEG process. These processes are applicable to many chlorinated organics such as PCBs, dioxins, solvents, pesticides, and other halogenated organics.

In the Acurex process, the treatment stream is filtered and then transferred to a reaction tank, where it is mixed with a mixture of a sodium reagent and a proprietary constituent. The products of this reaction are a sodium hydroxide stream and another nontoxic effluent. The Acurex reaction process is performed under a "nitrogen blanket" to minimize air emissions.

The Sunohio PCBX process, unlike the Acurex process, is a continuous treatment operation. It uses a proprietary reagent to convert the PCB molecules to metal chlorides and polyphenyl compounds. PPM is a batch process and uses a proprietary sodium reagent to dechlorinate organic molecules. A solid polymer is generated, which, although regulated, can be more easily disposed of than chlorinated organics.

The APEG process uses polyethylene glycols or their derivatives that have been reacted with alkali metals or their hydroxides. Dioxin and PCBs can be destroyed in soil using a series of reagents prepared from potassium and polyethylene glycols (KPEG). However, moisture adversely influences the rates of reaction. A heated slurry process has subsequently been developed to negate the influence of moisture. APEG is a batch process and is controlled at operating temperatures ranging from 75° to 150° C. The reaction products associated with this process include potassium chloride, nontoxic organics, and other dechlorinated materials.

Supercritical Fluid Extraction

In supercritical fluid extraction, as in liquid-liquid extraction, an organic-containing aqueous feed is contacted by a solvent in a countercurrent extraction column. The solvent is CO_2, either a supercritical fluid or a near critical liquid, and the feed is an aqueous solution of organics. The resulting extract, solute in solvent, is reduced in pressure and sent to a solvent-stripping system at forty to fifty atmospheres. A CO_2 vapor stream is recovered overhead, and the bottom is substantially enriched by the extracted organic.

The CO_2 vapor from the still is compressed adiabatically to extractor pressure (sixty-five atmospheres), increasing its temperature. From this higher temperature, heat is released by cooling and condensing the vapor in the reboiler tubes to boil up the reboiler bottoms, and the condensed CO_2 is returned as solvent recycle to the extractor. The product stripped of most of the CO_2 solvent is let down in pressure in sequential flashes. The raffinate is similarly flashed, and CO_2 is recovered from both streams, re-compressed, and returned to the solvent system.

A qualitative comparison can be made with two major established separation processes: distillation and normal-liquid solvent extraction. Distillation, or stripping, is used for separating a range of organics from water, where such organic chemicals are manufactured in aqueous systems. Examples include volatile alcohols, ketones, and the like, which are high-volume solvents and chemicals. Other examples include heavy, high-boiling liquids from which water must be distilled. In both sets of examples, energy requirements are substantial. Normal-liquid solvent extraction has minimal energy requirements. However, the solvent must then be separated from the extracted solute, generally by distillation, which normally requires vaporization of the entire solvent volume (low volatility mixtures)—at high energy costs.

Several additional benefits arise from the favorable kinetic properties of critical fluids as solvents, which may be important factors in improving process economies. The low viscosities of the solvent streams reduce pressure drops and thus pumping requirements. Improved diffusion characteristics can lead to higher separation efficiencies in mass transfer equipment, often reducing the volume and cost of such equipment.

Supercritical water oxidation is the destruction of refractory organic compounds using supercritical water at a temperature and pressure of at least 374.2° C and 218.3 atmospheres, respectively. It is a developing technology, which takes advantage of the greatly increased solubility of immiscible organics in water when an aqueous mixture reaches the supercritical state. Chlorinated pesticides and other high-molecular-weight organic compounds are reported to be completely oxidized to CO_2, H_2O, and inorganic salts under these conditions (Josephson 1982). This reaction has been performed in a pressurized reactor.

Commercial application of this technology to refractory organics (including solvents, chlorinated pesticides, and dioxins) and cyanides seems possible. However, no commercial-scale supercritical unit is currently operating. Until such an installation becomes operative and destruction efficiencies and system reliability are verified, this technology must be viewed as experimental.

Resource Recovery and Incineration

The 1984 survey by the Chemical Manufacturers Association (1986) showed that 278.5 million tons of hazardous wastes were treated and dis-

This section was prepared by Adel Sarofim and David Gordon Wilson.

posed of by responding companies. These results reported by 50 percent of the CMA member companies, including thirty-seven of the top fifty chemical companies by sales, are summarized in figure 9.14. Most of the wastes are liquid, involving dilute streams used to transport and wash chemicals or to transfer heat in heat exchangers. A significant fraction of the liquid wastes consists of dilute aqueous streams, which are not readily amenable to resource recovery or incineration. In this section, the focus is on solid wastes and liquid organic wastes.

In addition to wastes disposed of on site by the manufacturers, themselves, wastes are disposed of by independent disposal operators who collect them from a variety of waste generators. The latter wastes vary widely in chemical and physical composition and come often from small-volume generators, including commercial research laboratories and universities. They are often packaged in fifty-five-gallon fiber or steel drums ("lab packs") containing a variety of smaller containers imbedded in an inert absorbent, such as fuller's earth or vermiculite. Because of the highly heterogeneous nature of this waste, the only practical resource recovery is the energy from the incinerator. Thus recycling is restricted to the premises of the waste generator, who has control of the composition of the recycled streams. Recycling operations are composition and site specific. A few examples are provided below.

Figure 9.14. Treatment of hazardous waste by 725 plants.

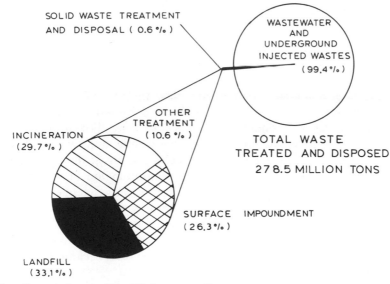

Note: Percents do not add to 100 due to rounding.

▌ The Reuse, Recovery, and Recycling of Hazardous Wastes

In reuse, wastes are brought back into the supply stream in substantially their original form (e.g., spilt mercury can be picked up, decontaminated, and reused). In recovery, components are recovered from the waste stream, purified, and put back into the supply stream (e.g., in solvent recovery). And in recycling, wastes are recovered from the waste stream and put to a different use, often in a different form (e.g., used solvents might be burned in a steam-raising boiler). Many wastes are suitable for these treatments, generally those that are merely potentially hazardous (those that pose no life-threatening risk so long as they do not get into the air, food, or water supplies).

A few wastes, however, are so hazardous that only the safest possible method of disposal should be contemplated. An extreme example is old nerve-gas shells and canisters, which require the most stringent handling procedures—robotic wherever possible—before being destroyed in a high-temperature furnace. Even in this case, the end product is a stream of hot inert gas whose energy could theoretically be recycled in a waste-heat boiler, for instance.

Waste materials can be categorized as solid, gaseous, or liquid, with subcategories of vapors and sludges. Another categorization is pure materials and compounds. And a third form is organics and inorganics. The complexity of these forms of division is greatly reduced when it is realized that liquids and sludges are by far the major form of hazardous wastes, both in terms of mass flow and in nuisance potential. We therefore use the first category.

Solids

METALS

Beryllium and uranium, the most toxic of the pure metals, are used in nuclear reactors. Their high value and high toxicity have together ensured that their recovery rate is high. For instance, numerically controlled turret lathes used for the production of jet-engine turbine disks are totally enclosed except for access panels to tool and stock areas; the lathe bed is inclined close to the vertical so that the cuttings drop into a trough; and a moving conveyor takes the cuttings to a closed recovery container. The cutting oils are also separately recovered and processed.

POWDERS

Pesticide powders are not presently recovered. In the steel and nonreferrous metals industries there is some recovery from accumulated dusts taken from pollution control equipment.

Gases and Vapors

Solvent recovery has been an established process in a wide range of industries for many years. In a review of solvent waste management applied to a range of new materials and products, Kaufman (1984) pointed out that Polaroid has in recent years changed its policy from that of choosing the materials on the basis of product use and leaving the disposal problems to subcontractors to one of considering the recovery or safe disposal of materials from the beginning. Kaufman lists the solvents Polaroid recovers and recycles in house, those treated by second parties, and those disposed of without recovery:

Solvents recovered and recycled on site
1. Toluene
2. Naphtha (110° C)
3. Anhydrous isopropanol (solvent of choice)
4. Diethylene glycol dimethylether
5. Trifluoroethanol
6. Methylene chloride
7. Methanol
8. Acetone
9. N-Propanol

Solvents recovered by second parties
1. Orthodichlorobenzene
2. Dimethylsulfoxide
3. Methylene chloride
4. 2-Pentanone

Solvents disposed of without recovery
1. Ethyl acetate
2. Methyl ethyl ketone
3. Acetic acid
4. Dimethyl formamide
5. Xylene

Solvents being phased out of production
1. Ethylene glycol monomethyl ether
2. Benzene

The chlorofluorocarbons (e.g., Freons) have also undergone changes leading toward recovery, principally because they are suspected of leading to long-term depletion of stratospheric ozones (National Academy of Sciences 1979).

Liquids and Sludges

LIQUIDS

These wastes may be divided into organic and inorganic categories. Present U.S. regulations allow hazardous materials having calorific values higher than that of coal, and having no significant quantities of halogens or sulfur, to be burned for heat recovery. Thus they can be treated as a minor component of the fuel in steam generators, diesel engines, and gas turbines. (Internal-combustion turbines seem especially effective, given that the coldest surfaces immediately downstream of the combustor in a modern gas turbine are the nozzle-vane and rotor-blade surfaces at about 1,250 K, while the gas temperature is of the order of 1,500 K and above.)

Materials of a lower calorific value than coal must be incinerated. More stringent regulations, including the requirement of a rigid test firing for each type and composition of hazardous waste, apply to these materials. However, from an environmental point of view, combustion is probably the method of choice for the destruction of virtually all organic compounds, as well as for some wastes that contain inorganic substances (National Research Council 1983). Incineration therefore, is not strictly recovery, though there seems no reason why the hot gaseous products of incineration should not be passed over heat-recovery surfaces. (Additional information on combustion of wastes is provided in the section on incineration.)

Mercury is a special case of an inorganic liquid that is normally recovered because of its value and because its vapors and compounds are toxic. An established industry exists to purify mercury from its contaminated condition when it is recovered from spills and from zinc amalgam or mercuric sulfide, to which forms mercury can be easily converted.

SLUDGES

These form the by-products of many primary methods of pollution treatment, including those for sewage and steel-furnace emissions. While most sludges are put in landfills, the costs of doing so with secure containment of leachates and drainings is rapidly increasing. Steel-furnace emissions, containing large quantities of iron oxides, can be processed within the industry. The predominant practice of discharging sewage sludges at sea is being increasingly discouraged, and discharge to the land in reserved forest areas has several disadvantages: hepatitis organisms, enteroviruses (poliomyelitis, ECHO, Coxsackie), and parasites are not killed; and heavy metals, principally lead, pass into the soil. Incineration of sewage sludge is safe but expensive. A less-costly method of partial recycling, which has been successfully developed under NSF sponsorship, is the production of bricks from sewage sludge, which appears to entail no environmental hazards (Alleman 1983; Bryan 1984).

▌ Incineration

Incineration in 1983 accounted for the disposal of about 2.8×10^6 tons per year of hazardous wastes, of which 2.4×10^6 tons per year were handled on site (Sweet et al. 1985). In addition, 3.8×10^6 tons per year of possibly hazardous industrial wastes (1981 estimate, Olexsey et al. 1985) were burned as fuels in industrial processes. As much as 25×10^6 tons per year of the hazardous wastes generated in the United States may be capable of being incinerated, according to EPA estimates (Olexsey et al.). Advantages of incineration or combustion, compared with disposal in a secure landfill, include the following:

1. With proper emission controls, wastes are converted into innocuous products.
2. There is no commitment to long-term containment of hazardous materials, except for the solid residue (see below).
3. Release of contaminants as a consequence of malfunction can be corrected relatively quickly and inexpensively. Malfunction of a secure landfill (e.g., leakage into groundwater) can usually be detected less readily and rapidly and is more costly to remedy.
4. Incinerators can handle most of those reactive wastes not allowed in landfills.

Incineration has some disadvantages relative to disposal in a secure landfill:

1. A costly test burn procedure is required for a permit for a hazardous-waste incinerator.
2. Emissions to the atmosphere must be controlled.
3. Ash must usually be disposed of in a secure landfill. Such ash is defined by EPA regulation as hazardous unless it is specifically exempted, based on a showing that it regularly does not meet any of the criteria for a hazardous waste.
4. Incineration equipment is relatively expensive to install and to maintain; hence incineration is more costly to the user than landfill disposal.
5. Incinerators operate best on a well-defined feed with known combustion heat.

Criteria for Thermal Destruction of Wastes

Most wastes can be destroyed essentially completely (with an efficiency greater than 99.99 percent) by high-temperature oxidation. Some oxidation products, such as SO_x, NO_x, HCl, and metal oxides, may be noxious. Emission of SO_x corresponds approximately to the stoichiometric conversion of sulfur in the waste to SO_2, with smaller amounts of SO_3. Nitrogen oxides are formed by oxidation of organically bound nitrogen in the waste, by decomposition of nitrates, and by thermal fixation of atmospheric nitrogen. Halogens in the waste produce a mixture of the hydrogen halide and gaseous halogen; for chlorine-containing material, the predominant product is HCl, which is favored over chlorine at incineration temperatures. Inorganic constituents, depending on their volatility, may either form solid residues or vaporize and recondense to form a submicrometer-sized aerosol. Emissions of the latter may be acceptable, depending on the types and quantities of metal ions they contain, or they may be reduced to acceptable levels by appropriate air pollution control devices.

Incinerators must be designed to provide the conditions necessary to achieve complete oxidation: a supply of air in excess of the stoichiometric requirement, adequate mixing of air and waste, and sufficiently high temperature to complete oxidation in the time available. These requirements are often designated the 3 Ts of incineration: temperature, time, and turbulence.

TEMPERATURE AND TIME REQUIREMENTS

The high-temperature oxidation of wastes proceeds through a multistep, free-radical process; the factors that control the rate of oxidation are many and are not completely understood (Tsang and Shaub 1981). The rates increase rapidly with increases in temperature. The oxidation may be inhibited by free-radical scavengers such as halogens (Senkan 1984; Wilson et al. 1969). Temperatures for gas-phase reaction range from 1,250 K to the adiabatic flame temperature, which may be over 2,750 K—or higher if the air is enriched with oxygen.

The time required for complete reaction decreases with increasing temperature, from the order of two seconds at 1,250 K to the order of fifty milliseconds at 2,750 K. However, the short reaction times attainable at higher temperatures are often precluded by the problems encountered with low-cost refractory materials above 1,550 K or with high-alumina refractories above 1,750 K.

Although the temperature histories required to achieve complete destruction of a waste are a function of whether the waste is injected either into a flame that contains a high concentration of free radicals or downstream of a flame, where the destruction mechanism is mainly thermal, some guidance for the selection of conditions for incinerator operation can be obtained from laboratory-scale pyrolysis and oxidation experiments. Several experimental reactors have been developed for determining the ease of destruction or incinerability of chemicals, for possible use in screening chemicals for trial-burn selection (Dellinger et al. 1984; K. Lee et al. 1972). The chemicals to be tested are vaporized and premixed with an excess of air and passed through a quartz tube heated to a known temperature in an electric furnace. The destruction efficiency, measured by analysis of the product gases, can be determined as a function of temperature and residence time in the reactor.

The effect of temperature on the destruction of chloroform in air for residence times of one to six seconds is shown in figure 9.15. Results such as these have been used to derive kinetic parameters for estimating the temperatures required to achieve a given destruction efficiency for any given residence time. Results for the temperatures required to attain a measurable destruction, 99 percent destruction, and 99.99 percent destruction are presented for selected chemicals in table 9.4 for a residence time of two seconds. The activation energies for decomposition are also shown, permitting extrapolation of the results to other residence times. The temperature T_2 for any residence time t_2 which gives the same destruction efficiency as that reported for a temperature T_1 and residence time t_1 (= 2 seconds) is given by the equation in the table, where R is the gas constant (1.98 kcal/mol), and the temperatures are in degrees Kelvin. Application of the equation shows that, whereas 2 seconds are required to obtain 99.99 percent destruction of acetonitrile at 950° C (1,223 K), only 0.13 seconds are required at 1,200° C (1,473 K). A destruction efficiency

Figure 9.15. Thermal decomposition profiles for chloroform in flowing air.

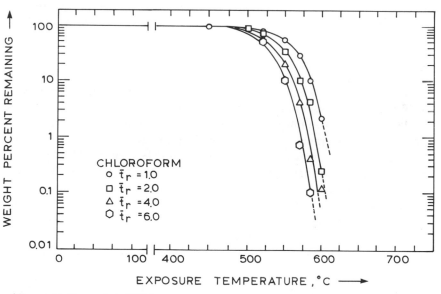

(*Source:* Dellinger et al. 1984.)

Table 9.4. Temperature required for destruction in two seconds, twenty selected chemicals

Chemical Compound	Degrees Centigrade for Destruction			Activation Energies (kcal/±mol)
	Measurable	99%	99.99%	
Acetonitrile	760	900	~950	39 ± 23
Tetrachloroethylene	660	850	920	33 ± 5.0
Acrylonitrile	650	830	860	31 ± 21
Methane	660	830	870	48 ± 3.0
Hexachlorobenzene	650	820	880	41 ± 22
1,2,3,4-Tetrachlorobenzene	660	800	850	30 ± 18
Pyridine	620	770	840	24 ± 7.0
Dichloromethane	650	770	780	62 ± 52
Carbon tetrachloride	600	750	820	26 ± 4.0
Hexachlorobutadiene	620	750	780	55 ± 13
1,2,4-Trichlorobenzene	640	750	790	39 ± 13
1,2-Dichlorobenzene	630	740	780	40 ± 13
Ethane	500	735	785	24 ± 8.0
Benzene	630	730	760	39 ± 6.0
Aniline	620	730	750	71 ± 19
Monochlorobenzene	540	710	780	23 ± 15
Nitrobenzene	570	670	700	64 ± 7.0
Hexachloroethane	470	600	640	30 ± 6.0
Chloroform	410	590	620	49 ± 8.0
1,1,1-Trichloroethane	390	570	600	32 ± 4.0

Source: Dellinger et al. 1984.

Note: $\exp\left[-\dfrac{E}{R}\left(\dfrac{1}{T_2} - \dfrac{1}{T_1}\right)\right] = \dfrac{t_1}{t_2}.$

of greater than 99.99 percent is attainable in a residence time of two seconds at temperatures of greater than 1,250 K (977° C or 1,791° F).

These are only rough guidelines to temperatures and times because of differences in free-radical concentrations encountered in different incinerators. For example, incineration in a flame would be facilitated by the high reactivity of flame-generated oxygen radicals and hydroxyl radicals. Conversely, chlorinated compounds, although readily degraded thermally because of the weak carbon-chlorine bond, may be difficult to burn because the chlorine radicals inhibit flame reactions. In an incinerator, temperatures somewhat higher than the 850 to 1,150 K indicated by the small-scale tests would be required to compensate for the time needed to vaporize and mix the chemicals.

Because it is difficult to apply the results of small-scale experiments to full-scale units, the performance of incinerators is now determined by direct measurement. In addition, the destruction of waste compound injected into an incinerator is an incomplete measure of performance, since chemical intermediates as toxic or more toxic than the parent compound may be produced. Well-known examples of such transformations are the production of the polychlorinated dibenzo dioxin from polychlorinated phenols and the formation of polychlorinated dibenzofurans from polychlorinated biphenols. These intermediates are also unstable at high temperatures, so that incinerators should be designed to meet their emission standards. The absence of toxic products of incomplete combustion (PICs) must, however, be established by measurements independent of the destruction efficiency of the waste constituents.

No systematic study of the composition and concentration of PICs emitted by hazardous waste incinerators has been conducted. A measure of the problems that may be encountered can be inferred from the recent extensive effort to determine the emissions of polychlorinated dibenzo-p-dioxins (PCDDs) and polychlorinated dibenzofurans (PCDFs) from municipal solid waste incinerators (McInnes and Hunt 1986).

PCDDs and PCDFs were first reported in 1977 in the fly ash captured in an electrostatic precipitator of an incinerator. They have since been measured in the ash and stack gases of at least thirty-five municipal solid waste incinerators in nine countries. The concentration of total PCDDs and PCDFs emitted in the stack gases ranges widely among units—from about 1 to 10 thousand ng/m^3. Although part of this difference may be attributable to differences in analytical and sampling procedures, the high emissions are undoubtedly a consequence of poor design and operating practices, particularly involving flames from the burning refuse impinging on and being quenched by the water-cooled walls used for energy recovery. PCDDs and PCDFs consist of complex mixtures of the different congeners (homologues containing from one to eight chlorine atoms) and of the isomers of the congeners. The available data indicate that the PCDFs on average are present in roughly twice the concentrations of the PCDDs and that the highly toxic 2,3,7,8-tetrachlorinated congener represents only 0.3 percent of the total PCDD concentration. Determination of total toxicity requires estimates of the concentration and relative toxicities of all isomers, making the problem of evaluating toxicity a formidable one.

The source of PCDDs and PCDFs in the emissions from municipal solid waste incinerators is unknown, but it is speculated that they are derived from polychlorinated phenols (PCPs) and polychlorinated biphenyls (PCBs) either present in the waste or formed in the flames. The study of emissions of PCDDs and PCDFs from municipal waste incinerators illustrates the complexity of obtaining data sufficiently detailed for a risk assessment, even when the problem is constrained to an examination of the small subset of the total organic emissions of concern. The data indicate, however, that concentration of PCDDs and PCDFs can be very low in well-operated and well-designed incinerators.

TURBULENCE REQUIREMENTS

Most incinerators are used for the disposal of liquid and solid wastes. Incinerators designed for injection of liquids must provide for atomizing the liquids into droplets small enough (less than 150 μm in diameter) that vaporization times are short relative to residence or mixing times in the combustion chamber. Solids in an incinerator are usually supported by either a hearth or a grate. On heating, the solids release volatile products and leave a carbonaceous residue, which is subsequently oxidized by reaction with oxygen.

Mixing on the scale of the cross-section of the combustion chamber must be achieved between the combustible vapors (produced by vaporization of liquids or pyrolysis of solids) and air in order to avoid pockets of gases starved for oxygen. In addition, sufficient mixing energy and sufficient time must be provided to enable large-scale eddies to break down to a scale small enough to permit mixing on a molecular level. In practice, gross-scale mixing is achieved by (1) tailoring injection of waste and air for uniform distribution in the combustion chamber; (2) using high velocities to ensure high turbulence; (3) using baffles and cross jets to promote mixing; and (4) using air in excess of the stoichiometric requirement, to compensate for imperfect mixing.

LEGISLATIVE REQUIREMENT

Incinerators used for destruction of hazardous waste must have an EPA permit. The granting of such a permit is contingent on a demonstration through trial burn tests that the incinerator meets EPA performance standards. These tests can cost up to $100 thousand (*Chemical and Engineering News* 1982). The three substantive requirements are (1) a destruction and removal efficiency of 99.99 percent; (2) a particulate emission below 180 milligrams per dry standard cubic meter when corrected to 50 percent excess air; and (3) control of emissions of HCl from the stack, or 99 percent removal, or an emission rate of 1.8 kilograms per hour of HCl, whichever is less stringent. Furthermore, specific requirements that must be met before an incinerator may be operated include identification of key fuel elements and principal organic hazardous constituents (POHCs). The destruction and removal efficiency for POHCs must be demonstrated at the 99.99 percent level by means of trial burns. Removal efficiency refers to the incinerator system as a whole and includes the scrubber as well as the combustion unit. Fuel rates, temperature, carbon monoxide level, and oxygen content of the incinerator must be monitored.

The selection of POHCs is based on the ease of destruction and the relative amounts of the materials to be incinerated in a given unit. A permit for an incinerator can be granted on the basis of a trial burn, with a

contrived waste composed of up to six compounds deemed the most difficult to destroy of those compounds the incinerator is intended for. Once an
incinerator has been granted a permit on the basis of such a trial burn, it is
deemed qualified to incinerate any compound that is less difficult to destroy than those used in the trial burn. The EPA has tentatively proposed a
hierarchy of relative incinerability based on heats of combustion, but other
criteria are also being considered.

Incinerator Designs

Usually, incinerators must be operated within a relatively narrow temperature range, with the lower end established by the temperature needed
to ensure adequate destruction of the waste (as high as 1,450 K for some
halogenated compounds) and the upper bound by materials of construction (as low as 1,550 K for some refractory surfaces). A burner fired with
auxiliary fuel can provide the energy both for heating the incinerator to the
desired temperature and for maintaining it at temperature for burning
wastes of low heat content. However, the potential exists for rapid temperature excursions, and explosive surges of gas evolution may occur when
solids of high volatility are burned, unless the solids are fed into the incinerator slowly. Incinerated metal containers may explode because of pressure buildup in them.

Cold surfaces in an incinerator will quench combustion reactions and
lead to emission of unburned or partially burned materials. This potential
source of undesirable emissions is greatest in small units, which have a
high surface-to-volume ratio. The problem of wall quenching can be mini-

Table 9.5. Incinerator design and capacity

Design	Number of Units	Air Pollution Control Equipment (percent)	Capacity[a] (million Btu/hr)	Utilization (percent)[b]	Capacity (million Btu/hr)
Rotary kiln	42	90	58.7	77	570
Liquid injection	95	42	36.1	55	1,540
Fume	25	40	29.5	94	40
Hearth	32	38	22.5	62	270
Other	14	...	23.8	...	110
Total or average	208	50	37.6	67	2,530

Source: Vogel et al. 1986.
[a] 181 incinerators reported.
[b] 90 incinerators reported.

mized by using hot refractory surfaces. Waste should not be fed into an incinerator during start-up and shutdown, when the walls are below operating temperature.

There are many incinerator designs, but the design of most existing incinerators can be classified as rotary kilns, liquid injection, fume, and hearth (see table 9.5). Incinerators typically consist of one or two combustion chambers, an air pollution control device, and a gas quench or heat recovery section. The latter reduce the temperature of the gases leaving the combustion chamber to the levels that can be tolerated by the gas clean-up equipment. Brief descriptions of some of the designs follow.

ROTARY KILNS

Rotary kilns have the advantage of being able to handle a wide variety of solid wastes, including containerized wastes in steel or fiber drums. The rotation of the kiln provides a tumbling action, and the inclination of the drum provides the motion toward the discharge end (see figure 9.16). The gas leaving the kiln passes through a secondary combustion chamber and then to an air pollution control device (of varying design). The temperatures and times in the primary and secondary combustion chambers are typically in the range of 1,200 to 1,500 K, and the residence times are selected to provide the desired destruction efficiency but typically are one to

Figure 9.16. Schematic of a rotary kiln incinerator.

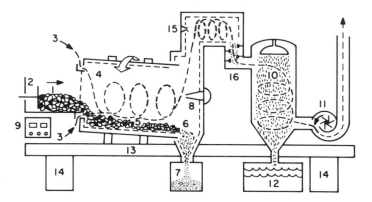

Note: 1. Waste to incinerator; 2. Autocycle feeding system: feed hopper, pneumatic feeder, slide gates; 3. Combustion air in; 4. Refractory-lined, rotating cylinder; 5. Tumble-burning action; 6. Incombustible ash; 7. Ash bin; 8. Autocontrol burner package: programed pilot burner; 9. Self-compensating instrumentation controls; 10. Wet scrubber package: stainless steel, corrosion-free wet scrubber; gas quench; 11. Exhaust fan and stack; 12. Recycle water, fly-ash sludge collector; 13. Support frame; 14. Support piers; 15. Afterburner chamber; 16. Precooler. (*Source:* National Research Council 1983.)

two seconds. The EPA has built a mobile rotary kiln incinerator on three semitrailers (Brugger et al. 1982). It has been tested at Times Beach, Missouri.

LIQUID INJECTION

Incinerators designed to dispose of liquid wastes often consist of a single refractory-lined combustion chamber. It is brought up to temperature using a burner fired by a conventional fossil fuel, which can also be used as an auxiliary burner to maintain the incinerator at the desired temperature at all times. Fine sprays of the waste are injected into the chamber, usually using a twin fluid atomizer, in which air or steam is used to desintegrate the waste streams into droplets of 100 μm or less. A schematic of a liquid-injection incinerator is shown in figure 9.17. The volume of the refractory-lined chamber downstream of the burners is designed to provide the desired residence time. The gaseous effluent is then cooled with a gas quench and passed through a scrubber. The design shown is for a high-chlorine-

Figure 9.17. Schematic of a liquid-injection incinerator.

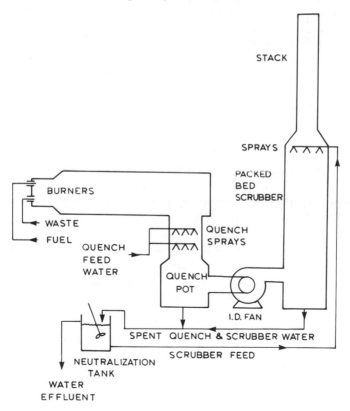

content waste, so that the scrubber fluid needs to be neutralized before disposal. Liquid-injection incinerators have been built on oceangoing vessels such as the *Vulcanus*.

OTHER DESIGNS

The degradation of molecules to innocuous compounds can be achieved by a multiplicity of devices that can provide the necessary temperature, time, and turbulence. Combustion systems used for this purpose include (1) stokers, in which the waste is supported on a grate through which part of the combustion air is passed; (2) single-hearth and multi-hearth units, in which the waste is supported on a hearth provided with a rotating rabble arm to provide agitation of the solids; (3) fluidized beds, in which the waste is injected into a hot inert bed of solids fluidized by air that comes through a distributor plate at the base of the bed; (4) fast-circulating fluidized beds, in which the air-flow rate is high enough to blow the solids out of the bed, to which they are recycled after capture in a cyclone. In combustors, the energy required to attain the high temperatures needed to destroy the waste is provided by the energy released on oxidation of the waste itself, possibly supplemented by a fossil fuel. Operating conditions for several incinerator designs are shown in table 9.6, together with the waste used in a trial burn. An alternative method of attaining high temperatures is by electrical heating, for example, by use of a plasma arc (Barton 1984). Such units rely on pyrolysis rather than oxidation to destroy the waste. More detailed process descriptions may be found in Sittig 1979.

Incinerator Performance

The efficiency of destruction of a variety of wastes has been tested in incinerators, boilers, and process furnaces. With few exceptions, these efficiencies were in excess of the regulatory limit of 99.99 percent. In boilers cofired with hazardous wastes, however, emissions of other products of incomplete combustion exceeded the residue of the waste (Castaldini et al. 1984). Some of the over 200 incinerators that have been permitted may also have emissions of unmonitored toxic trace compounds. Furthermore, performance under trial-burn conditions may not represent average operation, particularly for units subject to wide variations in operating conditions or to surges in emissions following the charging of volatile solid wastes. Although the operation of hazardous waste incinerators has produced no known adverse consequences to the public health or the environment, the uncertainties of the data and the potential risks from the dispersal of stack emissions has resulted in a recommendation by the EPA Science Advisory Board (1985b) that a more complete characterization of the emissions and effluents of incinerators be obtained.

Incineration has the advantage over secured landfills of destroying toxic wastes. The largest obstacle to implementing this technology is pub-

Table 9.6. Wastes, incinerators, and results of trial burns

Waste and Incinerator	Temperature (K)	Residence Time (seconds)	Waste Feed Rate (kg/h)	Auxiliary Fuel Rate (kg/h)	Excess Air (percent)
Altrazine: multiple chamber					
Trial 1	1,343	2.7	3.63	8.3	43
Trial 2	1,243	2.2	4.50	8.5	125
Trial 3	873	5.6	3.40	2.7	146
Trial 4	1,243	2.7	4.30	6.9	71
Trial 5	923	6.8	...	...	...
DDT (20%) in distillate oil; PCB (1.7%) in waste oil: liquid injection; thermal oxidizer					
Trial 1	1,144	...	4.70	2.5	111
Trial 2	1,144	3.4	300	0	169
Trial 3	1,144	2.9	300	0	157
Trial 4	1,255	3.0	330	0	163
Trial 5	1,255	4.0	330	0	123
Hexachlorocyclopentadiene: liquid injection					
All trials	1,621–51	0.17–0.18	290	0	123
Methyl methacrylate (34%), phenols (13%): fluidized bed					
Bed, all trials	1,047–661	12	40–90	120–70	...
Freeboard, all trials	1,097–116	12	~1,800	~3,600–4,600	11.6–13.4
Nitrochlorobenzene: liquid injection					
Trial 1	1,580	2.3	...	...	...
Trial 2	1,605	2.3	~404	~90,000	...
Polychlorinated biphenyls: rotary kiln					
Trial 1	1,143	2.3	~350	~80,000	...
Trial 2 (all trials)	1,253–363	2.3	845	1,780–2,250	75–140

Source: Corini et al. 1980.

lic concern with the siting of land-based units and with the transport and storage of wastes for oceangoing units. It is important to resolve uncertainties about the health and environmental effects of the effluents—gaseous, liquid, and solids—in order to allay such concerns.

References

Acar, Y. B., and R. K. Seals. 1984. Clay barrier technology for shallow land waste disposal facilities. *Hazardous Wastes* 1:167–81.

Alexander, M. 1973. Nonbiodegradable and other recalcitrant molecules. *Biotechnology and Bioengineering* 15:611–47.

———. 1984. Ecological constraints on genetic engineering. In *Genetic Control of Environmental Pollutants*, ed. G. C. Omenn and A. Hollaender. New York: Plenum.

Alleman, J. E. 1983. Beneficial use of sludge in building components. NTS PB84179498.

American Institute of Chemical Engineers. 1986. Hazardous Waste Task Force Report. *Technological Need for Improved Management of Hazardous Waste*. Washington, D.C.: AICE.

American Society for Testing and Materials. 1981. *Permeability and Groundwater Contaminant Transport*. ASTM STP 746. Philadelphia: ASTM.

———. *Hydraulic Barriers for Soil and Rock*. ASTM STP 874. Philadelphia: ASTM.

Barton, G. T. 1984. *Hazardous Wastes* 1:237–47.

Belton, T., R. Hazen, B. Ruppel, K. Lockwood, R. Mueller, E. Stevenson, and J. Post. 1985a. *A Study of Dioxin (2,3,7-8 Tetrachlorodibenzo-p-dioxin) Contamination in Select Finfish, Crustaceans and Sediments of New Jersey Waterways*. Trenton: New Jersey Department of Environmental Protection.

Belton, T., B. Ruppel, K. Lockwood, S. Shiboski, G. Bukowski, R. Roundy, N. Weinstein, D. Wilson, and H. Whelan. 1985b. *A Study of Toxic Hazards to Urban Fishermen and Crabbers*. Trenton: New Jersey Department of Environmental Protection.

Bend, J., and C. L. Foureman. 1984. Variation of hepatic aryl hydrocarbon hydroxylase (AHH) activity and 7-ethoxyresorufin 0-diethylase (7-ERD) activities in marine fish from Maine: Evidence that monooxygenase activities of only a few species are induced by environmental exposure to polycyclic aromatic hydrocarbon (PAH)-type compounds. *Marine Environmental Resources* 14:405–6.

Bend, J., and M. O. James. 1978. Xenobiotic metabolism in marine and freshwater species. In *Biochemical and Biophysical Perspectives in Marine Biology*, ed. D. Malins and J. Sargent. Vol. 4. New York: Academic Press.

Bitton, G., and C. P. Gerba. 1984. Groundwater pollution microbiology: The emerging issue. In *Groundwater Pollution Microbiology*, ed. Bitton and Gerba. New York: John Wiley & Sons.

Bopp, L. H., D. L. Bedard, and M. L. Haberl. 1986. Bacterial degradation of individual polychlorinated biphenyl congeners in an assay mixture is influenced by the other congeners present. *Abstracts of the Annual Meeting of the American Society of Microbiologists* 61:294.

Borquin, A., P. Pritchard, W. Walker, and P. Parrish, eds. 1985. *Proceedings of the Workshop: Biodegradation Kinetics*. Technical Report EPA-600/9-85-018. Washington, D.C.: U.S. Environmental Protection Agency.

Bowders, J. J., D. E. Daniel, G. P. Broderick, and H. M. Liljestrand. 1986. Methods for testing the compatibility of clay liners with landfill leachate. In *Proceedings of the Fourth International Symposium on Hazardous and Industrial Solid Waste Testing*. Washington, D.C.: American Society for Testing and Materials.

Brink, R. H. 1981. Biodegradation of organic chemicals in the environment. In *Environmental Health Chemistry,* ed. J. McKinney. Ann Arbor: Ann Arbor Press.

Brown, K. W., and D. C. Anderson. 1983. *Effects of Organic Solvents on the Permeability of Clay Soils.* EPA-600/2-83-016. Cincinnati: U.S. Environmental Protection Agency, Hazardous Waste Engineering Research Laboratory.

Brugger, J. E., J. J. Yezzi, Jr., I. Wilder, F. J. Freeston, R. A. Miller, and C. Pfrommer, Jr. 1982. *Proceedings of the 1982 Conference on Hazardous Material Spills,* Milwaukee (April 19–22) p. 116.

Bryan, E. H. 1984. *Research Supported by National Science Foundation Related to Treatment of Waste Water and Management of Residual Sludges.* EPA-600/9-84-021. Washington, D.C.: U.S. Environmental Protection Agency.

California Department of Health Services. 1984. *Alternative Technology for Recycling and Treatment of Hazardous Waste.* Sacramento: CDHS.

Callahan, M., M. Slimak, N. Gabel, I. May, C. Fowler, J. Freed, P. Jennings, R. Durfie, F. Whitmore, B. Maestri, W. Maybey, B. Holt, and C. Gould. 1979. *Water-Related Fate of 129 Priority Pollutants.* Vol. 2. EPA 440/4-79-029B. Washington, D.C.: U.S. Environmental Protection Agency.

Canney, P. J., and P. T. Schaefer. 1983. Detoxification of hazardous industrial wastewaters by wet air oxidation. Paper presented at AICHE meeting, Houston, March.

Castaldini, B., H. B. Mason, R. J. De Rosier, and S. Unnasch. 1984. Field tests of industrial boilers cofiring hazardous wastes. *Hazardous Wastes* 1:159–65.

Cerniglia, C. E. 1984. Microbial transformation of aromatic hydrocarbons. In *Petroleum Microbiology,* ed. R. M. Atlas. New York: Macmillan.

Chatterjee, D. K., and A. M. Chakrabarty. 1981. Plasmids in the biodegradation of PCBs and chlorobenzoates. In *Microbial Degradation of Xenobiotics and Recalcitrant Compounds,* eds. T. Leisinger, R. Hutter, A. M. Cook, and J. Nuesch. London: Academic Press.

Chemical Engineering. 1984a. Bioreclamation: The treatment of contaminated soil or groundwater. *Chemical Engineering* 91:19.

———. 1984b. First commercial PCB destruction via microorganisms has been completed. *Chemical Engineering* 91:20.

Chemical and Engineering News. 1982. June 28, p. 7.

———. 1985. Bhopal report. February 11.

Chemical Manufacturers Association. 1983. *CMA Hazardous Waste Survey for 1981 and 1982.* Washington, D.C.: CMA.

Chemical Manufacturers Association and Engineering Science. 1986. *Results of the 1984 CMA Hazardous Wastes Survey.* Austin: Engineering-Science.

Clayton, J., S. Pavlou, and N. Breitner. 1977. Polychlorinated biphenyls in coastal marine zooplankton: Bioaccumulation by equilibrium partitioning. *Environmental Science Technology* 11:676–81.

Colwell, R. R., and G. S. Sayler. 1978. Microbial degradation of industrial chemicals. In *Water Pollution Microbiology,* ed. R. Mitchell. New York: John Wiley & Sons.

Conney, A. H. 1982. Induction of microsomal enzymes by foreign chemicals and carcinogenesis by polycyclic aromatic hydrocarbons. *Cancer Research* 42:4875–917.

Connolly, J., and R. Winfield. 1984. *A User's Guide to WASTOX: A Framework for Modelling the Fate of Toxic Chemicals in Aquatic Environments.* Part 1, *Exposure Concentration.* Technical Report EPA-600/3-84-077. Washington, D.C.: U.S. Environmental Protection Agency.

Corini, J., C. Day, and E. Temrowski. 1980. *Trial Burn Data.* Draft Report. Washington, D.C.: U.S. Environmental Protection Agency, Office of Solid Waste.

Cralley, L. V., and L. F. Cralley, eds. 1983. *Industrial Hygiene Aspects of Plant Operations,* vol. 1. New York: Macmillan.

Cullinane, M. J., and L. W. Jones. 1985. *Technical Handbook for Stabilization/Solidification of Hazardous Waste.* Cincinnati: U.S. Environmental Protection Agency, Hazardous Waste Engineering Research Laboratory.

Daniel, D. E., and S. J. Trautwein. 1986. Field permeability test for earthen liners. In *Proceedings, In-Situ '86: ASCE Specialty Conference on Use of In-Situ Tests of Geotechnical Engineering,* Blacksburg, Va.

Dellinger, B., J. L. Torres, W. A. Ruby, D. L. Hall, J. L. Graham, and R. A. Carnes. 1984. *Hazardous Wastes* 1:137-57.

DeRenzo, D. J., ed. 1978. *Unit Operations for Treatment of Hazardous Industrial Wastes.* Park Ridge, N.J.: Noyes Data Corporation.

Deshpande, S. D., et al. 1985. Biological treatability of m-aminophenol plant wastewater containing structural isomers of benzene with different substituents. *Water Resources* 19:293.

Doull, J., C. Klaassen, and M. Amdur. 1980. *Toxicology: The Basic Science of Poisons.* New York: Macmillan.

Evans, W. C. 1977. Biochemistry of the bacterial cetabolism of aromatic cpds in anaerobic environments. *Nature* 270:17-25.

Fewson, C. A. 1981. Biodegradation of aromatics with industrial relevance. In *Microbial Degradation of Xenobiotics and Recalcitrant Compounds,* ed. T. Leisinger, R. Hutter, A. M. Cook, and J. Nuesch. London: Academic Press.

Fogel, S., R. L. Lancione, and A. E. Sewall. 1982. Enhanced biodegradation of methoxychlor in sod under sequential environmental conditions. *Applied and Environmental Microbiology* 44:113-20.

Federal Regulation. 1981. 46 FR 7666. Code of Federal Regulations, January 23.
———. 1982. 47 FR 27516. Code of Federal Regulations, June 24.

GCA Corporation. 1984. *Technology Technical Assistance of Treatment Alternatives for Wastes Containing Halogenated Organics.* Cincinnati: U.S. Environmental Protection Agency, Hazardous Waste Engineering Research Laboratory.

Ghosal, D., I.-S. You, D. Chatterjee, and A. Chakrabarty. 1985. Microbial degradation of halogenated compounds. *Science* 228:135-42.

Gibson, D. T. 1976. Microbial degradation of polycyclic aromatic hydrocarbons. In *Proceedings of the Third International Biodegradation Symposium,* ed. J. M. Sharpley and A. M. Kaplan. London: Applied Science Publishers.

Gibson, D. T., and V. Subramanian. 1984. Microbial degradation of aromatic hydrocarbons. In *Microbial Degradation of Organic Compounds,* ed. D. T. Gibson. New York: Marcel Dekker.

Gmur, D., and U. Varanasi. 1982. Characterization of benzo(a)pyrene metabolites isolated from muscle, liver and bile of a juvenile flatfish. *Carcinogenesis* 3:1397-1403.

Goode, D. J., and P. A. Smith. 1984. *Procedure for Modeling Flow through Clay Liners to Determine Required Liner Thickness.* Draft Report EPA-530-SW-84-001. Washington, D.C.: U.S. Environmental Protection Agency.

Guiney, P., and R. Peterson. 1980. Distribution and elimination of a polychlorinated biphenyl after acute dietary exposure in yellow perch and rainbow trout. *Archives Environmental Contamination and Toxicology* 9:667-74.

Guthrie, M. A., et al. 1984. Pentachlorophenol biodegradation anaerobic. *Water Resources* 18:451.

Hakulinen, R., and M. Salkinoja-Solonen. 1982. Treatment of pulp and paper industry wastewater in an anaerobic fluidized bed reactor. *Process Biochemistry* (March/April): 18-25.

Hamelink, J., R. Wybrant, and R. Ball. 1971. A proposal: Exchange equilibria control the degree chlorinated hydrocarbons are biologically magnified in lentic environments. *Transactions of the American Fish Society* 100:207-14.

Haxo, H. E. 1983. *Lining of Waste Impoundment and Disposal Facilities*. EPA SW-870. Washington, D.C.: U.S. Environmental Protection Agency.

Haxo, Jr., H. E., R. S. Haxo, N. A. Nelson, R. M. White, and S. Dakession. 1984. *Liner Materials Exposed to Hazardous and Toxic Wastes*. EPA-600/2-84-169. Cincinnati: U.S. Environmental Protection Agency, Hazardous Waste Engineering Research Laboratory.

Hayaishi, O. 1962. History and scope. In *Oxygenases*, ed. Hayaishi. New York: Academic Press.

Herget, W. F., and S. P. Levine. 1986. Preliminary test of FTIR spectroscopy for monitoring semiconductor process gas emissions. *Journal of Applied Industrial Hygiene* 2:110-12.

Hertzbrun, P. A., R. L. Irvine, and K. C. Malinowski. 1985. Biological treatment of hazardous waste in sequencing batch reactors. *Journal—Water Pollution Control Federation* 57:1163-67.

Hickman, G. T., and J. T. Novak. 1984. Acclimation of activated sludge to pentachlorophenol. *Journal—Water Pollution Control Federation*.

Hutzinger, O., D. Nash, S. Safe, A. DeFreitas, R. Norstrom, D. Wildish, and V. Zitko. 1972. Polychlorinated biphenyls: Metabolic behavior of pure isomers in pigeons, rats and brook trout. *Science* 178:312-14.

Johnson, L. M., and J. M. Thomas. 1984. Biodecontamination of a full-scale formaldehyde spill. In *Genetic Control of Environmental Pollutants*, ed. G. S. Omenn and A. Hollaender. New York: Plenum Press.

Josephson, J. 1982. Supercritical fluids. *Environmental Science Technology* 16:548A-51A.

Kapoor, I. P., R. Metcalf, R. Nystrom, and G. Sangha. 1970. Comparative metabolism of methoxychlor, methiochlor, and DDT in mouse, insects and in a model ecosystem. *Journal of Agriculture and Food Chemistry* 18:1145-52.

Karns, J. S., J. J. Kilbane, D. K. Chatterjee, and A. M. Chakrabarty. 1984. Microbial degradation of 2,4,5-trichlorophenoxyacetic acid and chlorophenols. In *Genetic Control of Environmental Pollutants*, ed. G. S. Omenn and A. Hollaender. New York: Plenum Press.

Kaufman, N. 1984. Solvent waste management in a high technology corporation. *Hazardous Wastes* 1:83-92.

Keenan, J. D., R. L. Steiner, and A. A. Fungaroli. 1984. Landfill leachate treatment. *Journal—Water Pollution Control Federation* 56:27-33.

Khan, M. 1977. Elimination of pesticides by aquatic animals. In *Pesticides in Aquatic Environments*, ed. Khan. New York: Plenum Press.

Khan, M., F. Korte, and J. Payne. 1977. Metabolism of pesticides by aquatic animals. In *Pesticides in Aquatic Environments*, ed. Khan. New York: Plenum Press.

Kiang, Y-H, and A. Metry. 1982. *Hazardous Waste Processing Technology.* Ann Arbor: Ann Arbor Science Publishers.

Klotz, A. V., and J. J. Stegeman. 1984. Multiple isozymes of hepatic cytochrome P-450 from the marine teleost fish (Stenotomus chrysops). *Marine Environmental Research* 14:402–4.

Klotz, A. V., J. J. Stegeman, and C. Walsh. 1983. An aryl hydrocarbon hydroxylating hepatic cytochrome P-450 from the marine fish Stenotomus chrysops. *Archives of Biochemistry and Biophysics* 226:578–92.

Knackmuss, H. J. 1981. Degradation of halogenated and sulfonated hydrocarbons. In *Degradation of Xenobiotics and Recalcitrant Compounds,* ed. T. Leisinger, R. Hutter, A. M. Cook, and J. Nuesch. London: Academic Press.

Kopecky, A. 1984. Biological degradation of polychlorinated biphenyls by mutant organisms. In *Genetic Control of Environmental Pollutants,* ed. G. S. Omenn and A. Hollaender. New York: Plenum Press.

Kosson, D. S., and R. C. Ahlert. 1984. In-situ and on-site biodegradation of industrial landfill leachate. *Environmental Progress* 3:176.

Krahn, M., M. Myers, D. Burrows, and D. Malins. 1984. Determination of metabolites of xenobiotics in bile of fish from polluted waterways. *Xenobiotics* 14:633–46.

Lech, J., and J. Bend. 1980. Relationship between biotransformation and the toxicity and fate of xenobiotic chemicals in fish. *Environmental Health Perspective* 34:115–31.

Lech, J., and R. Peterson. 1983. Biotransformation and persistence of polychlorinated biphenyls (PCBs) in fish. In *PCBs: Human and Environmental Hazards,* ed. F. D'Itri and M. Kamrin. Ann Arbor: Ann Arbor Science Publishers.

Lee, K., N. Morgan, J. L. Hansen, and G. M. Whipple. 1972. Revised model for the projection of the time-temperature requirements for thermal destruction of dilute organic vapors and its usage for predicting compound destructability. Paper presented at the 75th annual meeting of the Air Pollution Control Association, New Orleans, June.

Lee, R., R. Sauerheber, and G. Dobbs. 1972. Uptake, metabolism and discharge of polycyclic aromatic hydrocarbons by marine fish. *Marine Biology* 17:201–8.

Levine, S. P., and W. F. Martin, eds. 1985. *Protecting Personnel at Hazardous Waste Sites.* Stoneham, Maine: Butterworths, Ann Arbor Science Publishers.

Levine, S. P., et al. 1985a. Air monitoring at the drum bulking process of a hazardous waste remedial action site. *American Industrial Hygiene Association Journal* 46:192–96.

———. 1985b. Air monitoring during a hazardous waste remedial action at a drum bulking unit process. *Hazardous Wastes* 1:573–80.

Lutton, R. S. 1982. *Evaluating Cover Systems for Solid and Hazardous Waste.* EPA SW-867. Washington, D.C.: U.S. Environmental Protection Agency.

McAneny, C. C., and A. W. Hatheway. 1985. *Design and Construction of Covers for Uncontrolled Landfill Sites.* Draft Report. Washington, D.C.: U.S. Environmental Protection Agency.

McInnes, R. G., and G. T. Hunt. 1986. Critical criteria in the development of a toxic air emissions inventory for municipal solid waste incinerators. Paper presented at the spring 1986 conference of the New England Section, Air Pollution Control Association, Providence, April.

Mackay, D. 1982. Correlation of bioconcentration factors. *Environmental Science Technology* 16:274–78.

Mackay, D., and A. Hughes. 1984. Three-parameter equation describing the uptake of organic compounds by fish. *Environmental Science Technology* 18:439–41.

McMurtry, D. C., and R. O. Elton. 1985. New approaches to in-situ treatment of contaminated groundwater. *Environmental Progress* 4:168.

Malins, D. 1977. Metabolism of aromatic hydrocarbons in marine organisms. *Annals of the New York Academy of Sciences* 298:482–96.

Malins, D., T. Collier, L. Thomas, and W. Roubal. 1979. Metabolic fate of aromatic hydrocarbons in aquatic organisms. *International Journal of Environmental Analytical Chemistry* 6:55–66.

Malins, D., M. Krahn, D. Brown, L. Rhodes, M. Myers, B. McCain, and S.-L. Chan. 1985. Toxic chemicals in marine sediment and biota from Mukilteo, Washington: Relationships with hepatic neoplasma and other hepatic lesions in English sole (Parophrys vetulus). *Journal of the National Cancer Institute* 74:487–94.

Mason, H. 1957. Mechanisms of oxygen metabolism. *Advances in Enzymology and Related Areas of Molecular Biology* 19:79.

Matthews, H. 1983. Metabolism of PCBs in mammals: Routes of entry, storage and excretion. In *PCBs: Human and Environmental Hazards,* ed. F. D'Itri and M. Kamrin. Ann Arbor: Ann Arbor Science Publishers.

Melancon, M., and J. Lech. 1976. Isolation and identification of a plar metabolite of tetrachlorobiphenyl from bile of rainbow trout exposed to 14-C tetrachlorobiphenyl. *Bulletin of Environmental Contamination and Toxicology* 15:181–87.

———. 1983. Dose-effect relationship for induction of hepatic monooxygenase activity in rainbow trout and carp by Aroclor 1254. *Aquatic Toxicology* 4:51–61.

Melius, J. M., and W. E. Halperin. 1982. Medical screening of workers at hazardous waste disposal sites. In *Hazardous Waste Disposal: Assessing the Problem,* ed. E. Highland. Ann Arbor: Ann Arbor Science Publishers.

Michelson, D. L., et al. 1984. In-situ biological oxidation of hazardous organics. *Environmental Progress* 3:103.

Moese, M. 1986. Bioaccumulation and disposition of dietary phenanthrene in blue crabs (Callinectes sapidus): A pharmacokinetic approach. Ph.D., diss., New York University.

Mocse, M., and J. O'Connor. 1985. Phenanthrene kinetics in blue crab from dietary sources. *Marine Environmental Research* 17:254–57.

Moore, C. A. 1983. *Landfill and Surface Impoundment Performance Evaluation.* EPA SW-869. Washington, D.C.: U.S. Environmental Protection Agency.

Moriarty, F. 1976. *Persistent Organic Pollutants.* New York: Academic.

Nakatsugawa, T., and M. Morelli. 1976. Microsomal oxidation and insecticide metabolism. In *Insecticide Biochemistry and Physiology,* ed. C. Wilkinson. New York: Plenum Press.

National Academy of Sciences. 1979. *Protection against Depletion of Stratospheric Ozone by Chlorofluorocarbons.* Washington, D.C.: NAS.

National Research Council. 1983. *Prudent Practices for Disposal of Chemicals from the Environment.* Washington, D.C.: National Academy Press.

Neal, R. A. 1985. Mechanisms of the biological effects of PCBs, polychlorinated dibenzo-p-dioxins and polychlorinated dibenzofurans in experimental animals. *Environmental Health Perspectives* 60:41–46.

Nelson, N. 1972. PCBs: Environmental impact. *Environmental Research* 5:249–62.

New York Times. 1985. January series—The Bhopal disaster: How it happened.

Nisbet, I., and A. Sarofim. 1972. Rates and routes of transport of PCBs in the environment. *Environmental Health Perspectives* 1:21–38.

Norstrom, R., A. McKinnon, and S. DeFrietas. 1976. A bioenergetics based model for pollutant accumulation by fish: Stimulation of PCB and methylmercury residue levels in Ottawa River yellow-perch. *Journal of Fishery, Research Board of Canada* 33:248–67.

O'Connor, J. M., and T. J. Kneip. 1986. *Human Health Effects of Waste Disposal.* Washington, D.C.: U.S. Congress, Office of Technology Assessment.

O'Connor, J., and J. Pizza. 1986. Pharmacokinetic model for the accumulation of PCBs in marine fish. In *Wastes in the Ocean,* ed. I. Duedall. Vol. 9. New York: Academic Press.

———. In press. PCB dynamics in Hudson River striped bass: III-Tissue disposition and routes for elimination. *Estuaries.*

Olexsey, R. A., H. M. Freman, and R. E. Mournigham. 1985. *Hazardous Waste to Energy.* Cincinnati: U.S. Environmental Protection Agency, Hazardous Waste Engineering Research Laboratory.

Olishifski, P. E., and F. E. McElroy, eds. 1977. *Fundamentals of Industrial Hygiene.* Chicago: National Safety Council.

Oliver, B., and A. Miimi. 1985. Bioconcentration factors of some halogenated organics for rainbow trout: Limitations in their use of prediction of environmental residues. *Environmental Science and Technology* 19:842–49.

Phillipi, M., V. Krasnobajew, J. Zeyer, and R. Hutter. 1981. Fate of TCDD in microbial cultures and in soil under laboratory conditions. In *Microbial Degradation of Xenobiotics and Recalcitrant Compounds,* ed. T. Leisinger, R. Hutter, A. M. Cook, and J. Nuesch. London: Academic Press.

Pizza, J., and J. O'Connor. 1983. PCB dynamics in Hudson River striped bass: II-Accumulation from dietary sources. *Aquatic Toxicology* 3:313–27.

Poiger, H., and H. Buser. 1983. Structure elucidation of mammalian TCDD-metabolites. In *Human and Environmental Risks of Chlorinated Dioxins and Related Compounds,* ed. R. Tucker, A. Young, and A. Gray.

Poland, A., and E. Glover. 1977. Chlorinated biphenyl induction of aryl hydrocarbon hydroxylase activity: A study of the structure-activity relationship. *Molecular Pharmacology* 13:335–56.

Poland, A., W. Greenlee, and A. Kende. 1979. Studies on the mechanism of action of the chlorinated dibenzo-p-dioxins and related compounds. *Annals of the New York Academy of Sciences* 320:214–30.

Puskar, M. A., et al. 1986. Computerized infrared spectral identification of compounds frequently found at hazardous waste sites. *Analytical Chemistry* 58:1156–62.

Reineke, W. 1984. Microbial degradation of halogenated aromatic compounds. In *Microbial Degradation of Organic Compounds,* ed. D. T. Gibson. New York: Marcel Dekker.

Risebrough, R., P. Reichle, S. Herman, D. Peakall, and M. Kirven. 1968. Polychlorinated biphenyls in the global ecosystem. *Nature* 220:1098–1102.

Roberts, D. W. 1984. *Soil Properties, Classification and Hydraulic Conductivity Testing.* Draft Report SW-925. Washington, D.C.: U.S. Environmental Protection Agency.

Roy, W. R., R. A. Griffin, S. F. J. Chou, and I. G. Krupac. 1985. *Batch Soil Procedure to Design Clay Liners for Pollutant Removal.* Draft Report. Washington, D.C.: U.S. Environmental Protection Agency.

Ryan, D., P. Thomas, D. Korzeniowski, and W. Levin. 1979. Separation and characterization of highly purified forms of liver microsomal cytochrome P-450 from rats treated with polychlorinated biphenyls, phenobarbital and 3-methylcholanthrene. *Journal of Biological Chemistry* 254:1365-74.

Ryan, D., P. Thomas, and W. Levin. 1980. Hepatic microsomal cytochrome P-450 from rats treated with isofarole: Purification and characterization of four enzymic forms. *Journal of Biological Chemistry* 225:7941-55.

———. 1982. Purification and characterization of a minor form of hepatic microsomal cytochrome P-450 from rats treated with polychlorinated biphenyls. *Archives of Biochemistry and Biophysics* 216:272-88.

Safe, S. 1983. 2,3,7,8-TCDD: Biochemical effects. *Chemosphere* 12:447-52.

———. 1984a. Microbial degradation of polychlorinated biphenyls. In *Microbial Degradation of Organic Compounds,* ed. D. T. Gibson. New York: Marcel Dekker.

———. 1984b. Polychlorinated biphenyls (PCBs) and polybrominated biphenyls (PBBs): Biochemistry, toxicology and mechanism of action. *CRC Critical Reviews in Toxicology* 13:319-93.

Sawahata, T., J. Olson, and R. Neal. 1982. Identification of metabolites of 2,3,7,8-tetrachlorodibenzo-p-dioxin (TCDD) formed on incubation with isolated rat hepatocytes.

Schroeder, P. R., J. M. Morgan, T. M. Walski, and A. C. Gibson. 1984. *Hydrologic Evaluation of Landfill Performance (HELP) Model.* EPA-530-SW-84-009 and EPA-530-SW-84010. Washington, D.C.: U.S. Environmental Protection Agency.

Schwartz, P., S. Jacobson, G. Fein, J. Jacobson, and H. Price. 1983. Lake Michigan fish consumption as a source of polychlorinated biphenyls in human cord serum, maternal serum and milk. *American Journal of Public Health* 73:293-96.

Schwope, A. D., et al. 1981. *Guidelines for the Selection of Chemical Protective Clothing.* Cincinnati: American Conference of Governmental Industrial Hygienists.

Senkan, S. M. 1984. *Combustion Science and Technology* 38:197.

Shreve, R. N., and J. A. Brink. 1977. *Chemical Process Industries.* New York: McGraw-Hill.

Shuckrow, A. J., A. P. Pajak, and C. J. Touhill. 1983. *Management of Hazardous Waste Leachate.* EPA SW-871. Washington, D.C.: U.S. Environmental Protection Agency.

Sittig, M. 1979. *Incineration of Industrial Hazardous Wastes and Sludges.* Pollution Technology Review 63. Park Ridge, N.J.: Noyes Data Corporation.

Spacie, A., and J. Hamelink. 1982. Alternative models for describing the bioconcentration of organics in fish. *Environmental Toxicological Chemistry* 1:309-21.

Stegeman, J. J. 1981. Polynuclear aromatic hydrocarbons and their metabolites in the marine environment. In *Polycyclic Hydrocarbons and Cancer,* ed. H. Gelboin and P. T'so. Vol. 3. New York: Academic Press.

———. 1983. Hepatic microsomal monooxygenase activity and the biotransformation of hydrocarbons in deep benthic fish from the Western North Atlantic Can. *Journal of the Fish Aquatic Science* 40 (suppl. 2): 78-85.

Stegeman, J., R. Binder, and A. Orren. 1979. Hepatic and extrahepatic microsomal electron transport components and mixed function oxidases in the marine fish Stenotomus versicolor. *Biochemical Pharmacology* 28:3431-39.

Stegeman, J., B. Woodin, S. Park, P. Kloepper-Sams, and H. Gelboin. 1985. Microsomal cytochrome P-450 function in fish evaluated with polyclonal and monoclonal antibodies to cytochrome P-450E from scup Stenotomus chrysops. *Marine Environmental Research* 17:83–86.

Stegeman, J., P. Kloepper-Sams, and J. Farrington. 1986. Monooxygenase induction and chlorobiphenyls in the deep sea fish Coryphaenoides armatus. *Science* 231:1287–89.

Stein, J., T. Hom, and U. Varanasi. 1984. Simultaneous exposure of English sole (Parophrys vetulus) to sediment-associated xenobiotics: I-Uptake and disposition of 14-C polychlorinated biphenyls and 3-H benzo(a)pyrene. *Marine Environmental Research* 13:97–119.

Stone, R. B., K. A. Covell, T. R. Moran, L. W. Weyand, and C. U. Sparkman. 1985. *Using Mined Space for Long-Term Retention of Nonradioactive Hazardous Waste.* Vols. 1 and 2. EPA-600/2-85-021. Cincinnati: U.S. Environmental Protection Agency.

Sulfita, J., A. Horowitz, D. R. Shelton, and J. M. Tiedje. 1982. Dehalogenization: A novel pathway would be anaerobic biodegradation of haloaromatic compounds. *Science* 218:1115–17.

Sweet, W. E., R. D. Ross, and G. V. Velde. 1985. Hazardous waste management. *JAPCA* 35:138–43.

Thakker, D., H. Yagi, D. Whelan, W. Levin, A. Wood, A. Conney, and D. Jerina. 1981. Metabolic formation and reactions of bay-region diol epoxides: Ultimate carcinogenic metabolites of polycyclic aromatic hydrocarbons. In *Environmental Health Chemistry*, ed. J. McKinney. Ann Arbor: Ann Arbor Science Publishers.

Thomann, R., and J. Connolly. 1984. Model of PCBs in the Lake Michigan lake trout food chain. *Environmental Science Technology* 18:65–71.

Tsang, A., and W. Shaub. 1981. Chemical processes in the incineration of hazardous materials. Paper presented at 182d national meeting of the American Chemical Society, New York, August.

Union Carbide. 1985. *Bhopal MIC Incident.* Investigation Team Report, March. Danbury, Conn.: Union Carbide.

Unterman, R., D. L. Bedard, L. H. Bopp, M. J. Brennan, C. Johnson, and M. L. Haberl. 1985. *Microbiol Degradation of Polychlorinated Biphenyls.* EPA-600/9-85-025. Washington, D.C.: U.S. Environmental Protection Agency.

U.S. Congress. 1984. *The Hazardous and Solid Waste Amendments of 1984.* Public Law 98–616.

———. 1985. General Accounting Office. *Cleaning Up Hazardous Wastes: An Overview of Superfund Reauthorization Issues.* GAO/RCED-85-69. Gaithersburg, Md.: GAO, Document Handling and Information Services Facility.

U.S. Department of Health, Education, and Welfare. 1976. *The Industrial Environment: Its Evaluation and Control.* Washington, D.C.: DHEW National Institute of Occupational Safety and Health.

U.S. Department of Health and Human Services. 1984. *Personal Protective Equipment for Hazardous Materials Incidents: A Selection Guide.* PHS/CDC/NIOSH 84-114. Washington, D.C.: DHHS.

———. 1985. *Occupational Safety and Health Guidance Manual for Hazardous Waste Activities.* NIOSH/OSHA/USCG/EPA Interagency Task Group. PHS/CDC/NIOSH 85-115. Washington, D.C.: U.S. DHHS.

U.S. Environmental Protection Agency. 1982. *Superfund: What It Is, How It Works.* EPA WH-562A. Washington, D.C.: EPA Office of Solid Waste and Emergency Response.

CLEANUP OF CONTAMINATED SITES   279

————. 1983. *Treatability Manual.* Vols. 1–5. EPA-600/2-82-001. Washington, D.C.: EPA.

————. 1984a. *Environmental Progress and Challenges: An EPA Perspective.* Washington, D.C.: EPA Office of Management Systems and Evaluation.

————. 1984b. *Ground-Water Protection Strategy.* Washington, D.C.: EPA Office of Ground-Water Protection.

————. 1984c. *Interim Standard Operating Safety Procedures.* Revised. Washington, D.C.: EPA Office of Emergency and Remedial Response.

————. 1985a. *Construction Quality Assurance for Hazardous Waste Disposal Facilities.* Public Comment Draft. EPA-530-SW-85-021. Washington, D.C.: EPA.

————. 1985b. *Report on the Incineration of Liquid Hazardous Wastes, Environmental Effects, Transport and Fate.* Washington, D.C.: EPA Science Advisory Board.

————. 1986. *Hazardous Waste Treatment Technology.* Cincinnati: EPA Hazardous Waste Engineering Research Laboratory.

Van Veld, P. 1980. Uptake, distribution, metabolism and clearance of kepone by channel catfish (Ictralurus punctatus). Masters thesis, College of William and Mary.

Varanasi, U., and D. Gmur. 1981. Hydrocarbons and metabolites in English sole (Parophrys vetulus) exposed simultaneously to (3-H) benzo(a)pyrene and (14-C) naphthalene in oil-contaminated sediment. *Aquatic Toxicology* 1:49–67.

Varanasi, U., W. Reichert, J. Stein, D. Brown, and H. Saanborn. 1985. Bioavailability and biotransformation of aromatic hydrocarbons in benthic organisms exposed to sediment from an urban estuary. *Environmental Science Toxicology* 19:836–41.

Vogel, G. A., A. S. Goldfarb, R. E. Zver, A. Jewell, and I. Licis. 1986. Incinerator and cement kiln capacity for hazardous wastes treatment. Paper presented at U.S. Environmental Protection Agency, 12th Annual Research Symposium: Land Disposal, Remedial Action, Incineration, and Treatment of Hazardous Waste, Cincinnati, April.

Venkataramani, E. S., and R. C. Ahlert. 1984. Raid aerobic biostabilization of high strength industrial landfill leachate. *Journal—Water Pollution Control Federation* 56:1178.

Vogel, T., and P. M. McCarty. 1985. Biotransformation of tetrachloroethylene to trichloroethylene, dichloroethylene vinyl chloride and carbon dioxide under methanogenic conditions. *Applied and Environmental Microbiology* 49:1080–84.

Walker, C. H. 1975. Variations in the intake and elimination of pollutants. In *Organochlorine Insecticides: Persistent Organic Pollutants,* ed. F. Moriarty. New York: Academic Press.

Wassermann, M., L. Tomatis, and D. Wassermann. 1975. World map of the storage of organochlorine insecticides in humans. *Pure Applied Chemistry* 42:189–208.

Wassermann, M., D. Wassermann, S. Cucos, and H. Miller. 1979. World PCBs map: Storage and effects in man and his biologic environment in the 1970's. *Annals of the New York Academy of Sciences* 320:69–124.

Williams, D. E., and D. R. Buhler. 1983. Multiple forms of cytochrome P-448 and P-450 purified from B-naphthoflavone fed rainbow trout. *Federal Proceedings* 42:910.

Wilson, W. E., J. T. O'Donovan, and R. M. Fristrom. 1969. In *Twelfth International Symposium on Combustion.* Pittsburgh: Combustion Institute.

Young, L. Y. 1984. Anaerobic degradation of aromatic compounds. In *Microbial Degradation of Organic Compounds,* ed. D. T. Gibson. New York: Marcel Dekker.

10. Regulating Toxic Chemicals in the Environment

LESTER B. LAVE AND ARTHUR C. UPTON

A great deal of progress has been made in understanding the scientific aspects of dealing with toxic chemicals in the environment. The foregoing chapters detail the reasons for release of these chemicals into the environment, the levels of releases that can be expected, the chemical and physical transformations that occur in the environment, the resulting human exposures and associated diseases, and the opportunities and difficulties associated with cleaning up waste dumps. Scientific knowledge exists to control any particular emission, to clean up any particular dump, and to protect people against any particular route of exposure. Unfortunately, these actions are generally expensive and time consuming, so that all cannot be accomplished simultaneously. The principal uncertainties lie not in the scientific issues but rather in the policy issues, such as setting priorities, determining how clean is clean enough, and how much ought to be spent on keeping chemicals out of the environment. Lave and Upton provide an introduction to these policy issues.

For more than a decade, the public has been concerned about toxic chemicals in the environment and about the attempts of Congress and the Environmental Protection Agency to regulate them. To date, however, too little has been accomplished. Large quantities of toxic chemicals are being dumped into sites that are declared hazardous as soon as dumping ceases. Then these materials become subject to a macabre game of musical chairs, involving shifting them from one dump to another. Large amounts of money are being spent to little or no gain; and there is not even an outline for a sound policy.

Finding solutions has been impeded by four elements: (1) Congress and the public sometimes have sought unrealistic goals and so have set out on fruitless courses (Lave 1981). As Ayres, McMichael, and Rod demonstrate in chapter 3, human activity inevitably produces toxic chemicals.

Corking the smokestacks or the wastewater outlets is not possible—instead, a materials balance framework can delineate what is possible and what approaches are likely to be fruitful. (2) Public pressure, media attention, and political shifts have led to disjointed, start-and-stop, often frenetic behavior. (3) Billions of dollars have been spent to halt emissions, establish reporting procedures, and clean up waste dumps, with little reduction in human risks. (4) Current legislation and EPA regulations are not a sound basis for a long-term solution. In fact, current legislation and regulation are part of the problem. They tend to take a narrow view of the problems, ignoring problems that cross national boundaries. Unfortunately, once toxic chemicals start migrating in the environment, there are no visa restrictions.

Several fundamental difficulties have led to these problems. First, there is no adequate agreement on what constitutes an adverse health effect. Scientists need to determine and validate the significance of such markers as chromosomal aberrations and DNA adducts and to specify primary health effects, secondary health effects, physiological changes that bear watching, and those that do not represent health problems.

Second, there is no agreement on what is possible and desirable, given the price tag. A goal like zero emissions into the environment is not possible. And although the price of cleaning up will be paid by corporations initially, these costs will be passed on to everyone. Rather than reaching for a simplistic goal such as banning all pesticides, for example, society needs to consider which pesticides are relatively benign to humans and the environment and how they should be used to ensure they remain benign.

Third, there is no agreement on what chemicals are dangerous, in what concentrations, and in what mixtures. Analytic chemistry has gotten to the point where it can discover the presence of chemicals in concentrations of parts per billion or trillion, far lower than amounts known to cause a risk to human health. Society must decide what concentrations are dangerous and what are not worthy of concern.

Fourth, there is a failure to distinguish risks to human health from risks to the environment. Priorities must be set and thinking should be clarified.

Fifth, the public must be educated about risks so that they will support evolving, enlightened policy (Fischhoff et al. 1981; Ruckleshaus 1984). While there is vast uncertainty in current scientific knowledge, there is agreement that many past circumstances were not as dangerous as the public was led to believe.

This book is focused on only some of the scientific issues concerning toxic chemicals in the environment. Our focus in this chapter is on a few of the issues essential to improving the scientific basis for regulating chemicals in the environment. We begin by attempting to define the priorities for investigating potentially toxic chemicals.

Setting Testing Priorities among Toxic Chemicals

Chemical production has increased rapidly in recent years, both in volume and variety. The worldwide boom in this industry is due to the prominant role played by chemicals in economic and social development, such as increased food production, improved health care, and provision of many amenities of modern-day life. In the United States alone, more than 50,000 commercial chemicals are produced, including some 3,350 pesticides, 1,815 pharmaceutical drugs, 8,627 food additives, and 3,410 cosmetic ingredients (National Academy of Sciences/National Research Council 1984). The Environmental Protection Agency estimates that 2,000 new chemical substances are introduced into the market each year.

A major difficulty in controlling the hazards associated with chemicals is the inability to identify the substances that pose the greatest risk. Reliance cannot be placed on epidemiological studies, since they disclose risks only after human injury has occurred. Instead, toxicological testing is needed to identify in advance the most toxic chemicals in order to prevent disease by limiting exposure.

The science of toxicological testing has advanced considerably in recent decades, particularly in the development of short-term *in vivo* and *in vitro* tests. These tests are far more rapid and sensitive than those available only a few years ago. However, the definitive tests for many forms of toxicity continue to require time-consuming, costly assays in rodents. The standard test for carcinogenicity, for example, involves life-long observation of rats and mice, takes three to five years to complete, and costs nearly a million dollars per chemical tested. World wide, only about 300 chemicals can be introduced into testing facilities each year. Since this is far less than the number of new chemicals introduced, there is a need for a priority ranking of chemicals to be tested.

The potential harm from a chemical is related to both its toxicity and the exposure or dose to the target organ. Exposure depends on both concentration at the point of exposure and the number of people exposed. Often the principal exposure is indirect, through ingesting food or touching materials. While acute health effects may be easier to detect, chronic health effects probably cause more harm. Unfortunately, chronic disease might result from a number of individual factors or interactions among factors.

Criteria and strategies for setting priorities among chemicals to be tested are based on the principles of decision theory and involve a sequential protocol that starts with inexpensive screening tests and that reserves the elaborate, expensive tests for the doubtful cases (Lave et al. 1983, 1986; NAS/NRC 1984). The systematic development and validation of such multistage toxicological evaluation protocols is worthy of increased attention and support. The creation of the National Toxicological Program in 1986 and the passage of the Toxic Substances Control Act and other relevant legislation are a promising beginning to addressing these issues. The problem is so large and difficult, however, that no solution is in sight.

One indication of the size of the problem is that, of the large number of chemicals in use, relatively few have been tested comprehensively for toxicological effects. Little is known about current human exposures. The National Academy of Sciences (1984) evaluated the information available on chemicals for assessing health risk. It found that the best information is available for drugs, where complete health hazard assessment is possible for 18 percent of the chemicals, and at least some toxicity information is available for 75 percent of the chemicals. The least information is available on commercial chemicals, for which complete health hazard assessment is possible for less than 1 percent; toxicity information is totally unavailable for almost 80 percent.

Although the EPA is in charge of a premanufacturing notification process, which allows it to require testing before a new chemical can be introduced, the EPA has not elected to set out a comprehensive testing protocol as has the Organization for Economic Co-operation and Development (OECD 1985). Section 5 of the Toxic Substances Control Act requires manufacturers of new chemicals for commercial production to submit a premanufacture notice (PMN) to the EPA, which has the authority to require testing if it is concerned that the chemical *may* present unreasonable risk of injury to human health or the environment and to restrict or ban the substance if it is concerned that the chemical *will* present unreasonable risk of injury to human health or the environment. Each PMN should identify the chemical, project its uses and by-products, estimate its production volumes and number of workers exposed, and describe methods for its disposal. Any other information that a manufacturer has on the chemical's physical and chemical properties and health and environmental effects also should be submitted. Exemptions to this process include low-volume chemicals, polymers, and site-limited intermediate chemicals.

Less than 10 percent of PMNs are subject to detailed review (U.S. Congress, Office of Technology Assessment 1982). The EPA frequently resorts to structure-activity analysis (assuming that chemicals with similar structures have similar properties) in making decisions on chemicals. Decisions on introducing new chemicals in the United States are therefore based on few data. There is reason to be concerned that requiring expensive, time-consuming testing would lower the rate of introducing new chemicals and slow innovation. However, a better balance is needed between protection and innovation.

Estimating Health Effects of Toxic Chemicals

Existing knowledge does not permit precise estimation of the total health effect of toxic chemicals in air, water, food, consumer products, and the workplace, although it is clear that the effect is not small. A good deal of work has been done to quantify the risks associated with various hazards (see Lave 1982; U.S. Office of Science and Technology Policy 1985). Some of the major problems complicating estimation of the health effect are the following:

1. *Difficulty in determining causality.* In contrast to acute intoxication, in which the causative agent is often relatively easy to identify, the cause-effect relation in most other situations is more difficult to determine. The reasons for this include the following: (1) For many diseases or health effects, there are a large number of possible causes, any one of which may obscure the contribution of another. (2) A long time may elapse between the onset of exposure to a chemical and the appearance of the resulting harm. (3) Human beings typically are exposed to complex and varying mixtures of chemicals, which generally are not well characterized.
2. *Paucity of relevant toxicological data.* As discussed in the previous section, less than 1 percent of the chemicals known to man have been characterized toxicologically.
3. *Varying susceptibility.* The human population is heterogenous in susceptibility. The basis for this lies in inherited age and sex variations in metabolism and homeostasis, as well as in vulnerabilities associated with specific disease states (e.g., asthma, cirrhosis of the liver, chronic renal disease, hypertension). Because of these variations, dose-effect relationships differ markedly among individuals; however, the extent of such differences has been studied to only a limited degree thus far.

Although the overall effect of toxic chemicals on human health is highly uncertain, acute effects occasionally have been dramatic. For example, 3,000–4,000 people were poisoned by the grain fungicide hexachlorobenzene in Turkey in the 1950s; 10,000 people were poisoned by cooking oil contaminated with cresyl phosphate in Morocco in 1959; 50,000 people were poisoned by grain impregnated with methyl mercury fungicide in Iraq in 1971; 2,800 people were poisoned by the pesticide malathion in Pakistan in 1976; 12,600 people were poisoned by chemically contaminated cooking oil in Spain in 1981; tens of thousands of people were poisoned by methyl isocyanate in Bhopal, India, in 1984; and 9,000 people currently die each year from pesticide poisoning in various countries of the world (Weiss and Clarkson 1986). These are but a few of the many thousands of injuries that happen; most cases of environmentally related disease go unrecognized. For example, many of the cancers that result from exposure to asbestos, arsenic, radon, cigarette smoke, or other environmental agents are not attributed to their actual causes (Doll and Peto 1981). Similarly, many other environmentally related diseases, such as impairments in intelligence and stature caused by excessive exposure to lead during childhood, are not recognized as such. Without more complete understanding of the relationship between health and the environment and without more adequate monitoring of human exposure, the total health effect of environmental chemicals will remain uncertain.

What Is an Adverse Health Effect?

When exposure to a substance results in an almost immediate reaction that is life threatening, that significantly limits function, or that causes disease, there is a clear adverse health effect. When exposure produces or expedites the production of a serious chronic disease, such as cancer, there is also an adverse health effect, although cause and effect are less clear and, in fact, difficult to detect.

A difficult case concerns impairment of a physiological reaction or adaptive response. For example, residents of Los Angeles exhibit a smaller response to ozone than people living in a less-polluted environment (Hackney and Linn 1985). Furthermore, exposure to many chemicals tends to compromise the immune response. If this means that these exposed individuals are unaffected except under severe stress, they might either never experience the effect or experience only a fatal effect.

Toxic chemicals produce a range of reactions, from those that are clearly adverse to health to those that merely compromise the ability to perform some normal function under extreme conditions; it is senseless to equate an acute reaction causing death to a minute reduction in fertility in a middle-aged person. It makes more sense to think of a spectrum of effects, from those that are immediately life-threatening to a small, subtle effect under unusual and extreme conditions. The focus of research and regulation should begin at the life-threatening end of this spectrum.

Some Major Unsolved Problems

▌Exposure Thresholds

For most toxic chemicals, practical exposure thresholds can be demonstrated. But for some, there may be no threshold. This is the case, for example, with direct-acting alkylating agents, which induce mutations at almost any dose (Ehling et al. 1983). For certain carcinogenic agents, there are likewise epidemiological, experimental, and theoretical grounds for postulating a nonthreshold dose-incidence relationship, although the existence of a threshold cannot be rigorously excluded (Peto 1977; Scherer and Emmelot 1979; Hoel et al. 1983; U.S. OSTP 1985). Clastogenic effects and certain teratogenic effects also fall into this category.

If some agents have no level of exposure totally without risk, the question is whether any risk is small enough to be acceptable. The answer to this question depends on quantifying benefits and risk, which poses formidable technical problems in our present state of knowledge.

▌ Quality Assurance

To assure the quality of both the risk data and the methods of evaluating them, systematic peer review and well-defined criteria to guide the review are important. The review should also consider the treatment of uncertainty, since without its explicit treatment, the assessment cannot be complete. For credibility, the process should be open to public scrutiny and comment.

▌ Monitoring

For epidemiological evaluation of risks and for identification of individuals who are at increased risk, precise information about human exposure to toxic chemicals is needed. The growing availability of biological and biochemical markers of exposure (e.g., DNA adducts) should improve the effectiveness of exposure assessment. Monitoring for these markers of susceptibility to chemical-induced injury, as well as for indices of preclinical injury, should help to protect persons against harm.

However, most such markers require further validation at this time. Furthermore, their use raises policy issues, e.g., whether susceptible persons should receive special consideration in employment and whether preclinical evidence of injury may constitute grounds for special restrictions or compensation.

Acceptable Risk

Because it is not possible to eliminate toxic chemicals in the environment, society must decide which risks require immediate attention, which risks can be dealt with in the future, and which risks are acceptable. This is a controversial subject since it involves value judgments and a great deal of uncertainty about the level of risk and who is at risk. Much has been written about this subject, and we allude only to the main points here (Schwing and Albers 1980; Fischhoff et al. 1981; Ruckleshaus 1984; MacGregor and Slovic 1986).

People think about risk in a complicated way. They are more comfortable with familiar risks and consequences than with unfamiliar ones; they are more comfortable when they believe they have individual control than when they feel they do not; and they are more comfortable when they see a direct benefit from taking the risk. This cognitive structure leads some people to reject situations that experts believe pose tiny risks (e.g., living near nuclear power plants or toxic waste dumps) and to accept situations that have demonstrably large risks (e.g., highway travel or occupational exposure to toxic chemicals). Toxic chemicals in the environment tend to have the characteristics that make people most apprehensive: they are unfamiliar, they are out of the individual's control; and they confer no direct benefit. Thus it is not surprising that people express great concern over toxic chemicals in the environment and protest when measurable amounts are detected. Unfortunately, the public does not differentiate between large and small risks. Unless it can learn to discern a genuine threat to health from a trivial risk, there can be no intelligent public discussion.

In an attempt to aid decision making, some analysts have tried to put risks into perspective. The Supreme Court (1980) thought it feasible to classify some risks as trivial, or de minimis, as if this were intuitively obvious to any reasonable person. Unfortunately, there is little agreement on what level of risk is so trivial as to be not worth considering. Another approach is to compare a risk to the risks associated with everyday life (riding in an automobile, drinking water, eating food). Many everyday risks are quite high, as evidenced by the number of injuries and illnesses and by the fact that everyone dies eventually. Thus the assumption is that risks that seem trivial compared to those routinely accepted are unworthy of consideration.

A slight variation on this approach has been to focus on the decisions of federal regulatory agencies (Milvy 1986; Byrd and Lave 1987). Analysis of the risks of both activities not chosen for regulation and those that are reveals a wide range of risk levels, making it clear that these federal agencies have established no consistent level for acceptable risk. Nonetheless, patterns emerge: for example, when the risk to the general public is less than one cancer in a hundred thousand lifetimes, agencies rarely regulate; but residual risk once regulation is undertaken is frequently larger than one cancer in a hundred thousand lifetimes and almost never smaller than one cancer in a million lifetimes.

Science and Public Decisions

The role of science and scientists in public decisions concerning environmental chemicals is complicated (Crandall and Lave 1981). Many congressmen and agency heads believe that scientists emphasize the gaps and uncertainties in current knowledge; that scientists always want to study situations more; that scientists do not worry that preliminary answers might not emerge for years; and that scientists disagree with each other. Because policy makers feel impelled to make immediate decisions on matters involving great public controversy, they want scientists to speak definitively and with one voice to tell them what must be done.

Scientists complain that policy makers do not understand the nature of science and the time and resources needed for inquiry and for arriving at a consensus. Since the decision makers want detailed, certain advice, scientists must either guess or give the spotlight to charlatans, whose assertions have little or no scientific basis.

Since the public generally has less education than policy makers and gives less attention to particular situations, it becomes even more confused about what is scientifically supportable. One of the best examples is the health effects associated with the toxic waste dump at Love Canal. Two scientists used their own studies to assert that residents in this area had suffered great harm from exposure to the chemicals; one of the studies was done on behalf of the EPA (Picciano 1980). More careful analysis has shown both studies to be flawed; a great deal of work has failed to show any health effects among residents that can be attributed conclusively to the exposure (Heath 1983; Heath et al. 1984).

Policy makers realize that taking no action amounts to a decision; waiting for more information and analysis means that people will continue to be exposed. Thus policy makers are content with much less certainty than scientists in coming to a judgment. Unfortunately, many congressmen know little about science and have based legislation on false premises. For example, the Clean Air Act implicitly assumes that there is a threshold for the effects of air pollutants. The EPA is instructed to set primary ambient air quality standards that will "protect the most sensitive group in the population with an ample margin of safety." This legislation has led EPA and many scientists to try to define a health effect (is it any physiological response?) and to perform studies to determine the lowest concentration at which such measurable responses can be detected.

Although there probably are effective thresholds in the numbers of molecules required to cause a reaction in an individual cell, there may not be thresholds at the concentrations of interest. Some extremely sensitive individuals will display a physiological reaction at an extremely low concentration. Probably it is not feasible to rid the air of pollutants to the point that the most sensitive individuals will not react at all. For carcinogens, furthermore, a single molecule is assumed to be capable of causing cancer, and so the assumption is that no threshold exists. Unfortunately, the EPA is stuck with enforcing some legislation that makes no scientific sense.

Scientists find that funding, and thus much of their research agenda, is defined by legislation and by agency decisions. For example, several statutes require that the carcinogenicity of chemicals be determined, which has led to a great deal of work on long-term bioassays, on short-term *in vivo* and *in vitro* tests for carcinogenicity, and on inquiries into predicting a chemical's toxicity by its structural similarity to another toxic chemical. At the same time, scientific findings do influence agency policy and legislation. For example, the Food and Drug Administration no longer bans carcinogenic food additives if the predicted risks they pose are less than one cancer per million lifetimes.

Regulators unfortunately tend to focus on areas where scientists are most uncertain. For example, in setting an ambient air-quality standard for ozone, regulators characterized neither the health effects at ten parts per million, a level known to produce large health effects in humans, nor at one part per trillion, a level at which there is no presumption of health risk. Instead, they focused on the 0.06-to-0.14 parts-per-million range, precisely where scientific uncertainty is greatest. Thus regulators inevitably ask questions that scientists have the most difficulty answering and that are the most controversial.

The above point must not obscure the fact that science has contributed much to the discussion of the health effects of toxic chemicals. While scientists may have little to say about 0.12 versus 0.14 parts of ozone per million, they can say that 0.30 parts is likely to produce many problems. In the end, it is the scientific process—with its challenges, replications, new theories, and new experiments—that will resolve these uncertainties. The inherent limits of science must be recognized, but we are very far from those limits in formulating policies for toxic substances in the environment.

An understanding on the part of scientists and policy makers of the constraints the other group is under will help each group formulate realistic objectives and help in the development and use of scientific information. The risk associated with toxic chemicals in the environment is basically a scientific question. Until we gain a better understanding of the science, there is no hope of settling a host of difficult, controversial issues.

Adverse Health Effects on an Individual Level

One of the most difficult and litigous issues has been determining whether a disease manifest in an individual is due to a particular exposure he or she received some time in the past (Gough 1986). This has been the central issue in much litigation involving exposure to agent orange and asbestos.

Perhaps the most celebrated cases involve civilians exposed to ionizing radiation from weapons fallout and soldiers exposed directly during atomic bomb tests in the 1940s and 1950s. Some of these individuals have asked for compensation when diseases such as cancer appeared decades later. The departments of Energy and Defense have resisted these claims, and Congress finally ordered the Department of Health and Human Services to produce a report, with tables specifying the estimated probability that a particular cancer in such an individual could be assumed to be caused by exposure to radiation from government activities. The result is a report that draws on the full range of what is known about radiation carcinogenesis to infer the extent to which a given cancer can be reasonably attributed to a given dose of ionizing radiation received at a particular time (Rall et al. 1985). This approach, although highly uncertain, can be used to determine what share this exposure should be assigned, compared to other possible causes, in contributing to the subsequent occurrence of cancer in an individual.

While ionizing radiation is unique in terms of what is known about the mechanisms of injury and causation, this report is a watershed in applying risk analysis to sorting out the claims of individuals with disease. A comparable approach has since been suggested for asbestos (Chase et al. 1985). Although there are a host of difficulties with the approach, from uncertainty in the calculation of relative share to whether compensation based on this share would be equitable (see Lagakos and Mosteller 1986, and following comments), this approach holds promise for resolving one of the most intractable problems to date.

Conclusion

Rapid progress is taking place in determining health effects from toxic chemicals in the environment and in lowering the risks of such effects. Much has been learned in the last decade, and much more will be learned in the next decade. These scientific developments have shaped public attitudes and federal government policy—although not always for the best. For example, the dramatic improvements in the ability to detect toxic substances in minute quantities has served to raise public anxiety.

But intelligent policy cannot be made without the foundation of scientific knowledge, and scientific research is often shaped by the needs of policy makers.

The relevant questions are inherently complicated. What toxic substances are present in the environment? Where do they come from, especially when they cross political boundaries? How do they change in chemical composition and location? How are people exposed? How toxic is each chemical individually and in combination with other chemicals? What can be done to lower levels of exposure? What are the risks of current exposures?

Previous chapters list a number of extremely useful tools to answer these questions, such as the materials balance framework, models to examine the migration and transformation of chemicals in the environment, and DNA adducts as markers of exposure and precursors of disease. Some of these tools are already standard in the analysis of toxic chemicals in the environment, some are growing in use, and some promise to add greatly to understanding the problems in the future.

Unfortunately, these tools are not being routinely applied now. There is a large gap between what we know how to do and what is being done. It seems anomalous that decisions requiring large investments of resources, and potentially affecting the health of many people, should be made with so little preparation. This book lays out important and helpful concepts and tools, which are the basis of better analyses and policies on toxic chemicals in the environment.

References

Byrd, D., and L. Lave. 1987. Significant risk is not the antonym of de minimis risk. In *De Minimis Risk*, ed. Chris Whipple. New York: Plenum.

Chase, G. R., P. Kotin, K. Crump, and R. S. Mitchell. 1985. Evaluation for compensation of asbestos-exposed individuals. *Journal of Occupational Medicine* 27:189-98.

Crandall, R., and L. Lave. 1981. *The Scientific Basis of Health and Safety Regulation*. Washington, D.C.: Brookings.

Doll, R., and R. Peto. 1981. The causes of cancer: Quantitative estimates of avoidable risk of cancer in the United States today. *Journal of the National Cancer Institute* 66:1192-1308.

Ehling, U. H., D. Averbeck, P. A. Cerutti, J. Friedman, H. Grlem, A. C. Kolbye, Jr., and M. L. Mendelsohn. 1983. Review of the evidence for the presence or absence of thresholds in the induction of genetic effects by genotoxic chemicals. *Mutation Research* 123:281-341.

Fischhoff, B., S. Lichtenstein, P. Slovic, S. Derby, and R. Keeny. 1981. *Acceptable Risk*. New York: Cambridge University Press.

Gough, M. 1986. *Dioxin, Agent Orange: The Facts*. New York: Plenum.

Hackney, J., and W. Linn. 1985. Controlled exposures of humans to air pollutants. In

Risk Assessment and Risk Assessment Methods: The State of the Art. Washington, D.C.: National Science Foundation.

Heath, C. W., Jr. 1983. Field epidemiologic studies of population exposed to waste dumps. *Environmental Health Perspectives* 48:3-7.

Heath, C. W., Jr., M. R. Nadel, M. M. Zack, A. T. Chen, M. A. Bender, and R. J. Preston. 1984. Cytogenetic findings in persons living near the Love Canal. *Journal of the American Medical Association* 251:1437-40.

Hoel, D. G., N. L. Kaplan, and M. W. Anderson. 1983. Implication of nonlinear kinetics on risk estimation in carcinogenesis. *Science* 219:1023-37.

Lagakos, S. W., and F. Mosteller. 1986. Assigned shares in compensation for radiation-related cancers. *Risk Analysis* 6:345-58.

Lave, L. 1981. *The Strategy of Social Regulation.* Washington, D.C.: Brookings.

———. 1982. *Quantitative Risk Assessment.* Washington, D.C.: Brookings.

Lave, L., G. Omenn, K. Heffernan, and G. Dranoff. 1983. A model for selecting short-term tests of carcinogenicity. *Journal of the American College of Toxicology* 2:125-30.

Lave, L. B., and G. S. Omenn. 1986. Cost-effectiveness of short-term tests for carcinogenicity. *Nature* 324:29-34.

MacGregor, D., and P. Slovic. 1986. Perceived acceptability of risk analysis as a decision-making approach. *Risk Analysis* 6:245-56.

Milvy, P. 1986. A general guideline for management of risk from carcinogens. *Risk Analysis* 6:69-80.

National Academy of Sciences/National Research Council. 1984. *Toxicity Testing: Strategies to Determine Needs and Priorities.* Washington, D.C.: National Academy Press.

Organization for Economic Co-operation and Development. 1985. *Administrative and Legislative Aspects of Chemicals Control: Comparative Analysis of Selected Issues.* Paris: OECD.

Peto, R. 1977. Epidemiology, multistage models and short-term mutagenicity tests. In *Origins of Human Cancer,* ed. H. H. Hiatt, J. D. Watson, and J. A. Winsten. Cold Spring Harbor, N.Y.: Cold Spring Harbor Laboratory.

Picciano, D. 1980. Pilot cytogenetic study of the residents living near Love Canal, a hazardous waste site. *Mammalian Chromosome News Letter* 21:86-93.

Rall, J. E., G. W. Beebe, D. G. Hoel, S. Jablon, C. E. Land, O. F. Nygaard, A. C. Upton, R. S. Yalo, and V. H. Zeve. 1985. *Report of the National Institutes of Health Working Group to Develop Radioepidemiological Tables.* NIH Publication 85-2748. Washington, D.C.: Government Printing Office.

Ruckleshaus, W. D. 1984. Risk in a free society. *Issues in Science and Technology* 4:157-62.

Scherer, E., and P. Emmelot. 1979. Multihit kinetics of tumor cell formation and risk assessment of low doses of carcinogen. In *Carcinogens: Identification and Mechanisms of Action,* ed. A. C. Griffin and C. R. Shaw. New York: Raven Press.

Schwing, R., and W. Albers. 1980. *Societal Risk Assessment: How Safe Is Safe Enough?* New York: Plenum.

Supreme Court of the United States. 1980. *Industrial Union Department, AFL-CIO vs. American Petroleum Institute.* 448, U.S. 607.

Weiss, B., and T. W. Clarkson. 1986. Toxic chemical disasters and the implication of Bhopal for technology transfer. *Milbank Quarterly* 64:216-40.

Whelan, E. E. 1985. *Toxic Terror: The Truth about the Cancer Scare.* Ottawa, Ill.: Jameson Books.

U.S. Congress, Office of Technology Assessment. 1982.

U.S. Office of Science and Technology Policy. 1985. Chemical carcinogenesis: A review of the science and its associated principles. *Federal Register* 50:10372–442.

Index

RNA binding, in biotransformation, 237
Rotary kiln, solid waste incineration, 265–67

Safe Drinking Water Act, 29
Sampling, for environmental monitoring, 73–84
SCEs (sister chromatid exchanges), reflecting DNA damage, 162
Scintillation counter, in alpha particle measurement, 83
Selenium: adult daily intake, 98; in drinking water, 76; from petroleum refining, 12; prohibited from landfills, 239
Silica: in air samples, 81; dust and alveolar clearance, 128; spectrophotometric measurement of, 90
Silver: in drinking water, 76; uses and emissions of, 55–59
Skin: cancer and sunlight, 9; cancers of, 176; exposure to contaminants, 131–32; xenobiotic permeability of, 175–77
Sludge: sampling and analysis of, 79; waste treatment, 258
Sodium hydroxide, and epidermal alteration, 177
Soil-water partition coefficient, 100
Solid wastes, treatment of, 256–57
Solvents, waste management, 257
Sorption, chemical treatment of wastes, 246–47
Source-receptor modeling, materials balance application, 51
Source segregation, of toxic wastes, 20–21
Spectrophotometry, analysis by, 89–90
Spills, of toxic chemicals, 12–13
Steel, sulfur in manufacture of, 50–51
Strontium-89, in hazardous wastes, 83
Strontium-90, in hazardous wastes, 83
Structure-sensitivity analysis, basis of new chemical introduction, 283
Styrene, in air samples, 81
Sulfate: in drinking water, 77; spectrophotometric measurement of, 90
Sulfite, titrimetric measurement of, 90
Sulfur: in auto and industrial emissions, 82; in iron and steelmaking, 50–51; toxicity of, 42–43
Sulfur dioxide: in air samples, 81; and alveolar clearance, 128; in auto and

industrial emissions, 82; monitoring of, 91–92; spectrophotometric measurement of, 90; titrimetric measurement of, 90; toxicity of, 185–86
Sulfuric acid, and alveolar clearance, 128
Sunburn, changes in the skin, 176
Sunlight, and skin cancer, 9. See also Ultraviolet light
Sunohio PCBX process, waste dechlorination, 253
Supercritical fluid extraction, waste treatment, 253–54
Systemic poisons, toxic chemical class, 41–42

Target tissue: defined, 115; dose to, 114–41; kidney, 196
TCD (thermal conductivity detector), hazardous element analysis, 87
TCDD (tetrachlorodibenzo-p-dioxin), 43, 232–33; and chloracne, 177; resistance to biodegradation, 225; skin reaction to sun, 176; toxicity differences, 174. See also Dioxins
TCE (trichloroethylene), partitioning model application, 101–5
Teratogens, effects on fetus, 200
1,2,3,4-Tetrachlorobenzene, thermal destruction of, 262
Tetrachloroethylene, thermal destruction of, 262
Tetracyclins, effect on kidney function, 197
Tetraethyl lead, percutaneous absorption of, 131
Thalidomide, effects on fetus, 200
Thallium, prohibited from landfills, 239
Thermoplastic microencapsulation, of hazardous wastes, 247–48
Titrimetry, analysis by, 89–90
TOCP (triorthocresyl phosphate), and "dying-back syndrome," 199
Toluene: in air samples, 81; recycling of, 257; respiratory toxin, 184
Total Diet studies, 107; food contaminant monitoring, 98–100
Toxaphene, in drinking water, 76
Toxic chemicals: absorption of, 122–28, 130, 132–33; classification of, 41–44; cleanup, 3; consumer uses of, 13, 52–53, 55–59; control of, 5–35, cumulative

05   20